Enhancing Recovery

Preventing Underperformance in Athletes

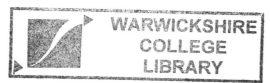

Michael Kellmann, PhD

University of Potsdam

Editor

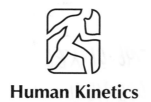

Human Kinetics

Library of Congress Cataloging-in-Publication Data

Enhancing recovery : preventing underperformance in athletes / Michael Kellmann, editor.
   p. cm.
  Includes bibliographical references and index.
  ISBN 0-7360-3400-5
   1. Sports--Psychological aspects. 2. Sports--Physiological aspects. 3. Physical
education and training. 4. Stress (Physiology) 5. Fatigue. I. Kellmann, Michael, 1965-

GV706.4.E54 2002
796'.01--dc21

                                    2002017184

ISBN: 0-7360-3400-5

Acquisitions Editor: Michael S. Bahrke, PhD; **Developmental Editor:** Melissa Feld; **Assistant Editor:** Susan C. Hagan; **Copyeditor:** Patsy Fortney; **Proofreader:** Sue Fetters; **Indexer:** Gerry Lynn Messner; **Permission Manager:** Dalene Reeder; **Graphic Designer:** Nancy Rasmus; **Graphic Artist:** Francine Hamerski; **Photo Manager:** Leslie A. Woodrum; **Cover Designer:** Kristin A. Darling; **Photographers:** Alberta Motor Association (p. 340, middle), Mark Fewster (p. 338, top), Foto Baldur (p. 337, top), Muza Hanina (p. 335, bottom), Petter Hassmén (p. 337, middle), Gerd Hoffmann (p. 337, bottom), Helena Kammerer (p. 333), Michael Kellman (p. 18), Göran Kenttä (p. 336, top), Nick Myers (p. 340, bottom), Tom Nicholson (p. 339, middle), Jorge Palafox (p. 338, middle), Benoit Pelasse (p. 334, bottom), Paula Smith Monthie (p. 336, bottom), Roland Strahl (p. 334, top), Peter Tittenberger (p. 334, middle), University of Alberta Photo Services (p. 336, middle), UNCG Photo Services (p. 335, middle), Valerie Viehoff (p. 340, top), Chris Wendt (p. 335, top), Clare Wilson (pp. 151, 152), Doug Woeppel (p. 339, bottom), Kevin Wright (p. 338, bottom); **Art Managers:** Carl D. Johnson and Kelly Hendren; **Illustrator:** Craig Newsom; **Printer:** Sheridan Books

Printed in the United States of America   10 9 8 7 6 5 4 3 2 1

Human Kinetics
Web site: www.humankinetics.com

United States: Human Kinetics
P.O. Box 5076
Champaign, IL 61825-5076
800-747-4457
e-mail: humank@hkusa.com

Canada: Human Kinetics
475 Devonshire Road Unit 100
Windsor, ON N8Y 2L5
800-465-7301 (in Canada only)
e-mail: orders@hkcanada.com

Europe: Human Kinetics
Units C2/C3 Wira Business Park
West Park Ring Road
Leeds LS16 6EB, United Kingdom
+44 (0) 113 278 1708
e-mail: hk@hkeurope.com

Australia: Human Kinetics
57A Price Avenue
Lower Mitcham, South Australia 5062
08 8277 1555
e-mail: liahka@senet.com.au

New Zealand: Human Kinetics
P.O. Box 105-231, Auckland Central
09-523-3462
e-mail: hkp@ihug.co.nz

To my wife, Helena

Contents

PART IV   TRANSFER TO RELATED AREAS

Foreword

The importance of recovery for elite athletes cannot be overemphasized. Effective recovery from intense training loads is becoming the difference between success and failure in sport. Over the latter part of the 20th century, athletes, coaches, and sport scientists have been creative and energetic in finding new ways to improve the quality and quantity of athletes' training. These efforts have consistently come up against the limiting factors of overtraining, fatigue, injury, illness, and even burnout.

These physiological and psychological limits dictate a need for a wealth of practical books on avoiding overtraining, maximizing recovery, and successfully walking the modern athlete's knife edge of high training loads. But there is not a wealth of practical books. Even if this book simply took all of the existing research and made it more practical, it would be significant. But *Enhancing Recovery* also breaks new ground in three ways: It is truly interdisciplinary, it focuses on underrecovery rather than overtraining, and it is practical and useful for coaches and athletes as well as scientists.

The field of overtraining has suffered from a lack of effective interdisciplinary work. The early groundbreaking work was done by physiologists who searched for a physiological marker to identify the overtrained athlete. Unfortunately, this search has not yet yielded a reliable early physical indicator of overtraining. Many researchers noted that although a simple physiological marker is not always present in the overtrained athlete, there may be some psychological markers that appear with some regularity early in the process. Psychologists began their own search for a psychological marker for overtraining. Physicians and trainers have become involved in working with athletes already broken down through poor adaptation to training. All of these efforts have lacked integration across disciplines.

As most elite sport scientists, elite coaches, and elite sports medicine groups have discovered, the problem of bad adaptation to training involves medical, physiological, psychological, environmental, and coaching issues. In *Enhancing Recovery*, Kellmann recruits and integrates these various perspectives into a theoretical and practical whole. A coach can hope to prevent an athlete's underrecovery by understanding all of the factors that lead to the condition.

Michael Kellmann and the other authors of this book intentionally focus on the dangers of *underrecovery* rather than the problem of *overtraining*. This is one case in which a change in language is more than mere semantics. Shifting the language helps us see a problem from a novel perspective, and it provides a considerable advantage to those who work on solving the problem. Coaches, who often feel condemned by the use of the term *overtraining,* intuitively grasp the importance of allowing adequate recovery for gaining the optimal benefits of training. In addition, the focus on underrecovery suggests important alternatives to reducing the training load of the elite athlete.

A new discipline of enhanced recovery is at the cutting edge of sport science, and specialists in this interdisciplinary area will become more essential for elite sport teams. (In fact, the United States Olympic Committee Sport Science program has begun talking about developing a position in this area.) The change in language from *overtraining* to *optimal recovery* shifts from the problem to the solution; this shift will help coaches, athletes, and sport scientists in their work.

Enhancing Recovery uses much of the latest scientific research as a foundation for developing practical training tactics for professionals in sport. Recovery is an essential part of training. Michael Kellmann drives home this point in the first chapter, and all of the contributors follow suit in the subsequent chapters. The text is based on real work with elite teams, and this lends authority to the authors' observations. There are several key chapters throughout the book. Chapter 12, which describes practical uses of the *Recovery-Stress Questionnaire for Athletes,* is helpful for anyone considering using this groundbreaking instrument. Yuri Hanin has always been at the forefront of efforts to individualize sport psychology services, and his chapter 11 highlights optimal recovery as an individual issue. Any coach or athlete who reads these chapters will understand that anything practical for the national team will also be practical for a club team.

I had the pleasure of working with Michael Kellmann on a panel on overtraining at a sport psychology conference in 1999. I knew then that he would contribute a great deal to the field of sport science. I simply didn't realize it would be so soon. The authors that Kellmann has brought together have written an important volume. I anticipate that coaches, athletes, and other sport scientists will find it a useful performance tool for many years to come.

Sean McCann

Preface

Enhancing Recovery: Preventing Underperformance in Athletes addresses recovery as a key factor of performance. The main assumption is that a constant lack of recovery or disturbed recovery turns into overtraining. Even being only slightly underrecovered over an extended period of time results in underperformance in athletes and nonathletes alike.

This book is written for coaches, athletes, and students as well as for the scientific community. It focuses on both research and applied counseling aspects to help readers enhance recovery and prevent subsequent underperformance. The broad approach of this book makes it appropriate not only for those working in the areas of sport psychology and sports medicine but also for those in other related fields in which the impact of recovery and underrecovery is important, such as health and ergonomics. The integration of empirical psychological and physiological research as well as the use of applied intervention and prevention strategies makes this book unique. Throughout almost all chapters case studies and examples are used to emphasize that recovery is an important factor in human life.

This book uses an interdisciplinary approach to describe fully the problem of underrecovery. Connections are made among medicine, physiology, periodization training, and psychology as well as motivation, health, and lifestyle. The analysis and debriefing of performance/training and the individual application of recovery will show the broad range of consulting and the impact recovery has on performance. Physicians, physiologists, and (sport) psychologists from Austria, Canada, Finland, Germany, Sweden, and the United States demonstrate the multilevel concept of recovery.

Cal Botterill, Dan Gould, Michael Kellmann, David Smith, Clare Wilson, and Craig Wrisberg served on the symposium Overtraining in Sport at the 1999 Annual Conference of the Association for the Advancement of Applied Sport Psychology in Banff (Canada). At that conference, the first contact with Mike Bahrke from Human Kinetics was made, and Human Kinetics expressed interest in publishing a book on recovery. To address fully the field of underrecovery, more international experts were invited to offer a broader perspective on the topic.

Overtraining is an important term in the literature, and recently two major publications have dealt with this topic (Kreider, R. B., Fry, A. C., & O'Toole, M. L. [Eds.]. [1998]. *Overtraining in sport.* Champaign, IL: Human Kinetics; Lehmann, M., Foster, C., Gastmann, U., Keizer, H., & Steinacker J.M. [Eds.]. [1999]. *Overload, fatigue, performance incompetence, and regeneration in sport.* New York: Plenum.). Although this book may at first seem similar to these two books, the *conceptualization and the underlying model is completely different.* This book is unique in its emphasis on recovery and intervention strategies from a psychological as well as from a physiological perspective. What can coaches, athletes, and supporting staff do to deal with overtraining or, even better, to prevent overtraining? Here the focus is on recovery as a necessary part of training and on the fact that underrecovery is a precursor of overtraining.

Because this book is intended for both athletes and coaches, practical examples and case studies have been included. One of the goals is to educate coaches and athletes about the need to integrate recovery time into practice. For example, when athletes understand that a weekend off training is part of the training schedule (which means that they should not train on their own or go for a heavy bike ride with friends), they take a huge step toward adequate recovery. In addition, the multilevel concept of this book also emphasizes that physical training is just one part of athletes' lives. Emotional worries or problems outside of the training environment (e.g., fights, parents' divorce) affect them heavily and often disturb their recovery times.

This book consists of four parts. In part I, Conceptualizing the Problem, Michael Kellmann differentiates between the concepts of underrecovery and overtraining, clarifies definitions, and provides everyday examples that support the assertion that underrecovery is often the precursor of overtraining (chapter 1). Dan Gould and Kristen Dieffenbach address the need for sport psychological overtraining research and intervention. They also explain that overtraining is a performance-influencing factor, a fact that was recently shown in several studies of high-performance athletes (chapter 2). Michael Kellmann addresses the need for optimal psychological assessment tools for underrecovery and overtraining in chapter 3. In chapter 4 Göran Kenttä and Peter Hassmén conceptualize the overtraining process. They differentiate among the types of stress that affect an athlete's performance and identify factors that contribute to overtraining, including the athlete's ability to adapt to physical training.

Determinants of underrecovery are addressed in part II. In chapter 5, Training Load and Monitoring an Athlete's Tolerance for Endurance Training, David Smith and Stephen Norris explain that athletes are constantly pushing the window of positive training adaptation to obtain a small improvement in performance. Smith and Norris discuss physiological factors that should be considered as indicators of overtraining in athletes. Jürgen Steinacker and Manfred Lehmann point out in chapter 6 the medical aspects of overreaching, overtraining, underrecovery, and resulting underperformance. They show that sickness and injury reports in training camps often correspond with the impact of the training load.

Applied intervention is discussed in part III. Stephen Norris and David Smith focus on the significance of correct competitive scheduling and training sequencing, which together underscore the processes leading to optimal performance (chapter 7). Cal Botterill and Clare Wilson report on overtraining experiences in Canadian National Team programs with special consideration of emotional and mental as well as physical factors. They discuss the role of emotional and mental factors in underrest as well as overtraining and outline plans and strategies for a monitoring and education study for several national and elite programs (chapter 8). Hap Davis, Cal Botterill, and Karen MacNeill present a model for identifying psychophysiological and emotional signs that the athlete is overstressed in training before illustrating how the sport psychologist can intervene within a multidisciplinary sport science model (chapter 9). John Hogg focuses on debriefing athletes after a competition as an important process designed to facilitate necessary change and progress toward the next level of performance. He discusses the various ways in which coach and athlete can interact to ensure that lessons are learned and future goals are set (chapter 10). Yuri Hanin points out that recovery strategies should match the personal situation and preferences of individuals. He advocates an intraindividual approach to finding the best individual recovery strategies (chapter 11). Michael Kellmann, Tom Patrick, Cal Botterill, and Clare Wilson highlight practical suggestions regarding assessment and monitoring of recovery and point out the experience they have gained working with the Recovery-Cue and the Recovery-Stress Questionnaire for Athletes (chapter 12).

Recovery and related areas are addressed in part IV. David Paskevich's chapter deals with recovery and health. He focuses on the relationship between recovery and both physical and psychological health, and he includes the importance of attitudes, beliefs, and perceptions (chapter 13). Craig Wrisberg and Matthew Johnson describe the role of recovery as a part of life quality. Taking time to rest and getting a break are often key factors in performance. In athletes' lives other factors such as performing in competition or getting along with family and friends are also important; these factors directly and indirectly influence their perceptions of quality of life (chapter 14). The importance of volitional processes supporting the actual and efficient realization of goals, especially when adverse conditions interfere with goal realization, is addressed by Jürgen Beckmann. Individuals have certain volitional self-regulation strategies at their disposal. Such strategies can help athletes achieve recovery when periods of rest are disturbed (chapter 15). Wolfgang Kallus points out the impact of recovery in different professions (e.g., flight controllers) and in everyday life. Naturally, we all hope that the people who are responsible for others take care of their own personal recovery (chapter 16).

Finally, Michael Kellmann summarizes the most important findings and statements of the previous chapters in chapter 17. He applies those topics to three performance groups: low density of performing (1-3 times a year), medium density of performing (1-34 or more games a year, such as a soccer season), and high density of performing (Cirque du Soleil with 400 shows a year).

Acknowledgments

I would like to acknowledge several people who provided me with outstanding support both personally and professionally at different stages of my career. Some of them served as contributors to this book. I explicitly would like to thank Wolfgang Kallus, Craig Wrisberg, Cal Botterill, John Hogg, and Jürgen Beckmann for their support.

I would like to thank all of the contributors to this volume. It was my pleasure to work with such dedicated professionals. Not only the quality of the chapters but also their delivery in a timely fashion made it a pleasure to edit this book. In the editorial process my research assistant Kim Raisner, who is an elite athlete, made great suggestions for how the quality of some chapters could be improved so that they have the maximum impact on athletes.

Appreciation is also expressed to Mike Bahrke for his continuous support and to Melissa Feld and Susan C. Hagan for their highly professional editorial work. Two anonymous reviewers provided helpful insight and suggestions for this book.

PART I

Conceptualizing the Problem

Kellmann, M. (2002). Underrecovery and overtraining: Different concepts—
similar impact? In M. Kellmann (Ed.), *Enhancing recovery: Preventing
underperformance in athletes* (pp. 3-24). Champaign, IL: Human Kinetics.

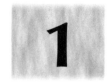

Underrecovery and Overtraining: Different Concepts—Similar Impact?

Michael Kellmann

The focus of this chapter is on the conceptualization of recovery and the close relationship between underrecovery and overtraining. An oversimplified description of underrecovery is the failure to fulfill current recovery demands. Underrecovery can be the result of excessively prolonged and/or intense exercise, stressful competition, or other stressors. However, being underrecovered over a longer period may not necessarily lead to overtraining, although it will lead to progressive fatigue and underperformance (Budgett, 1998). Optimal performance is only achievable if athletes recover after competition and optimally balance training stress and adequate recovery (Kuipers, 1998; Rowbottom, Keast, & Morton, 1998). Therefore, coaches and athletes need to regularly evaluate the relationship between training load and performance. Recovery, an essential component of athletic training and a counterbalance to training and nontraining stress, is too often overlooked.

The importance of focusing on training, competition, and nontraining stress factors will be illustrated by the following examples. A former NCAA Division I student-athlete described his college life:

The stress really started to get to me during the first month of my freshman year. Every morning I was up at 5:30 A.M. to lift weights and go for a one-hour training run. After that I showered, wolfed down some breakfast, and headed to morning classes.

Sometimes I'd eat a quick lunch and then take a nap. Other times I was so exhausted that I'd skip lunch and spend the whole time sleeping. Track practice was from 3:00 to 5:30 P.M. and after that I'd sometimes be so sore I'd have ice therapy and whirlpool treatments. Then I'd get a quick shower, have some dinner, and go to mandatory study hall, where I tried to complete my class readings and network assignments. By 11:00 P.M. I was "brain dead" and could not wait to get to bed. Sometimes I'd fall asleep right away, but other times I had trouble turning my mind off . . . worrying about classes, wondering what the coach was thinking, asking myself whether I belonged here or not. The next thing I knew, the alarm clock was buzzing and it was time to get up and do it all over again. I had no social life, nothing was any fun, and I was not doing anything very well—classes, weightlifting, practice, meets—I felt that I was just barely getting by.

It is just a small step from regular daily practice to a high frequency of competition. For example, in the midseason report for the professional German soccer club, Hertha BSC, the health situation was summarized as follows: "When over half of the 29 players are injured, the coach and manager have to think about practice, regeneration, and medical consultation" (Berliner Morgenpost, December 21, 1999). Hertha BSC played more games than any of the other German professional soccer teams in the first half of the 1999/2000 season—29 games in 18 weeks, an average of one game every

4.3 days including travel time. By midseason the players described themselves as physiologically and mentally drained. Similar or higher game frequencies occur in North American sports such as basketball, baseball, and hockey. For example, the NHL teams played 82 games during the regular season in 2000/2001. According to the official game schedule, the Colorado Avalanche, like any other NHL team, played an average of one game every 2.3 days, and reaching the play-offs added more games to the record. How much recovery time is allotted between games? As noted by Hollmann (1989) a decade ago, "in this way the athlete is rushed from one peak to the other and the recovery phases become too short in today's limits of human performance" (p. 79).

Underrecovery is not due only to a frequency of competitions that leaves no room for adequate recovery. It can also occur as a result of training mistakes such as (1) monotonous training programs, (2) more than three hours of training per day, (3) more than a 30% increase in training load each week, (4) ignoring the training principle of alternating hard and easy training days or by following two hard days with an easy day, (5) no training periodization and respective regeneration microcycles after two or three weeks of training, or (6) no rest days (Gastmann, Petersen, Böcker, & Lehmann, 1998; Lehmann, Foster, Gastmann, Keizer, & Steinacker, 1999a; Norris & Smith, this volume, chapter 7). A former top German track and field athlete indicated that too much training can also hurt performance: "The concept, to take a semester off because of the Olympic Games in 1972 did not work. The only thing I thought about was sports. I had trained up to three times a day and my performance diminished because I was totally overtrained in Munich" (Frankfurter Allgemeine Zeitung, May 12, 1999). In this context, Budgett (1998) stated that, "the cycle of partial recovery followed by hard training and recurrent breakdowns needs to be stopped" (p. 109).

Reframing the usual training regime is sometimes forced by injuries. A professional tennis player reported, "My recent successes are due to less tennis, more regeneration, and the enforced break (due to injuries); I am less exhausted and burnt out than the other players" (Neue Züricher Zeitung, 28 May, 1995). In this context, Froehlich (1993) stated that "it is not surprising that athletes sometimes perform better after a forced rest period that was caused by a mild illness or slight injury" (p. 68). At the 2001 World Championships two female German downhill skiers won medals, although they had been injured during the weeks prior to competition. Despite being unable to train, they performed far beyond expectations and reported later that they were able to replenish their resources and refocus on the competition. A similar story about a top female German speed skater demonstrates that sometimes injuries have a good side: "Now she had time for recovery and to make decisions for her future which she could not realize before due to the time constraints of training" (Süddeutsche Zeitung, November 13, 1999). Injuries sometimes provide athletes with an excuse for taking a break without feeling guilty. Some athletes may conceivably cause or feign injury, either consciously or unconsciously, in order to secure some much-needed rest.

An awareness of the importance of the recovery process often marks the difference between a mediocre and an outstanding athlete. According to the Associated Press (May 12, 1999) the only preparation Tiger Woods undertook for Part III of the PGA Tour in 1999 was *not* to touch a club for 10 days. He reported that he just "hung out" with friends and got away from the game. He had just finished playing four major tournaments and had felt really burned out. After getting away from golf for some days and doing what he liked, he looked fresh and relaxed at the next tournament.

A forced break, or realizing that high training load without adequate recovery is not the key for success, may lead to a change in training habits. A professional cyclist reported, "I am *better* this year, because I *train less;* in other years, I was already tired before the race" (Süddeutsche Zeitung, October 27, 1995). Athletes often arrive at competitions dead tired with sore legs and stiff muscles (see Botterill & Wilson, this volume, chapter 8). In those cases, optimal performance is almost impossible. Koutedakis and colleagues (1999) found that after a six-week postseason holiday a group of dancers had an increase in peak anaerobic strength, leg strength, and VO_2max over their prebreak levels. Budgett (1998) reported that athletes who have been underperforming for many months are often surprised by the good performance they can produce after 12 weeks of extremely light exercise.

The Problem of Underrecovery

In sports, the connection between the current recovery-stress state and performance in competition or training achievement is obvious (Kallus & Kellmann, 2000; Kellmann & Günther, 2000). To avoid overtraining and to optimize performance in sports, physiological and psychological recovery should be programmed as an integral component of training (Hooper & Mackinnon, 1995). Rowbottom and colleagues (1998) pointed out that "too often the recovery element is overlooked as an essential aspect of any training regime" (p. 57). Moreover, athletes need sufficient recovery during phases of intensive training to prevent overtraining. Within the training camp, when the extent and intensity of the training are deliberately increased, it is important to monitor the subjective view in order to assess recovery (Hooper & Mackinnon, 1995). If recovery is inadequate, psychological and physiological consequences may occur (e.g., Budgett, 1998; Foster, 1998; Hoffman et al., 1999; Kellmann & Günther, 2000; Kuipers, 1998; Lehmann, Foster, Dickhult, & Gastmann, 1998; Lehmann, Foster, & Keul, 1993; Lehmann et al., 1997). These negative effects are also a risk in programs that are too strenuous or critical competitive programs. Of course, appropriate training is the prerequisite to improve performance (e.g., Banister, Morton, & Clarke, 1997; Koutedakis & Sharp, 1998; Rowbottom, Keast, Garcia-Webb, & Morton, 1997). Uncertainty about the extent and content of training will often lead to inappropriate training responses in the athlete and insufficient competition results. It can also lead to overreaching and, in the long run, to staleness, the burnout syndrome, or the overtraining syndrome (Bruin, 1994; Gould & Dieffenbach, this volume, chapter 2; Gould et al., 1998; Kuipers & Keizer, 1988; Lehmann et al., 1993). Hoffman and colleagues (1999) pointed out that peak athletic performance depends on the proper manipulation of training intensity and volume as well as a provision for adequate rest and recovery between practice sessions. However, the exact point at which training becomes overtraining is difficult to define (Koutedakis et al., 1999). In conclusion, reducing the training load is not necessarily the answer to avoiding overtraining; rather, the training load may need to be individually determined in order to maximize performance (Budgett, 1998; Hooper & Mackinnon, 1995).

The next sections will focus on stress and recovery for a better understanding of overtraining and underrecovery. This is important because the approach by Lehmann and colleagues (Lehmann, Foster, Dickhult et al., 1998; Lehmann

et al., 1993, 1997, 1999a) defines overtraining as an imbalance between stress and recovery. The authors explicitly assert that stress encompasses all aspects of training, competition, and nontraining stress factors.

Stress

From a system point of view, stress is a destabilization or deviation from the norm in a biological/psychological system (psychophysical balance). The amount a particular system deviates from its optimal value (desired value) is influenced by specific standards and leads to a desired/actual value discrepancy (e.g., Boucsein, 1991). Deviations from the psychophysical balance are characteristics of demands that are either too high or too low. As a result, fatigue, sleepiness, psychological stress, monotony, or psychological saturation can occur (Hacker & Richter, 1984).

In the 1970s applied psychology separated the concepts of stress and strain. Stress is considered to be *objective factors, affecting people from the outside.* Strain is understood to be the result of these stressors on the person, that is, *its effect in people and on people* (Fletcher, 1988; Rohmert & Rutenfranz, 1975). Because of the limited use of the word *strain* in many areas of stress research, the term *stress* will be used to address the person side of the transaction ("strain"), and the term *stressor* will be used for the situational aspects. From a psychological point of view, the mediating subjective appraisal processes of a person play a predominant role in how a person deals with stress (e.g., Jerusalem, 1990; Lazarus, 1991; Lazarus & Launier, 1978). Depending on the subjective perception of objective facts, the same stressor can cause different degrees of stress. The individual is not passively exposed to the stressors, but can influence their quality and quantity depending on the goal of action and can even induce or avoid them.

Stress can have positive and negative effects on a person, depending on the state of the person and the recovery process. Stress, coping, and recovery determine the state of the person, which in turn determines the person's reactions to subsequent stressors (Kallus, 1992). Thus, the *recovery-stress state* plays a key role in the understanding of stress effects. The recovery-stress state takes into account the resources of the person, as they determine the "strength" of the person to cope with stressors and thus even determine the appraisal of stressors.

The intensity of stress is not the only important factor. The *duration,* the *distribution over time,* and the *nature* of stress are also crucial. The possible positive consequences of action latitude on stress are also discussed in modern action psychological models (Frese & Zapf, 1994; Schönpflug, 1983, 1987) and in publications on the biopsychology of stress (Janke & Wolffgramm, 1995).

According to the biopsychological stress model by Janke and Wolffgramm (1995), stress is an unspecific reaction-oriented syndrome that is characterized by a deviation from the biological homeostatic state of the organism. Stress is accompanied by emotional symptoms such as anxiety and anger, elevated activation in the central and autonomous nervous system, hormonal responses, changes in immune functions, and behavioral changes. Stress initiates processes of adaptation and coping. Therefore, stress, as a transactional process of time, can neither be examined nor validly diagnosed without the involvement of validation and assimilation processes, consideration of the individual observed recovery possibilities, and an involvement of feedback processes of the organism. Whereas many methods are already available for recording assimilation processes (Rüger, Blomert, & Förster, 1990), assessment of recovery processes is still insufficient (see Kellmann, this volume, chapter 3).

In contrast to stress, recovery is far less precisely defined. The editors of the *Handbook of Stress,* Goldberger and Breznitz (1993), stated that "a crucial but neglected area in understanding stress concerns the temporal characteristics of recovery from stressful encounters" (p. 5).

Recovery

A clear and sufficient definition of recovery can rarely be found in the literature. Authors discussing overtraining, especially in the field of sports medicine, often refer to recovery but do not provide detailed information on what physiological and psychological recovery is about. Mostly, recovery is defined as the compensation of deficit states of an organism (e.g., fatigue or decrease in performance) and, according to the homeostatic principle, a reestablishment of the initial state (e.g., Allmer, 1996; Hellbrügge, Rutenfranz, & Graf, 1960).

Allmer (1996) pointed out that the above recovery definitions always imply overly demanding situations. Hacker and Richter (1984) emphasized that stress can be initiated by underdemanding circumstances too, such as sleepiness, psycho-

logical stress, psychic saturation, or monotony, which also follow according to the above-defined recovery demands. This approach underlines that recovery is not only due to activity reduction but also is effected by an activity increase. Löhr and Preiser (1974) emphasized "that recovery does not always have to be relaxation, but can occasionally be tension too" (p. 579).

These definitions are all quite general and consider recovery as a counterpart to the disturbance in an initial state or a deficit condition of the organism that enables the individual to perform. Kellmann and Kallus (1999, 2000) stated that recovery encompasses active processes of reestablishing psychological and physiological resources and states that allow the individual to tax these resources again. This more precisely described the complex issue of recovery. But it is still not sufficient to understand recovery as an elimination of fatigue or a system restart. Only a differentiated and repeated observation indicates the complexity of an individual's recovery process.

Kallus (1995) and Kallus and Kellmann (2000) described the complex recovery process and proposed characteristics of a general psychophysiological concept. Those different recovery features will be outlined along with practical examples as well as reports from athletes and coaches.

- The recovery process is gradual and cumulative. The total recovery time depends on the previous activities and the type and duration of stress. In general, if practice is completed in a high-training-volume phase, recovery usually takes longer than if practice is completed in a taper phase (Hooper & Mackinnon, 1995, 1999; Hooper, Mackinnon, & Hanrahan, 1997; Hoffman et al., 1999; Raglin, 1993). A taper phase is a regeneration technique during which the physiological and psychological stressors of daily training are gradually reduced prior to competition in order to maximize the differences between the positive and negative effects of training. Runners, swimmers, and cyclists who taper show significant improvements in performance; muscular strength and power; and factors such as sleep disturbances, stress, fatigue, ratings of perceived exertion, and mood states (Hooper, Mackinnon, & Howard, 1999).

- According to the previous definitions and descriptions, recovery ends when a psychophysical state of restored efficiency and homeostatic balance is reached. The general training model is based on the idea that physical exercise leads to a disturbance in cellular homeostasis (Viru, 1984,

1994). These exercise-induced changes are assumed to be the main stimulus for initiating physiological responses to restore homeostasis and to induce training adaptations. As Kuipers (1998) and Norris and Smith (this volume, chapter 7) pointed out, it is often difficult to detect the exact time when the next training stimulus should optimally be set without initiating an impairment of performance.

• Recovery depends on a reduction of, a change of, or a break from stress. Although reduction of stress and a break from stress seem to be obvious, a change of stress may need more explanation because it coincides with the previous definitions. Following the perspective from Löhr and Preiser (1974) that recovery does not always have to be relaxation but occasionally can be tension too, recovery can also be initiated by activity changes that take place (for example, during changes of action). Activities that interfere with different systems may enhance recovery on one level while continuing to be stressful on another, when alternated with other activities. According to Selye (1974), these single stressful activities can be eu-stress (positive stress) related. By alternating physiological and psychological stress, athletes can increase the possibility of optimized recovery. The body can relax while reading a book or going to the movies. On the other hand, the psychological system can recover during physiological activity. The underlying mechanism is that one system rests while another is active. For example, housecleaning is not as stressful if the required activities can be alternated as soon as one body part gets tired. By alternating activities such as ironing, washing dishes, vacuuming, cutting grass, washing the car, people can work longer. In sports, this approach is systematically used in circuit training. While one muscle group is trained, the others can rest, which enhances the total training time. However, it has to be mentioned that during circuit training the whole body is stressed to a certain extent because of the all-around exercise activity. In summary, recovery takes place through an enhancement of activity (e.g., physical exercise), a reduction of activity (e.g., sleep), or a change of activity (e.g., circuit training).

• Recovery is specific to the individual and depends on individual appraisals. If 10 people were asked to name their "personal number one recovery strategy," seven or eight different answers would probably be given. A classroom exercise demonstrates this quite well. Each individual is asked to write down his or her "personal number one recovery strategy" and then to pass the paper to the next person. In almost all cases the personal favorite does not match the choice of the neighbor. In the sport context, this means that athletes have different recovery strategies and needs, and that the recovery activity selected by the coach does not necessarily lead to the desired result. After the same activity, one athlete is highly relaxed, whereas another does not feel recovered at all. For example, some athletes feel uncomfortable in a sauna—they perceive it as a stressor and consequently for them a sauna is not recovering at all.

Because recovery needs to be applied individually, each person should have more than one strategy available. Sometime, the first choice cannot be used or does not work because of external or internal circumstances. For example, running may work perfectly as a recovery strategy in a familiar environment at home. However, after crossing several time zones, running may stress the organism for a couple of days when the individual is still suffering from jet lag. Since the sudden shift of time zones is a disrupter of the sleep-wake cycle, athletes, especially those in high-performance sports, should arrive at competition sites at least one day per time zone prior to competition to adapt to the current time and conditions (Savis, 1994; Tschiene, 1999). This shows that a second, third, or fourth "backup" recovery strategy should be available and applied depending on current personal and situational factors.

• Recovery can be described on various levels. Kallus and Kellmann (2000) have discussed different levels on which recovery can be described (e.g., physiological, psychological, behavioral, social, environmental). On a physiological level, recovery takes place by restoring resources such as food, water, and minerals (Kenttä & Hassmén, 1998). The reestablishment of physiological fitness after injuries or in the hormonal and biological processes during sleep indicates other biological processes of recovery (Hollmann & Hettinger, 2000; Savis, 1994). Although, sleep affects the psychological aspect as well. However, the feeling of relaxation and the reestablishment of well-being and a positive mood demonstrate the psychological aspects of recovery. Behavioral aspects of recovery support the biological processes and result in recovery by changing the activity from one stressor to another or by engaging in leisure activities. Social aspects of recovery take place, for example, when people get together for the weekend for social events, such as dinners or parties. Interpersonal relationships, such as those with a friend or partner, demonstrate more private and intimate aspects of social recovery.

• Recovery processes involve various organismic subsystems that monitor our bodies and perform important functions before, during, and after physical exercise. The cardiovascular, hormonal, endocrine, or muscular subsystems, for example, are involved during, and of course after, exercise (Foster, 1998; Kuipers, 1998; Lehmann et al., 1997; Lehmann, Foster, Dickhult et al., 1998; Norris & Smith, this volume, chapter 7; Smith & Norris, 2000, this volume, chapter 5; Viru & Viru, 1999). For example, during exercise the muscular and cardiovascular subsystems are mainly stressed, whereas some parameters of the endocrine subsystem peak during night sleep. If night sleep, in particular when delta brain waves occur, is disturbed, it affects the restoration and rejuvenation of the body (Savis, 1994). Growth hormone and cell division are at their peak during delta sleep, while metabolic rate, respiration, core temperature, and heart rate are at their circadian lowest at that time. According to Savis (1994), delta sleep has been described as an "agent of recovery relative to the metabolic activity and energy expended by an individual" (p. 115), which underlines the importance of sufficient and good-quality sleep.

As indicated, the organismic subprocesses of recovery can be dissociated—the amount of time necessary for recovery from the stress of training may vary within and among the different organismic systems of the human body (e.g., Gabriel, Urhausen, Valet, Heidelbach, & Kindermann, 1998; Hackney, 1999; Steinacker et al., 2000; Urhausen, Gabriel, & Kindermann, 1995; Viru, 1985; Viru & Viru, 1997, 1999). Viru and Viru (1999) pointed out that the variability of hormonal responses is frequently caused by the combined influence of factors such as temperature, hypoxia, biorhythmus, diet, fatigue, and the initial hormone level. Misevaluation of hormonal responses can be avoided if those determinants and modulators are considered appropriately.

• Recovery can be divided into three approaches—passive, active, and proactive. Several studies have shown that recovery is faster when subjects exercise moderately instead of resting passively (Ahmaidi et al., 1996; Belcastro & Bonen, 1975; Bonen & Belcastro, 1974; Taoutaou et al., 1996; Thiriet et al., 1993; Wilmore & Costill, 1988). In sports, the term for moderate exercise during the recovery process is *active recovery,* and the term for sitting and lying quietly is *passive recovery* (Hollmann & Hettinger, 2000; Maglischo, 1993). Passive recovery also includes treatments such as massages, hot and cold baths, steam baths, and saunas, which initiate physiological reactions through physiological stimuli (heat, cold, pressure) affecting blood flow, respiration rate, and muscle tonus (Weineck, 1994). In summary, passive recovery includes automatic psychological and biological processes to restore the initial state. Unfortunately, activities referred to as passive recovery are often the only ones applied systematically.

Recovery, however, is also a *proactive self-initiated process* to reestablish psychological and physiological resources. Active recovery such as muscle relaxation and stretching are known as cool-down activities after practice and competition. The purpose of those exercises is to eliminate the results of fatigue through aimed physical activity. During cool-down, an increased blood circulation in the muscles results in a high state of metabolism; lactic acid does not have a chance to build up in the muscles, and the blood gases can more quickly sink to a normal level. Light exercise is superior to rest during recovery periods because a faster rate of blood flow is maintained. Thus, more lactic acid can be removed from muscles in less time. At lower levels of effort, including complete rest, the rate of removal is slower. If the effort is too high, however, additional lactic acid will be produced (Maglischo, 1993).

What makes sense regarding the physiological systems also applies to the general life of humans. When recovery includes a purposeful action, it can be defined as *proactive recovery.* A person is responsible for his own activities and can actively initiate the process. For example, going to a movie, visiting close friends, and going for a run can be *self-initiated* and proactively put a person in charge.

• Recovery is closely tied to situational conditions. Sometimes it is as simple as it sounds: "If my roommate snores, I won't get any sleep." The impact of situational conditions that affect recovery (e.g., sleep, quality of a bed, partner contact) is obvious. In Berlin-Grünau (Germany), for example, a very nice rowing facility was built for the 1936 Olympics. Although it still provides great training opportunities, old iron water pipes are still running through the building. If someone flushes the toilet on the top floor at night, everyone below gets disturbed during sleep. It is also important to consider how individuals appraise the obvious situational conditions. For example, if an athlete's accommodation is close to a loud street, her rest may be disturbed day and night. However, if an athlete is used to living in a loud neighborhood, she might have no problem sleeping through loud noises, but instead may get irritated by an absolutely quiet environment. Individuals' sensitivity to disturbing events depends on their own experiences.

Coaches have to be aware of those circumstances and should encourage athletes to communicate about disturbances in their surroundings. The coach is not in the same room when the water runs through the pipes or when the roommate snores. In addition, situational circumstances can often be changed easily if the coach/staff receives the necessary information soon enough (Kellmann, Kallus, Günther, Lormes, & Steinacker, 1997). Therefore, awareness and communication are the key elements in preventing underrecovery due to situational conditions (see also Botterill & Wilson, this volume, chapter 8).

• In addition to the criteria described by Kallus (1995) and Kallus and Kellmann (2000), recovery is a self-determined process, as pointed out by Botterill and Wilson (this volume, chapter 8). A dramatic change occurs when the individual's perception and self-awareness change. Suddenly, the supposed recovery strategy may have an opposite effect. Watching TV is probably one of the most common leisure-time activities in North America and Europe, and it is very often considered a recovery-related activity. In a way, it makes sense and fits the purpose if watching TV is consciously used to switch the mind off. It only has the status of a planned activity as long as the person is in control of the remote. But often, after a two- or three-hour TV session the individual realizes that the TV show is really not very interesting, or he is watching the same soap for the third or fourth time. After realizing the waste of time, the supposed recovering effect turns into disturbed recovery. This highlights how important control is in recovery. Another aspect is to know what type of recovery is best suited to the individual.

Kuhl and Beckmann (1994) also used the TV example to experimentally demonstrate the impact of self-determination in controlling one's activities. Their subjects first worked on a monotonous task without a sense of self-determination. Afterwards, when seated in front of a TV, they watched a program they considered boring for about 20 minutes before switching to a more interesting program. The authors assumed that the lack of self-determination during work alienated subjects from their own preferences when they were later watching TV. When subjects had experienced the training activity as self-determined and viewed this activity as meaningful, they immediately switched to a more attractive program when placed in front of the TV, demonstrating that they seemed to have better access to their preferences (Beckmann, this volume, chapter 15; Kuhl & Beckmann, 1994).

• Summarizing the features of recovery, three important aspects can be highlighted. (1) Recovery can be judged as an opposition to fatigue or an overdemanding situation. Here, recovery takes place through sleep or a reduction of activity. (2) Recovery can also be seen as an opposition to an underdemanding situation. In this case, recovery takes place through an activity increase, such as physical exercise. Finally, (3) recovery also occurs by varying the stressed systems through an activity change.

The following example demonstrates that determining what constitutes a recovery activity is not always simple and straightforward. The same activity can be considered a recovery activity and a stressor at the same time.

The coach of a Canadian male speed skating team planned a training schedule that included a day off as a key element for recovery purposes. The coach did not tell the athletes what to do for recovery, so they decided to go for a bike ride in the mountains. The purpose of the bike ride was to relax, be with the team, and get refreshed by the scenery of the Canadian Rocky Mountains. However, the athletes soon turned their relaxing bike ride into a competition that left no room for physiological recovery at all. Luckily, no one was injured.

This bike ride can now be judged from two perspectives. First, social recovery of the athletes took place when they went into a different environment and got mentally refreshed. On the other hand, the athletes created an additional training stressor that interfered with the training schedule of the coach. Since the athletes knew that the coach would not appreciate their bike ride competition, they did not tell him, and the next day practice continued based on the regular schedule. The next physiological stressor was set, and some days later the coach was surprised by the performance decline (Example provided by a coach of the Canadian Speed Skating Team in a team meeting, October 1999). In order to recover adequately, athletes must understand that a weekend off from training is part of the planned training schedule; they should not train additionally *without informing the coach,* not even just to go for a strenuous bike ride with friends.

Kellmann and Kallus (1999) pointed out that recovery is the overall concept that integrates the different physiological, subjective, as well as proactive action-oriented components including regeneration. Levels of recovery include

- psychological recovery,
- mood-related recovery,
- emotional recovery,
- behavioral recovery,
- social recovery, and
- physiological recovery (regeneration).

Regeneration encompasses all goal-directed processes, allowing the athlete to replenish psychophysiological resources for performance (Allmer, 1996; Renzland & Eberspächer, 1988).

As pointed out earlier, the description provided by Kellmann and Kallus (2000)—that recovery encompasses those processes of replenishing psychological and physiological resources and states that allow the athlete to tax these resources again—is not sufficient to fully define recovery. Based on the features of recovery (Kallus, 1995) and the previously discussed key elements, a more precise definition was developed:

> Recovery is an inter- and intraindividual multilevel (e.g., psychological, physiological, social) process in time for the re-establishment of performance abilities. Recovery includes an action-oriented component, and those self-initiated activities (proactive recovery) can be systematically used to optimize situational conditions and to build up and refill personal resources and buffers. (Kellmann & Kallus, 2001, p. 22)

Now that recovery has been defined, the terms *underrecovery* and *disturbed recovery* need to be clarified. Breaks (e.g., halftimes, time-outs) during practice and competition serve the purpose of psychological as well as physiological recovery for athletes and for their interaction with coaches or advisors (Anshel, 1990; Hagedorn, 1989). Athletes often receive more information from coaches than they can process during the recovery phase (Herzog, Voigt, & Westphal, 1985). Many coaches

are not aware of the importance of the recovery phase and are not aware of its correlation with the recovery process. This can result in underrecovery or disturbed recovery. *Underrecovery* can be the result of breaks that are too short, in which the psychological and physiological needs were not fulfilled and optimal recovery could not take place. If the requirements of adequate recovery are met, but the athlete is confronted with an emotional discussion with the coach, noise, or lack of or wrong debriefing of performance (Hogg, 1998; this volume, chapter 10), it can nevertheless result in *disturbed recovery*. In many laboratory experiments, Kallus (see Kallus & Krauth, 1995) found that during the regeneration phase, athletes experience a considerable increase in the amount of sensitivity to disturbances, annoyances, and irritations. Thus, slight interruptions in the normal situation during the break may have great effects on the athlete's performance.

Coaches' behavior also plays a central role in the structure of the breaks. In a survey of 76 professional coaches Kellmann (1997) found that highly stressed coaches describe their behavior during rest periods in competition as more directive and more angry compared to those in the low-stressed group. Age appears to be an important mediator for behavior, with older coaches showing more positive behavior during rest periods in competition than do their younger colleagues. In addition, performance expectations of coaches are another indicator for behavior during rest periods in competition. Coaches whose athletes fulfilled performance expectations show higher values in the Rest-Period Questionnaire for Coaches (Kellmann & Kallus, 1994, 1995) scales such as *Positive Coach-Athlete Relationship, Team-Atmosphere, Performance Feedback,* and *Goal-Orientation* than coaches whose expectations were not fulfilled.

Recovery-Stress State

Athletes in general are likely to not only differ from the general population but also show a broad range of inter- and intraindividual differences (Froehlich, 1993; Weinberg & Gould, 1999). This also applies to the training load. "Thus a particular training schedule may improve the performance of one individual, be insufficient for another, and be damaging for a third" (Raglin, 1993, p. 842). Raglin continues, "The outcome (i.e., either adaptation or maladaptation) may be influenced by the particular characteristics of the athlete (i.e., predisposition)."

The different effects of the same training stimulus may be explained by the individual *recovery-stress state*. The recovery-stress state represents the extent to which someone is physically and/or mentally stressed as well as whether the person is capable of using individual strategies for recovery and which strategies are used (Kallus & Kellmann, 2000; Kellmann & Günther, 2000; Kellmann & Kallus, 1999, 2000). From the perspective of a biopsychological stress model (Janke & Wolffgramm, 1995) recovery and stress should be treated using a multilevel approach, dealing with physiological, emotional, cognitive, behavioral, performance, and social aspects, considering these aspects both separately and together. The recovery-stress state can be changed positively either by stress reduction or, more important, by *self-initiated recovery activities,* which are outlined in the model describing the interrelations of stress states and recovery demands.

Stress States and Recovery Demands

Kellmann (1991, 1997) proposed a model describing the interrelations of stress states and recovery demands (see figure 1.1). The basic assumption is that with increasing stress, increased recovery is necessary. Limited resources (e.g., time) initiate a vicious cycle: under increased stress and unable to meet increased recovery demands, the athlete experiences more stress. People may be stressed to the point that they fail to find or make time to recover adequately, or to consider better ways of coping with the situation.

In this model, the simplest case is a symmetrical increase in stress and recovery demands: the two axes drift apart with elevated stress levels ("scissors" function). With intermediate levels of stress, one can find an area of optimal performance and thus an area of adequate recovery (solid arrows in figure 1.1). Beyond this point, one cannot meet recovery demands without additional recovery activities. Stress will accumulate, and without intervention, burnout symptoms are likely to develop. The state of balanced stress and recovery is related to optimal performance, and perhaps to the performance-related psychobiosocial states and their emotional correlations within the Individual Zones of Optimal Functioning (IZOF) model (Hanin, 1997, 2000).

In a state of adequate recovery, the individual can react appropriately and cope successfully with stress without additional recovery activities. A lack of recovery (Kellmann & Kallus, 1999) or underrecovery can trigger a process that leads to a state of elevated stress. As increasing stress limits the possibility of recovery, the athlete must be given special opportunities to recover in order to reestablish an optimal level of performance. In summary, the model suggests that it is not bad to be high on stress, as long as the individual knows how to recover optimally.

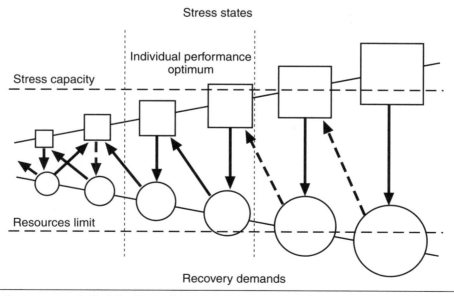

Figure 1.1 The "scissors model" of the interrelation of stress states and recovery demands.

Reprinted, by permission, from K.W. Kallus and M. Kellmann, 2000, Burnout in Athletes and Coaches. In *Emotions in sport,* edited by Y.L. Hanin (Champaign, IL: Human Kinetics), 212.

The underlying mechanism of Kellmann's scissors model can be compared to the health-oriented model of salutogenesis developed by Antonovsky (1979, 1987). The salutogenesis approach proposes a health ease/dis-ease continuum—also called a breakdown continuum—on which an individual can be located. The question is not whether someone is ill but rather how far away a person is from the end points. The person's position on the breakdown continuum depends on current resistance deficits and the availability of general resistance resources for tension management. Antonovsky's general resistance resources include positive factors and conditions from different areas (physiological, biochemical, artifactural-material, cognitive, emotional, valuative-attitudinal, interpersonal-relational, and macrosociocultural) that can be positively used to deal with possible negative events/stressors (resistance deficits). In other words, the model of salutogenesis includes factors that can be used to shift a person toward the positive end of the health ease/dis-ease continuum. Consequently, health is not defined as a lack of disease or illness but includes buffers that can be used to compensate for the appearance of negative physiological and psychological health-affecting conditions (see Paskevich, this volume, chapter 13).

Important principles of Antonovsky's model of salutogenesis match the introduced scissors model of the interrelation of stress states and recovery demands. Whereas the different stress states can be compared to personal resistance deficits, recovery activities—in Antonovsky's terms—can be labeled general resistance resources. Both models are dynamic and so a person can be located either on Antonovsky's breakdown continuum or on the *recovery-stress state* shown in figure 1.1. Most important, both models encompass various levels, including physiological, emotional, cognitive, behavioral, and social, considering these aspects both separately and together. Both models credit passive, active, and proactive recovery activities.

The Problem of Overtraining

The relevance, impact, and consequences of overtraining have been addressed in many medical and sport psychology articles (e.g., Berger et al., 1999; Lehmann, Foster, Dickhult et al., 1998; Lehmann et al., 1993, 1997, 1999a; Kellmann, 2000; Kenttä & Hassmén, 1998), book chapters (e.g., Raglin, 1993; Raglin & Wilson, 2000), and edited books (Kreider, Fry, & O'Toole, 1998a; Lehmann, Foster, Gastmann, Keizer, & Steinacker, 1999b). Silva (1990) reported that 66% of a research sample of athletes experienced overtraining and of those, 50% had bad memories. Morgan, O'Connor, Sparling, and Pate (1987) and Morgan, O'Connor, Ellickson, and Bradley (1988) found that 60% of females and 64% of males have been stale at least once during their running careers. Ninety-one percent of swimmers who were stale during their freshman year in college experienced staleness in the following years. Only 30% of athletes who did not become stale had those problems later on (Raglin & Morgan, 1989). Overtraining was seen in 21% of swimmers on the Australian National Team during a half-year season (Hooper, Mackinnon, Howard, Gordon, & Bachmann, 1995), in 33% of Indian national-level basketball players during a six-week training camp (Verma, Mahindroo, & Kansal, 1978), and in more than 50% of semiprofessional soccer players after a five-month competitive season (Lehmann, Schnee, Scheu, Stockhausen, & Bachl, 1992).

Raglin and Morgan (1989) reported that the most frequent causes of overtraining cited by athletes are (1) too much stress and pressure, (2) too much practice and physical training, (3) physical exhaustion and all-over soreness, (4) boredom because of too much repetition, and (5) poor rest or lack of proper sleep. Insufficient and/or lack of recovery time between practice sessions is the main cause of the overtraining syndrome (Fry, Morton, & Keast, 1991; Mackinnon & Hooper, 1991; Raglin, 1993). Factors such as nutrition, sleep deficit, sickness, travel, and competitions increase the negative effect of insufficient recovery (Costill et al., 1988; Kenttä & Hassmén, 1998). In the following paragraphs various definitions and indicators of overtraining are discussed.

Overtraining Defined

In general, overtraining is described as *an imbalance between training and recovery* (Kuipers & Keizer, 1988). However, according to Lehmann and colleagues (Lehmann, Foster, Dickhult et al., 1998; Lehmann et al., 1993, 1997, 1999a), overtraining is due to *an imbalance between stress and recovery,* that is, too much stress combined with too little regeneration. Both descriptions sound similar, but the definition by Lehmann and colleagues explicitly asserts that stress includes all training, competition, and additional *nontraining stress factors.* Social, educational, occupational, economical, nutritional, and travel factors; time stress; and the monotony of training act to increase the risk of developing an overtraining syndrome.

Most researchers probably agree with the overall description provided by Lehmann and colleagues (1993, 1997, 1999a) because the general description does not differentiate in detail between process and result and desired and undesired consequences of overtraining. However, the details describing the phenomenon of overtraining in the literature have created much confusion because of a lack of international standardized terminology and the absence of clear diagnosis criteria (Hooper & Mackinnon, 1995). Different terms have been used to describe overtraining: overwork, overreaching, staleness, burnout, overfatigue, short- and long-term overtraining, and so on (Kreider, Fry, & O'Toole, 1998b). Some authors clearly differentiate between overtraining and staleness and describe the different physiological and psychological effects (e.g., Hackney, Pearman, & Nowacki, 1990; Raglin, 1993), whereas others do not differentiate (e.g., McCann, 1995) or equate overtraining/staleness with burnout (e.g., Henschen, 1993; Mahoney, 1989; Rowland, 1986). In addition to the existing level of confusion, European researchers use the term *overtraining* differently in comparison with North Americans (Hooper & Mackinnon, 1995; Raglin, 1993; Raglin & Wilson, 2000). It should be noted that the terminology used also depends on the professional background (e.g., medical staff, sport psychologists). Moreover, an appropriate definition often loses its content in the translation or is interpreted differently. In summary, two rather diametrical approaches and a combined approach that possibly integrates both definitions (see table 1.1) are identified in the literature.

Approach I

The research group of Bill Morgan (University of Wisconsin, Madison, USA) has been dealing with the problem of overtraining for the past 15 to 20 years. In their probably most cited publication, Morgan, Brown, Raglin, O'Connor, and Ellickson

(1987) and Raglin (1993) differentiate between overtraining as a process and staleness as the undesirable consequence of overtraining.

> *Overtraining* is regarded as a stimulus consisting of a systematic schedule of progressively intense physical training of a high absolute and relative intensity. Moreover, overtraining is considered an integral and necessary aspect of endurance training, whereas *staleness* is regarded as an undesirable response that is a consequence or product of overtraining. (Raglin, 1993, p. 842)

From the authors' perspective this conceptualization avoids the confounding of cause (i.e., overtraining) with consequences (i.e., staleness), and the evaluation of the dose-response relationship between overtraining and staleness.

Exercise physiologist Hackney and colleagues came to a similar definition:

> *Overtraining:* An abnormal extension of the training process with the results culminating in the state of staleness or being overtrained. This term can be defined as "the process." *Staleness:* A state in which the athlete has difficulty maintaining standard training regimens and can no longer achieve previous performance results (i.e., performance decline). The terms "staleness" or "being overtrained" are commonly used interchangeably. This term can be defined as the end "result." (Hackney et al., 1990, p. 22)

Hackney's approach of judging overtraining as a "process" is similar to that of Raglin (1993). However, Hackney rates overtraining as an abnormal extension and not the regular training process. Both definitions consider overtraining as a normal or abnormal aspect of training. Staleness is the unwanted consequence of overtraining, which leads to a long-term and *uncontrolled* performance impairment. From their perspective the trick is to use overtraining but to avoid staleness.

Table 1.1 Comparison of Terminology

Approach I	Approach II	Combined approach
Overtraining	Overreaching	Short-term overtraining (overreaching)
Overtraining	Overtraining	Long-term overtraining (overtraining)
Staleness	Overtraining syndrome	Overtraining syndrome

Approach II

In contrast, Kreider and colleagues (1998b) define the key terms as follows:

[*Overreaching* is an] accumulation of training and non-training stress resulting in a short-term decrement in performance capacity with or without related physiological and psychological signs and symptoms of overtraining in which restoration of performance capacity may take from several days to several weeks. [*Overtraining* is an] accumulation of training and non-training stress resulting in a long-term decrement in performance capacity with or without related physiological and psychological signs and symptoms of overtraining in which restoration of performance capacity may take from several weeks to months. (Kreider et al., 1998b, p. viii)

Here, the main difference between overreaching and overtraining is a short-term vs. long-term performance decrement. In a state of overreaching the restoration of performance capacity may take from several days to several weeks; at the stage of overtraining, from several weeks to months.

Kreider and colleagues (1998b) differentiated between training that results in a short-term decrement of performance, and training that results in more prolonged decrements of performance. However, since they proposed the possible existence of a continuum "from under-training to optimal training, overreaching, or overtraining" (p. viii), overtraining cannot be judged as an integral and necessary aspect of training.

Combined Approach

A possible combination of the previous approaches was presented by Lehmann and colleagues (1999a), who developed a terminology that integrates both definitions. They distinguished between *short-term overtraining,* which lasts less than three weeks, and *long-term overtraining,* which lasts at least three weeks or more. The authors also point out that short-term overtraining (also called overreaching or supercompensation training) is a common part of athletic training, which leads to a state of overreaching in affected athletes. This state of overreaching is characterized by transient underperformance, which is reversible within a short-term recovery period of one to two weeks and can

be rewarded by a state of supercompensation (an increase in performance ability following one to two weeks of regeneration after a short-term phase of overtraining). Therefore, short-term overtraining or overreaching (terms that can be used synonymously) is a regular part of athletic training.

Nevertheless, when overreaching is too profound or is extended for too long, *short-term overtraining turns into long-term overtraining.* This occurs "if a necessary regeneration period is inappropriately short or recovery therefore remains incomplete and is additionally associated with too many competitions and non-training stress factors. The athlete clearly runs the risk of a resulting overtraining syndrome" (Lehmann et al., 1999a, p. 2).

With this approach Lehmann and colleagues (1999a) considered overreaching (and short-term overtraining) an integral and necessary aspect of training, as did Raglin (1993) and Hackney and colleagues (1990). Furthermore, the terms *staleness,* as the unwanted end result of overtraining (Raglin, 1993), and *overtraining syndrome* should have the same meaning. However, the tricky question remains of how to fine-tune the training process. At what stage of the training process does short-term overtraining turn into long-term overtraining, and how can this be prevented?

Accumulation and Interaction of Training and Nontraining Stressors

How complex the fine-tuning of a training process is can be highlighted by the accumulation and interaction of training and nontraining stressors. Performance abilities are influenced by many factors, such as *training* (e.g., stress/recovery relationship, training volume, intensity, methods, technique training, frequency of competitions), *lifestyle* (e.g., sleep, daily schedule, nutrition, alcohol consumption and smoking, housing conditions, leisure activities), *state of health* (e.g., cold, fever, gastric and intestinal diseases, infections), and *environment* (e.g., family, roommates, teammates, social contacts, job/school, coach).

Besides the integration of the previous approaches, Lehmann and colleagues' (1999a) definition includes training, competition, and additional nontraining stress factors. With this, the authors meet the requirements of the biopsychological stress model (Janke & Wolffgramm, 1995) using a multilevel approach. Psychological and physiological, emotional, cognitive, behavioral, performance, and social aspects are considered to be important. As hard as it may be for coaches to accept, athletes do have a life outside of sports. Emotional stress or fighting inside and outside of the training environment (e.g., illness, fights with friends or partners, parents' divorce) can affect them strongly. Problems and obligations at school, difficulties with time management (practice/school/friends), and other responsibilities can be pictured as a single package load. Often, individuals can easily handle those situations, but when a heavy training load is added to an already high "personal package load," the total impact on the systems simply gets too high. Although all components could easily be handled by themselves, the combination is overwhelming.

It is important not only to consider nontraining stressor overload but also to take a look at subsequent disturbing recovery effects. When an athlete worries about personal friendships or the family life is threatened by a divorce, all thoughts circle around that situation, and these thoughts increase at night while trying to sleep. According to Kellmann's model (figure 1.1), the lack of sleep or other recovery activities can be compensated for, for a limited time, but after a while the person is at risk of developing an overtraining syndrome. Consequently, athletes should actively try to fix disturbed relationships in their family and social environment and pay attention to getting enough rest and sleep. Coaches should provide a climate in which athletes can let them know about their personal situations. In a personal crisis, the impact of "regular training" is higher on athletes. Openness, communication skills, and a nonthreatening environment created by the coaches help athletes to overcome the noncommunication threshold.

Indicators and Types of Overtraining

During long-term overtraining, athletes are on a chronic performance plateau that cannot be influenced positively by short amounts of rest and recovery periods. Long-term overtraining can be characterized by an inability to train at customary levels. The symptoms include feelings of depression, general apathy, decreased self-esteem, emotional instability, impaired performance, lack of supercompensation, restlessness, irritability, disturbed sleep, weight loss, loss of appetite, increased resting heart rate, increased vulnerability to injuries, and hormonal changes (e.g., Barron, Noakes, Levy, Smith, & Millar, 1985;

Callister, Callister, Fleck, & Dudley, 1989; Flynn et al., 1994; Hackney et al., 1990; Hooper et al., 1995, 1997, 1999; Kuipers, 1998; Kuipers & Keizer, 1988; Lehmann, Foster, Dickhult et al., 1998; Lehmann et al., 1993, 1997, 1999a; Morgan et al., 1987; O'Connor, Morgan, & Raglin, 1991). An important clinical feature of overtraining syndrome is the increased susceptibility to infections with corresponding symptoms, suggesting some kind of impaired immune response (Foster, 1998; Froehlich, 1993; Lehmann et al., 1997; Steinacker & Lehmann, this volume, chapter 6; Steinacker et al., 1999).

According to Israel (1976), the sympathetic and parasympathetic type of overtraining syndromes are differentiated in the literature (see table 1.2). Lehmann et al. (1999a) reported that the parasympathetic type, which is characterized by a predominance in vagal tone or an adrenal insufficiency, is more frequent than the sympathetic type, which resembles a hyperadrenergic state or thyroidal hyperfunction.

The main symptoms of overtraining syndrome are restlessness and excitation (sympathetic form) or inhibition and depression (parasympathetic form), accompanied in both cases by a reduction in performance. According to Lehmann et al. (1993), the sympathetic form is rare; when found, it is more present in "anaerobic" types of sports that require activities such as sprinting, jumping, and throwing. The parasympathetic form is typically found in aerobic types of sports, such as long-distance running, swimming, road cycling, and so on (see also Israel, 1976). The characteristics of the parasympathetic type (e.g., good recovery capacity, low resting heart rate, no sleep disturbances) suggest excellent health and may be misleading (Kuipers, 1998). However, it has to be noted that some authors (e.g., Hooper, & Mackinnon, 1995; Lehmann, Foster, Dickhult et al., 1998; Lehmann et al., 1993) question the previous classification because of a lack of empirical support and experimental confirmation.

Overtraining and the Interrelations of Stress States and Recovery Demands

The model of stress states and recovery demands may explain how overtraining can develop (see figure 1.2). The axis of the stress states can be seen as a continuum of an increasing training load, which can be labeled at the end points "no training" and "overtraining" (similar to Kreider et al., 1998b). With an extended training load the

Table 1.2 Some Findings in Sympathetic- and Parasympathetic-Type Overtraining Syndromes

Sympathetic type	Parasympathetic type
Impaired performance	Impaired performance
Lack of supercompensation	Lack of supercompensation
Restlessness, irritability	Fatigue, depression, apathy
Disturbed sleep	Undisturbed sleep
Weight loss	No weight problems
Increased resting heart rate	Low resting heart rate
Increased resting blood pressure	Low resting blood pressure
Delayed recovery after exercise	Good recovery capacity
	Suppressed heart rate—exercise profile
	Suppressed glucose—exercise profile
	Suppressed lactate—exercise profile
	Suppressed neuromuscular excitability
	Suppressed sympathetic intrinsic activity
	Suppressed catecholamine sensitivity

Adapted, by permission, from M. Lehmann, C. Foster, N. Netzer, W. Lormes, J.M. Steinacker, Y. Lui, A. Opitz-Gress, and U. Gastmann, 1998, Physiological responses to short- and long-term overtraining in endurance athletes. In *Overtraining in sport,* edited by R.B. Kreider, A.C. Fry, and M.L. O'Toole (Champaign, IL: Human Kinetics), 21.

organismic recovery demands increase proportionally. A short-term planned sacrifice of recovery enhances long-term performance effects (e.g., supercompensation). If the training load and intensity increase over a longer time "without adequate recovery" or with merely "inappropriate recovery," the individual experiences long-term underrecovery, which may result in the overtraining syndrome. To reach the optimal recovery-stress state, athletes have to increase their self-initiated activities to fulfil their recovery demands. At each state of the model, recovery can work as a regulation mechanism, which is caused by an increasing distance between the two axes into a higher recovery debt (days to weeks). The higher a person is on the stress states or the more extensive the overtraining syndrome that occurs, the more recovery efforts are needed in order to reach the individual optimal recovery-stress state (Kellmann, 1997).

This approach is similar to that of Budgett (1998), who proposed that underrecovery, not necessarily too much training, leads to the over-

training syndrome. Like Kellmann, he focused on the relationship between training and recovery and stated that "eventually fatigue becomes so severe that recovery does not occur despite two weeks of relative rest" (p. 107).

Individual Differences

Athletes in general not only differ from the general population, but also exhibit a broad range of differences among themselves. To compare them, for example, with norm data of psychological or physiological tests may be misleading. Interindividual differences in recovery potential, exercise capacity, nontraining stressors, and stress tolerance may explain the different degrees of vulnerability experienced by athletes under identical training conditions (Lehmann et al., 1993). The key is to evaluate athletes individually, monitoring them regularly and comparing the obtained data longitudinally (Froehlich, 1993). Stress and recovery should be monitored during the training process to prevent overtrain-

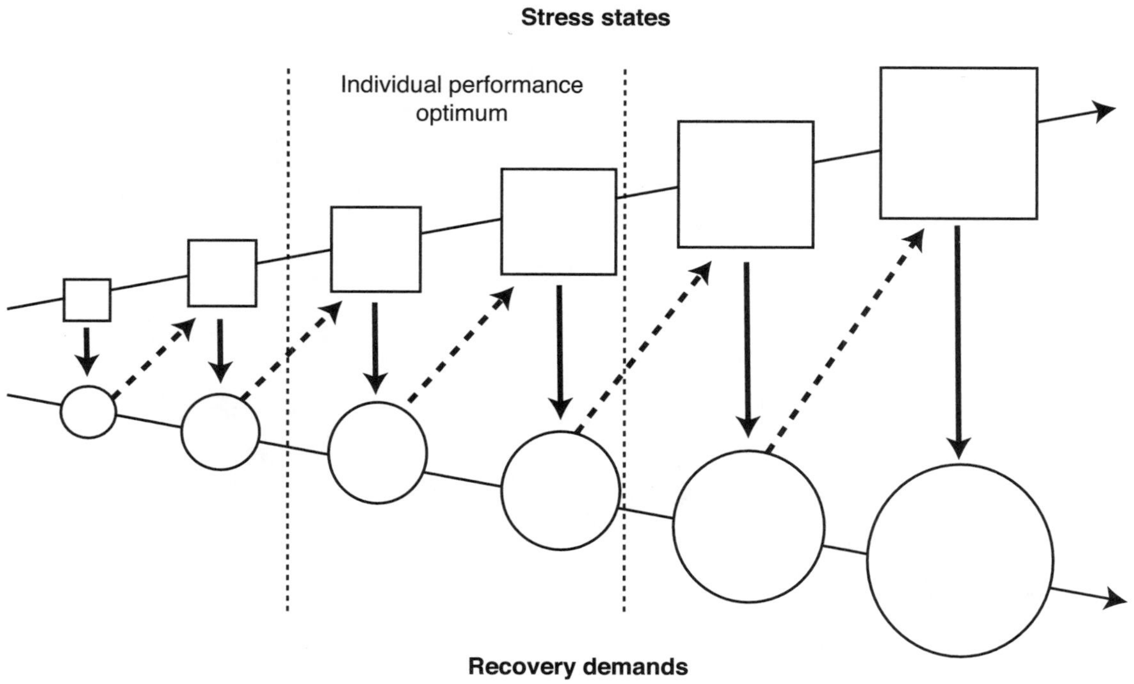

Stress states

Figure 1.2   The "scissors model" and increasing stress states.

ing (e.g., Berglund & Säfström, 1994; Hooper, Mackinnon, et al., 1999; Kellmann, 2000; Kellmann, Altenburg, Lormes, & Steinacker, 2001; Kellmann & Günther, 2000). Recognizing that different athletes have different thresholds for overtraining, Hooper and Mackinnon (1995) recommended that training be individualized. When working with teams or a group of athletes, coaches may find individualization of training difficult. But especially in weight- and strength-training sessions, this can easily be achieved. Reductions or increases of rounds and sets during weight- and strength-training sessions, and specific instructions regarding exercise intensity, can serve to individualize training. However, when training is individualized, it should be clearly communicated to the athletes that it is done to achieve individual optimal training results. If the individual training is not explained, the situation for athletes with the lower training volume may become awkward.

Younger athletes especially show earlier symptoms related to overtraining but do not relate those to the training process. Goss (1994) reported that mood disturbances are related to age. Older swimmers possessed fewer mood disturbances than younger swimmers did. Therefore, monitoring is important for everybody but espe-

cially for younger athletes such as juniors. The variability of psychological and physiological characteristics is higher with younger athletes than with older athletes because of the incomplete developmental process. As an example, figure 1.3 shows the 1998 Rowing Junior World Champions of the women's quad scull.

Obviously, the physiological characteristics of the rowers in the women's quad scull differ, and this also may affect the amount of training athletes can receive at certain times. Every athlete has an important function in moving the boat. In this case, the second female from the left was on the stroke, which is the leading position in a boat. Obviously, the athlete with the best rowing rhythm and the skills to lead the boat in the race—not the physically strongest athlete—should be on the stroke position. As already stated, the individual adaptation or resistance to training is quite different, and also depends on the physiological constitution. At a certain stage, one athlete can be very tired, whereas another shows almost no effects. The main purpose of the intervention approach for the German Junior National Rowing Team is to identify athletes during the training camp whose recovery-stress states do not correspond with changes in the training schedule (Kellmann & Günther, 2000; Kellmann et al., 1997,

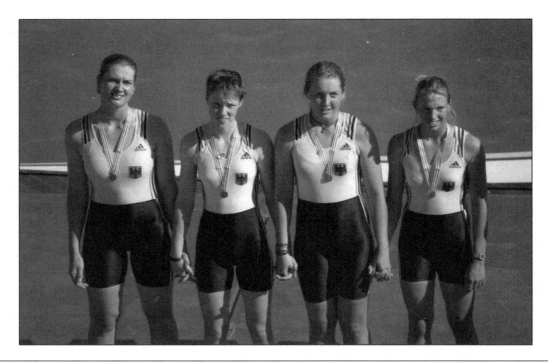

Figure 1.3   1998 Junior World Champions in the women's quad scull.

2001). Through early intervention, individual training can be adapted in order to help the athlete deal with training stress and to prevent overtraining (Botterill & Wilson, this volume, chapter 8; Hooper et al., 1995; Kellmann, Patrick, Botterill, & Wilson, this volume, chapter 12).

Treatment of Overtraining

A commonly accepted view in the literature is that the best treatment for overtraining is rest and recovery phases from two to six weeks (sometimes longer) depending on the seriousness of overtraining. In selected cases of an overtraining syndrome, athletes may require months without any training and without any physical activity in order to recover completely (Hackney et al., 1990; Lehmann et al., 1993; Raglin, 1993; Raglin & Morgan, 1994). Even after six months of recovering, Barron and colleagues (1985) reported that some athletes had disturbances of neuroendocrine functions.

Changes in training can also unburden the practice routine. A reduction of training load, a change of intensity, or technique training provides different input for the athletes. This additional variability positively affects athletes. When a coach suspects that an athlete is showing signs of overtraining, he should suggest a doctor's visit to reduce the risk of injuries and overstrain damage. If diagnosed, an additional treatment with electrolytes can be considered.

Active and proactive recovery is the best treatment to "work against the overtraining syndrome." Lying down and doing nothing can be part of the treatment, but different physical exercises such as gymnastics, games, regenerative runs, or swimming as well as a balanced and healthy diet play an important role in the recovery process (Kenttä & Hassmén, 1998; this volume, chapter 4). Environment and climate changes can also help athletes get a break both physically and mentally. Activities denied because of the rigid training regime can be important too, and psychoregulative techniques, such as relaxation or imagery, can accelerate the recovery process. However, it is best to prevent overtraining in the first place.

Sometimes Less Is More

The concept that sometimes "less is more" is often ignored in the daily training regime. Even in leisure sports the "no-excuse, feel-the-burn, more-is-better" theory of working out is rampant. However, the focus should be on the quality instead of the quantity of training. When performance plateaus occur, athletes often increase their efforts and increase the training load (Counsilman, 1971), which initiates a vicious cycle and, after continuation, can turn into a heavy overtraining syndrome. In this context, Raglin (1993) stated: "Coaches who are aware of those athletes who are suffering from distress could intervene by reducing training or providing short rest periods, and this would theoretically lead to enhanced performance" (p. 832). Consequently, overtraining can be prevented but it is frequently overlooked as a result of the lack of understanding on the part of coaches and athletes. The risk of overtraining syndrome can be reduced, if not eliminated, through careful periodization of training (Norris & Smith, this volume, chapter 7).

Adequate rest and recovery, especially during the heaviest training periods, is crucial. Coaches may have to enforce rest because some athletes are unwilling to reduce training for fear of becoming detrained. Similarly, coaches may need to prevent athletes from trying to get back into shape too quickly after a break. Overtraining can be effectively treated by rest or prevented outright by not training hard, but these obviously are not desirable options for the competitive athlete (Hackney et al., 1990; Kenttä & Hassmén, 1998; Lehmann et al., 1993; Raglin, 1993). Most athletes should be discouraged from doing additional workouts simply because they feel particularly good during training. Often, *rest* to athletes is just a four-letter word.

During a symposium titled Overtraining in Sports (Kellmann et al., 1999), Sean McCann (1999), the head sport psychologist of the U.S. Olympic Committee, stated that sometimes athletes have to be called lazy when they *do not rest*. Humans tend to do what they are good at and not what they should focus on to get better. For athletes it means that they focus on training and quite often ignore recovery. Sean McCann emphasized that adequate recovery is an important part of the optimal training process (see Davis, Botterill, & MacNeill, this volume, chapter 9).

In the real training world the concept of less is more seems to be hard to sell. Most coaches feel that coaching is their job, and it is the duty of their athletes to follow their regimes. In addition, when coaches back off too much, performance may decrease. This shows that there is a careful balance between practice and recovery. Practice is important to improve performance, but the *focus should be on the quality rather than on the quantity of training*. During long and hard training sessions athletes tend to take "hidden rests," for example, by going at a slower pace during the

exercises. A thoughtful variation of the training exercises includes a recovering element. An increase of the overall quality of training occurs when the standard regular training routine is modified, when new exercises are introduced, or simply when different types of training are applied.

Summary

Underrecovery and overtraining: different concepts—similar impact? This question can clearly be answered with a yes and a no. Yes, they have the same impact—performance declines; No, they are not similar—*underrecovery is the precursor/cause of overtraining*. Consequently, the key to prevent overtraining is an active and proactive enhancement of recovery. Coaches and athletes need to be educated about the importance of optimal recovery and its impact on performance. When athletes understand that a weekend without training is part of the planned training schedule, which implies that they should not train on their own or go for a heavy bike ride with friends, they take a huge step toward adequate recovery. In addition, the multilevel concept of stress and recovery emphasizes that physical training is just one part of athletes' lives (Wrisberg & Johnson, this volume, chapter 14). Emotional worries outside of the training environment may disturb the recovery process as well. Consequently, athletes' self-initiated activities and coaches' knowledge about individual preferences for recovery strategies (Hanin, this volume, chapter 11) are important elements in avoiding overtraining and subsequent underperformance—not only in sports but also in life (Kallus, this volume, chapter 16).

References

Ahmaidi, S., Granier, P., Taoutaou, Z., Mercier, B., Dubouchaud, H., & Prefaut, C. (1996). Lactate kinetics during passive and active recovery in endurance and sprint athletes. *European Medicine and Science in Sports and Exercise, 28,* 450-456.

Allmer, H. (1996). *Erholung und Gesundheit: Grundlagen, Ergebnisse und Maßnahmen* [Recovery and health: Basics, results and interventions]. Göttingen, Germany: Hogrefe.

Anshel, M.H. (1990). *Sport psychology: From theory to practice.* Scottsdale, AZ: Gorsuch Scaribrick.

Antonovsky, A. (1979). *Health, stress, and coping.* San Francisco: Jossey-Bass.

Antonovsky, A. (1987). *Unraveling the mystery of health.* San Francisco: Jossey-Bass.

Associated Press (1999, May 12). Woods is rested and ready to compete at the Nelson. *Golfweb Wire Services* [Online]. Retrieved May 30, 2001, from http://cbs.sportsline.com/u/ce/multi/0,1329,1025913_64,00.html

Banister, E.W., Morton, R.H., & Clarke, J.R. (1997). Clinical dose-response effects of exercise. In J.M. Steinacker & Ward, S.A. (Eds.), *The physiology and pathophysiology of exercise tolerance* (pp. 297-309). New York: Plenum.

Barron, J.L., Noakes, T.D., Levy, W., Smith, C., & Millar, R.P. (1985). Hypothalamic dysfunction in overtrained athletes. *Journal of Clinical Endocrinology and Metabolism, 60,* 803-806.

Belcastro, A.N., & Bonen, A. (1975). Lactic acid removals during controlled and uncontrolled recovery exercise. *Journal of Applied Physiology, 39,* 932-937.

Berger, B.G., Motl, R.W., Butki, B.D., Martin, D.T., Wilkinson, J.G., & Owen, D.R. (1999). Mood and cycling performance in response to three weeks of high-intensity, short-duration overtraining, and a two-week taper. *The Sport Psychologist, 13,* 444-457.

Berglund, B., & Säfström, H. (1994). Psychological monitoring and modulation of training load of world-class canoeists. *Medicine and Science in Sports and Exercise, 26,* 1036-1040.

Bonen, A., & Belcastro, A.N. (1974). Comparison of self-selected recovery methods on lactic acid removal rates. *Medicine and Science in Sports and Exercise, 8,* 176-178.

Boucsein, W. (1991). Arbeitspsychologische Beanspruchungsforschung heute—eine Herausforderung an die Psychologie [Work psychological stress research—A challenge for psychology]. *Psychologische Rundschau, 42,* 129-144.

Bruin, D. (1994). Adaptation and overtraining in horses subjected to increasing training loads. *Journal of Applied Physiology, 76,* 1908-1913.

Budgett, R. (1998). Fatigue and underperformance in athletes: The overtraining syndrome. *British Journal of Sport and Medicine, 32,* 107-110.

Callister, R., Callister, R.J., Fleck, S.J., & Dudley, G.A. (1989). Physiological and performance responses to overtraining in elite judo athletes. *Medicine and Science in Sports and Exercise, 22,* 816-823.

Costill, D.L., Flynn, M.G., Kirwin, J.P. Houmard, J.A., Mitchell, J.B., Thomas, R., & Park, S.H. (1988). Effects of repeated days of intensified training on muscle glycogen and swimming performance. *Medicine and Science in Sports and Exercise, 20,* 249-254.

Counsilman, J. (1971). Handling the stress and staleness problems of the hard training athletes. *Proceedings of the International Symposium on the Art and Science of Coaching* (pp. 15-22). Toronto, Canada.

Fletcher, B. (1988). The epidemiology of occupational stress. In C.L. Cooper & R. Payne (Eds.), *Causes, coping, and consequences of stress at work* (pp. 3-52). Chichester, U.K.: Wiley.

Flynn, M.G., Pizza, F.X., Boone, J.B., Andres, F.F., Michaud, T.A., & Rodriguez-Zayas, J.A. (1994). Indices of training stress during competitive running and swimming seasons. *International Journal of Sport Medicine, 15,* 21-26.

Foster, C. (1998). Monitoring training in athletes with reference to overtraining syndrome. *Medicine and Science in Sports and Exercise, 30,* 1164-1168.

Frese, M., & Zapf, D. (1994). Action as the core of work psychology. A German approach. In H.C. Triandis, M.D. Dunnette, & L.M. Hough (Eds.), *Handbook of industrial and organizational psychology* (Vol. 4, pp. 271-340). Palo Alto, CA: Consulting Psychologists Press.

Froehlich, J. (1993). Overtraining syndrome. In J. Heil (Ed.), *Psychology of sport injury* (pp. 59-70). Champaign, IL: Human Kinetics.

Fry, R.W., Morton, A.R., & Keast, D. (1991). Overtraining in athletes: An update. *Sports Medicine, 12,* 32-65.

Gabriel, H.H.W., Urhausen, A., Valet, G., Heidelbach, U., & Kindermann, W. (1998). Training and overtraining: An introduction. *Medicine and Science in Sports and Exercise, 30,* 1151-1157.

Gastmann, U., Petersen, K.G., Böcker, J., & Lehmann, M. (1998). Monitoring intensive endurance training at moderate energetic demands using resting laboratory markers failed to recognize an early overtraining stage. *Journal of Sports Medicine and Physical Fitness, 38,* 188-193.

Goldberger, L., & Breznitz, S. (1993). Stress research at a crossroads. In L. Goldberger & S. Breznitz (Eds.), *Handbook of stress* (pp. 3-6). New York: The Free Press.

Goss, J. (1994). Hardiness and mood disturbances in swimmers while overtraining. *Journal of Sport & Exercise Psychology, 16,* 135-149.

Gould, D., Guinan, D., Greenleaf, D., Medbery, R., Strickland, M., Lauer, L., Chung, Y., & Peterson, K. (1998). Positive and negative factors influencing U.S. Olympic athletes and coaches: Atlanta Games assessment—final report: Executive summary. Oral presentation at the USA Softball, Fort Worth, TX.

Hacker, W., & Richter, P. (1984). *Psychische Fehlbeanspruchung* [Psychological over- and understrain]. Berlin: Springer.

Hackney, A.C. (1999). Neuroendocrine system: Exercise overload and regeneration. In M. Lehmann, C. Foster, U. Gastmann, H. Keizer, & J.M. Steinacker (Eds.), *Overload, fatigue, performance incompetence, and regeneration in sport* (pp. 173-186). New York: Plenum.

Hackney, A.C., Pearman III, S.N., & Nowacki, J.M. (1990). Physiological profiles of overtrained and stale athletes: A review. *Journal of Applied Sport Psychology, 2,* 21-33.

Hagedorn, G. (1989). Die Auszeit im Sportspiel [Time-out in sport games]. *Sportpsychologie, 3,* 26-28.

Hanin, Y.L. (1997). Emotions and athletic performance: Individual Zones of Optimal Functioning model. In R. Seiler (Ed.), *European Yearbook of Sports Psychology* (Vol. 1, pp. 29-72). St. Augustin, Germany: Academia.

Hanin, Y.L. (2000). Individual Zones of Optimal Functioning (IZOF) Model: Emotion-performance relationships in sport. In Y.L. Hanin (Ed.), *Emotions in sport* (pp. 65-89). Champaign, IL: Human Kinetics.

Hellbrügge, T., Rutenfranz, J., & Graf, O. (1960). *Gesundheit und Leistungsfähigkeit im Kindes- und Jugendalter* [Health and performance ability during childhood and adolescence]. Stuttgart, Germany: Thieme.

Henschen, K. (1993). Athletic staleness and burnout: Diagnosis, prevention, and treatment. In J. Williams (Ed.), *Applied sport psychology* (pp. 328-337). Mountain View, CA: Mayfield.

Herzog, K., Voigt, H.F., & Westphal, G. (1985). *Volleyball-Training: Grundlagen und Arbeitshilfen* [Volleyball Training: Fundamentals and Applied Examples]. Schorndorf, Germany: Hofmann.

Hoffman, J.R., Epstein, S., Yarom, Y., Zigel, L., & Einbinder, M. (1999). Hormonal and biochemical changes in elite basketball players during a 4-week training camp. *Journal of Strength Condition Research, 13,* 280-285.

Hogg, J.M. (1998). The post performance debriefing process: Getting your capable track and field athletes to the next level of performance. *New Studies in Athletics, 13,* 49-57.

Hollmann, W. (1989). Ethische Gefahren im Hochleistungssport—Reflexionen aus sportmedizinischer Sicht [Ethical dangers in elite sports—reflections from the medical perspective]. *Brennpunkte der Sportwissenschaft, 3,* 72-83.

Hollmann, W., & Hettinger, T. (2000). *Sportmedizin* [Sports medicine]. Stuttgart, Germany: Schlattauer.

Hooper, S.L., & Mackinnon, L.T. (1995). Monitoring overtraining in athletes. *Sports Medicine, 20,* 321-327.

Hooper, S.L, & Mackinnon, L.T. (1999). Monitoring regeneration in elite swimmers. In M. Lehmann, C. Foster, U. Gastmann, H. Keizer, & J.M. Steinacker (Eds.), *Overload, fatigue, performance incompetence, and regeneration in sport* (pp. 139-148). New York: Plenum.

Hooper, S.L., Mackinnon, L.T., & Hanrahan, S. (1997). Mood states as an indication of staleness and recovery. *International Journal Sport Psychology, 28,* 1-12.

Hooper, S.L., Mackinnon, L.T., & Howard, A. (1999). Physiological and psychometric variables for monitoring recovery during tapering for major competition. *Medicine and Science in Sports and Exercise, 31,* 1205-1210.

Hooper, S.L., Mackinnon, L.T., Howard, A., Gordon, R.D., & Bachmann, A.W. (1995). Markers for monitoring overtraining and recovery. *Medicine and Science in Sports and Exercise, 27,* 106-112.

Israel, S. (1976). Zur Problematik des Übertrainings aus internistischer und leistungsphysiologischer Sicht [The problem of overtraining from the internal and performance physiological perspective]. *Medizin und Sport, 16,* 1-12.

Janke, W., & Wolffgramm, J. (1995). Biopsychologie von Streß und emotionalen Reaktionen: Ansätze interdisziplinärer Kooperation von Psychologie, Biologie und Medizin [Biopsychology of stress and emotional reactions: Starting points of an interdisciplinary cooperation of psychology, biology, and medicine]. In G. Debus, G. Erdmann, & K.W. Kallus (Eds.), *Biopsychologie von Streß und emotionalen Reaktionen* (pp. 293-349). Göttingen, Germany: Hogrefe.

Jerusalem, M. (1990). *Persönliche Ressourcen, Vulnerabilität und Streßerleben* [Personal resources, vulnerability, and stress experience]. Göttingen, Germany: Hogrefe.

Kallus, K.W. (1992). *Beanspruchung und Ausgangszustand* [Strain and initial state]. Weinheim, Germany: PVU.

Kallus, K.W. (1995). *Der Erholungs-Belastungs-Fragebogen* [The Recovery-Stress Questionnaire]. Frankfurt, Germany: Swets & Zeitlinger.

Kallus, K.W., & Kellmann, M. (2000). Burnout in athletes and coaches. In Y.L. Hanin (Ed.), *Emotions in sport* (pp. 209-230). Champaign, IL: Human Kinetics.

Kallus, K.W., & Krauth, J. (1995). Nichtparametrische Verfahren zum Nachweis emotionaler Reaktionen [Non-parametric methods for the proof of emotional reactions]. In G. Debus, G. Erdmann, & K.W. Kallus (Eds.), *Biopsychologie von Streß und emotionalen Reaktionen* (pp. 23-43). Göttingen, Germany: Hogrefe.

Kellmann, M. (1991). *Die Abbildung des Beanspruchungszustandes durch den Erholungs-Belastungs-Fragebogen: Untersuchungen zur Leistungsprädiktion im Sport* [The assessment of the recovery-stress state by the Recovery-Stress Questionnaire: Studies dealing with performance prediction in sports]. Unpublished diploma thesis, University of Würzburg, Germany.

Kellmann, M. (1997). *Die Wettkampfpause als integraler Bestandteil der Leistungsoptimierung im Sport: Eine empirische psychologische Analyse* [The rest period as an integral part of optimizing performance in sports: An empirical psychological analysis]. Hamburg, Germany: Kovac.

Kellmann, M. (2000). Psychologische Methoden der Erholungs-Beanspruchungs-Diagnostik [Psychological methods for the assessment of recovery and stress]. *Deutsche Zeitschrift für Sportmedizin, 51,* 253-258.

Kellmann, M., Altenburg, D., Lormes, W., & Steinacker, J.M. (2001). Assessing stress and recovery during preparation for the World Championships in rowing. *The Sport Psychologist, 15,* 151-167.

Kellmann, M., Gould, D., Smith, D.J., Botterill, C., Blakeley, A., McCann, S.C., & Wrisberg, C.A. (1999). Overtraining in sport (Symposium). Abstract of the 14th Conference of the Association for the Advancement of Applied Sport Psychology (AAASP) from the 22-26 September 1999 in Banff, Alberta. *Abstracts* (pp. 12-13). Banff: AAASP.

Kellmann, M., & Günther, K.-D. (2000). Changes in stress and recovery in elite rowers during preparation for the Olympic Games. *Medicine and Science in Sports and Exercise, 32,* 676-683.

Kellmann, M., & Kallus, K.W. (1994). Interrelation between stress and coaches' behavior during rest periods. *Perceptual and Motor Skills, 79,* 207-210.

Kellmann, M., & Kallus, K.W. (1995). The Rest-Period Questionnaire for Coaches: Assessing the behavior of coaches during rest periods. In R. Vanfraechem-Raway & Y. Vanden Auweele (Eds.), *Proceedings of the 9th European Congress on Sport Psychology* (Part 1, pp. 43-50). Brussels, Belgium: FEPSAC/Belgian Federation of Sport Psychology.

Kellmann, M., & Kallus, K.W. (1999). Mood, recovery-stress state, and regeneration. In M. Lehmann, C. Foster, U. Gastmann, H. Keizer, & J.M. Steinacker (Eds.), *Overload, fatigue, performance incompetence, and regeneration in sport* (pp. 101-117). New York: Plenum.

Kellmann, M., & Kallus, K.W. (2000). *Der Erholungs-Belastungs-Fragebogen für Sportler; Handanweisung* [The Recovery-Stress Questionnaire for Athletes; manual]. Frankfurt, Germany: Swets Test Services.

Kellmann, M., & Kallus, K.W. (2001). *Recovery-Stress Questionnaire for Athletes; User manual.* Champaign, IL: Human Kinetics.

Kellmann, M., Kallus, K.W., Günther, K.-D., Lormes, W., & Steinacker, J.M. (1997). Psychologische Betreuung der Junioren-Nationalmannschaft des Deutschen Ruderverbandes [Psychological consultation of the German Junior National Rowing Team]. *Psychologie und Sport, 4,* 123-134.

Kenttä, G., & Hassmén, P. (1998). Overtraining and recovery. *Sports Medicine, 26,* 1-16.

Koutedakis, Y., Myszkewycz, L., Soulas, D., Papapostolou, V., Sullivan, I., & Sharp, N.C.C. (1999). The effects of rest and subsequent training on selected physiological parameters in professional female classical dancers. *International Journal of Sports Medicine, 20,* 379-383.

Koutedakis, Y., & Sharp, N.C.C. (1998). Seasonal variations of injury and overtraining in elite athletes. *Clinical Journal of Sport and Medicine, 8,* 18-21.

Kreider, R.B., Fry, A.C., & O'Toole, M.L. (Eds.). (1998a). *Overtraining in sport.* Champaign, IL: Human Kinetics.

Kreider, R.B., Fry, A.C., & O'Toole, M.L. (1998b). Preface. In R.B. Kreider, A.C. Fry, & M.L. O'Toole (Eds.), *Overtraining in sport* (pp. vii-ix). Champaign, IL: Human Kinetics.

Kuhl, J., & Beckmann, J. (1994). Alienation: Ignoring one's preferences. In J. Kuhl & J. Beckmann (Eds.), *Volition and personality* (pp. 375-390). Toronto: Hogrefe.

Kuipers, H. (1998). Training and overtraining: An introduction. *Medicine and Science in Sports and Exercise, 30,* 1137-1139.

Kuipers, H., & Keizer, H.A. (1988). Overtraining in elite athletes: Review and directions for the future. *Sports Medicine, 6,* 79-92.

Lazarus, R.S. (1991). *Emotion and adaptation.* New York: Oxford University Press.

Lazarus, R.S., & Launier, R. (1978). Stress-related transactions between person and environment. In R. Plutchik & M. Lewis (Eds.), *Perspectives in international psychology* (pp. 287-327). New York: Plenum.

Lehmann, M., Foster, C., Dickhult, H.-H., & Gastmann, U. (1998). Autonomic imbalance hypothesis and overtraining syndrome. *Medicine and Science in Sports and Exercise, 30,* 1140-1145.

Lehmann, M., Foster, C., Gastmann, U., Keizer, H.A., & Steinacker, J.M. (1999a). Definition, types, symptoms, findings, underlying mechanisms, and frequency of overtraining and overtraining syndrome. In M.J. Lehmann, C. Foster, U. Gastmann, H. Keizer, & J.M. Steinacker (Eds.), *Overload, fatigue, performance incompetence, and regeneration in sport* (pp. 1-6). New York: Plenum.

Lehmann, M., Foster, C., Gastmann, U., Keizer, H.A., & Steinacker, J.M. (Eds.). (1999b). *Overload, fatigue, performance incompetence, and regeneration in sport.* New York: Plenum.

Lehmann, M., Foster, C., & Keul, J. (1993). Overtraining in endurance athletes: A brief review. *Medicine and Science in Sports and Exercise, 25,* 854-861.

Lehmann, M., Foster, C., Netzer, N., Lormes, W., Steinacker, J.M., Lui, Y., Opitz-Gress, A., & Gastmann, U. (1998). Physiological responses to short- and long-term overtraining in endurance athletes. In R.B. Kreider, A.C. Fry, & M.L. O'Toole (Eds.), *Overtraining in sport* (pp. 19-46). Champaign, IL: Human Kinetics.

Lehmann, M., Lormes, W., Opitz-Gress, A., Steinacker, J.M., Netzer, N., Foster, C., & Gastmann, U. (1997).

Training and overtraining: An overview and experimental results in endurance sports. *Journal of Sports Medicine and Physical Fitness, 37,* 7-17.

Lehmann, M., Schnee, W., Scheu, R., Stockhausen, W., & Bachl, N. (1992). Decreased nocturnal catecholamine excretion: Parameter for an overtraining syndrome in athletes. *International Journal of Sport Medicine, 13,* 236-242.

Löhr, G., & Preiser, S. (1974). Regression und Recreation—Ein Beitrag zum Problem Streß und Erholung [Regression and recreation—A paper dealing with stress and recovery]. *Zeitschrift für experimentelle und angewandte Psychologie, 21,* 575-591.

Mackinnon, L.T., & Hooper, S. (1991). *State of the art review no. 26: Overtraining.* Canberra: Australian Sports Commission.

Maglischo, E.W. (1993). *Swimming even faster.* Mountain View, CA: Mayfield.

Mahoney, M.J. (1989). Sport psychology. In I.S. Cohen (Ed.), *The G. Stanley Hall lectures* (Vol. 9, pp. 101-134). Washington, DC: American Psychological Association.

McCann, S.C. (1995). Overtraining and burnout. In S.M. Murphy (Ed.), *Sport psychology interventions* (pp. 347-368). Champaign, IL: Human Kinetics.

McCann, S.C. (1999). The role of a sport psychologist when addressing overtraining in elite athletes. Abstracts of the 14th Conference of the Association for the Advancement of Applied Sport Psychology (AAASP) from 22-26 September 1999 in Banff, Alberta. *Abstracts* (pp. 13). Banff: AAASP.

Morgan, W.P., Brown, D.R., Raglin, J.S., O'Conner, P.J., & Ellickson, K.A. (1987). Psychological monitoring of overtraining and staleness. *British Journal of Sport Medicine, 21,* 107-114.

Morgan, W.P., O'Conner, P.B., Ellickson, K.A., & Bradley, P.W. (1988). Personality structure, mood states, and performance in elite distance runners. *International Journal of Sport Psychology, 19,* 247-263.

Morgan, W.P., O'Conner, P.B., Sparling, P.B., & Pate, R.R. (1987). Psychologic characterization of the elite female distance runner. *International Journal of Sport Medicine, 8,* 124-131.

O'Connor, P.J., Morgan, W.P., & Raglin, J.S. (1991). Psychobiologic effects of 3 d of increased training in female and male swimmers. *Official Journal of the American College of Sports Medicine, 23,* 1055-1061.

Raglin, J.S. (1993). Overtraining and staleness: Psychometric monitoring of endurance athletes. In R.B. Singer, M. Murphey, & L.K. Tennant (Eds.), *Handbook of research on sport psychology* (pp. 840-850). New York: Macmillan.

Raglin, J.S., & Morgan, W.P. (1989). Development of a scale to measure training induced distress. *Medicine and Science in Sports and Exercise, 21* (Supplement), 60.

Raglin, J.S., & Morgan, W.P. (1994). Development of a scale for use in monitoring training-induced distress in athletes. *International Journal of Sports Medicine, 15,* 84-88.

Raglin, J.S., & Wilson, G.S. (2000). Overtraining in athletes. In Y.L. Hanin (Ed.), *Emotions in sport* (pp. 191-207). Champaign, IL: Human Kinetics.

Renzland, J., & Eberspächer, H. (1988). *Regeneration im Sport* [Regeneration in sports]. Cologne, Germany: bps.

Rohmert, W., & Rutenfranz, J. (1975). *Arbeitswissenschaftliche Beurteilung der Belastung und Beanspruchung an unterschiedlichen industriellen Arbeitsplätzen* [Scientific rating on stress and strain in different industrial workplaces]. Bonn, Germany: Bundesminister für Arbeit und Sozialordnung.

Rowbottom, D.G., Keast, D., Garcia-Webb, P., & Morton, A.R. (1997). Training and overtraining: An introduction. *Medicine and Science in Sports and Exercise, 29,* 1233-1239.

Rowbottom, D.G., Keast, D., & Morton, A.R. (1998). Monitoring and preventing of overreaching and overtraining in endurance athletes. In R.B. Kreider, A.C. Fry, & M.L. O'Toole (Eds.), *Overtraining in sport* (pp. 47-66). Champaign, IL: Human Kinetics.

Rowland, T. (1986). Exercise fatigue in adolescents: Diagnosis of athlete burnout. *The Physician and Sportmedicine, 14,* 69-77.

Rüger, U., Blomert, A.F., & Förster, W. (1990). *Coping. Theoretische Konzepte, Forschungsansätze, Meßinstrumente zur Krankheitsbewältigung* [Coping. Theoretical concepts, research designs, and instruments for dealing with illness]. Göttingen, Germany: Verlag für Medizinische Psychologie im Verlag Vandenhoeck & Ruprecht.

Savis, J.C. (1994). Sleep and athletic performance: Overview and implications for sport psychology. *The Sport Psychologist, 8,* 111-125.

Schönpflug, W. (1983). Coping efficiency and situational demands. In R. Hockey (Ed.), *Stress and fatigue in human performance* (pp. 299-326). Chichester, U.K.: Wiley.

Schönpflug, W. (1987). Beanspruchung und Belastung bei der Arbeit—Konzepte und Theorien. Arbeitspsychologie [Strain and stress during work—concepts and theories]. In U. Kleinbeck & J. Rutenfranz (Eds.), *Enzyklopädie der Psychologie* (Part III/1, pp. 131-184). Göttingen, Germany: Hogrefe.

Selye, H. (1974). *Stress without distress.* Philadelphia: Lippincott.

Silva III, J. M. (1990). An analysis of the training stress syndrome in competitive athletics. *Journal of Applied Sport Psychology, 2,* 5-20.

Smith, D.J., & Norris, S.R. (2000). Changes in glutamine and glutamate concentrations for tracking training tolerance in elite athletes. *Medicine and Science in Sports and Exercise, 32,* 684-689.

Steinacker, J.M., Kellmann, M., Böhm, B.O., Liu, Y., Opitz-Gress, A., Kallus, K.W., Lehmann, M., Altenburg, D., & Lormes, W. (1999). Clinical findings and parameters of stress and regeneration in rowers before World Championships. In M. Lehmann, C. Foster, U. Gastmann, H. Keizer, & J.M. Steinacker (Eds.), *Overload, fatigue, performance incompetence, and regeneration in sport* (pp. 71-80). New York: Plenum.

Steinacker, J.M., Lormes, W., Kellmann, M., Liu, Y., Reißnecker, S., Opitz-Gress, A., Baller, B., Günther, K., Petersen, K.G., Kallus, K.W., Lehmann, M., & Altenburg, D. (2000). Training of junior rowers before World Championships. Effects on performance, mood state and selected hormonal and metabolic responses. *Journal of Sports Medicine and Physical Fitness, 40,* 327-335.

Taoutaou, Z., Granier, P. Mercier, B., Mercier, J., Ahmaidi, S., & Prefaut, C. (1996). Lactate kinetics during passive and active recovery in endurance and print athletes. *European Journal of Applied Physiology, 73,* 465-470.

Thiriet, P., Gozal, D., Wouassi, D., Oumarou, T., Gelas, H., & Lacour, J.R. (1993). The effect of various recovery modalities on subsequent performance, in consecutive supramaximal exercise. *Journal of Sports Medicine and Physical Fitness, 33,* 118-129.

Tschiene, P. (1999). Die unmittelbare Wettkampfvorbereitung [The preparation for competition]. In G. Thieß & P. Tschiene (Eds.), *Handbuch zur Wettkampflehre* (pp. 319-349). Aachen, Germany: Meyer.

Urhausen, A., Gabriel, H., & Kindermann, W. (1995). Blood hormones as markers of training stress and overtraining. *Sports Medicine, 20,* 251-276.

Verma, S.K., Mahindroo, S.R., & Kansal, D.K. (1978). Effect of four weeks of hard physical training on certain physiological and morphological parameters of basketball players. *Medicine and Science in Sports and Exercise, 18,* 379-384.

Viru, A. (1984). The mechanism of training effects: A hypothesis. *International Journal of Sport Medicine, 5,* 219-227.

Viru, A. (1985). *Hormones in muscular activity: Volume I—hormonal ensemble in exercise.* Boca Raton, FL: CRC Press.

Viru, A. (1994). Molecular cellular mechanism of training effects. *Journal of Sports Medicine and Physical Fitness, 34,* 309-322.

Viru, A., & Viru, M. (1997). Organism's activity in sports training. *Medicina Sportiva, 1,* 45-50.

Viru, A., & Viru, M. (1999). Evaluation of endocrine activities and hormonal metabolic control in training and overtraining. In M. Lehmann, C. Foster, U. Gastmann, H. Keizer, & J.M. Steinacker (Eds.), *Overload, fatigue, performance incompetence, and regeneration in sport* (pp. 53-70). New York: Plenum.

Weinberg, R., & Gould, D. (1999). *Foundations of sport and exercise psychology.* Champaign, IL: Human Kinetics.

Weineck, J. (1994). *Optimales Training* [Optimal training]. Erlangen, Germany: perimed.

Wilmore, J.H., & Costill, D.L. (1988). *Training for sport and activity: The physiological basis of the conditioning process.* Dubuque, IA: Wm. C. Brown.

Gould, D., & Dieffenbach, K. (2002). Overtraining, underrecovery, and burnout in sport. In M. Kellmann (Ed.), Enhancing recovery: Preventing underformance in athletes (pp. 25-35). Champaign, IL: Human Kinetics.

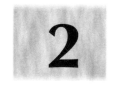

Overtraining, Underrecovery, and Burnout in Sport

Daniel Gould and Kristen Dieffenbach

Be careful in trying to "get the edge" that you don't overdo it and "lose the edge."

My coach is a real pusher, to the point where I think he pushes too hard. I think it would be better if I did not train as hard.

If 5 is good then 50 is better . . . the year before the Olympics, they [my athletes] would do sets of 50 jumpies and this year they are doing sets of 700 jumpies. If I can push them more and more, when they finally get there, they will be great. However, this pushing can blow up in your face—like you finally get to the Olympics and are exhausted.

I didn't have an option to choose not to do that event after making the team . . . the timing was very poor and that contributed to overtraining, and my performance was probably 80% at the Games due to fatigue and lack of recovery.

As these quotes from U.S. Olympic athletes and coaches reveal, the problem of overtraining in sport is becoming an increasing concern. In fact, Raglin and Wilson (2000) recently estimated that physical training loads increased 20% in the last decade. Athletes, then, especially elite athletes, are doing much more physical work in preparation for optimal performance. In a review of the sport burnout research, Gould (1996) also indicated that many people feel that athlete burnout is on the rise in part because of these increases in training loads. Given these assertions, a need exists to examine the factual base for such statements. Thus, this chapter is designed to examine the need for further sport research in the areas of psychological overtraining, underrecovery, and burnout, and to consider appropriate interventions.

Key Definitions

Before accomplishing this purpose, key terms must be defined. Unfortunately, overtraining, burnout, and related topics have not always been clearly delineated. Recently, however, a consensus definition of overtraining was derived as a result of extensive discussions by a special task force formulated by the U.S. Olympic Committee and composed of elite coaches and sport scientists studying the topic. Specifically, overtraining is a syndrome that results when excessive, usually physical, overload on an athlete occurs without adequate rest

(USOC, 1998; see also Kellmann, this volume, chapter 1). The excessive overload placed on the performer results in decreased performance and the inability to train.

Staleness and *burnout* are related terms. Staleness is an "initial failure of the body's adaptive mechanisms to cope with psychological and physiological stress" (Silva, 1990, p. 10). It is thought to result when overtraining occurs and performance decreases for several weeks. Burnout is more severe than staleness and is defined as a psychological, emotional, and physical withdrawal from a formerly pursued and enjoyable sport as a result of chronic stress (Smith, 1986). It is an exhaustive psychophysiological response exhibited as a result of frequent, sometimes extreme, and generally ineffective efforts to meet excessive physical training and psychological demands. It is also important to note that when athletes burn out on sport, they do not always discontinue involvement altogether. Some athletes who experience burnout remain active. They feel they cannot discontinue for various reasons (e.g., family pressure), and this "trapped" participation is characterized by lower motivation, emotional detachment, less satisfaction, and poor performance (Gould, Tuffey, Udry, & Loehr, 1996a; Raedeke, 1997). With these definitions in hand, the topics of overtraining, underrecovery, and burnout can now be addressed.

Evidence of Overtraining in Athletes

The importance of better understanding overtraining in athletes was recently demonstrated by Gould and his colleagues (Gould, Greenleaf, Dieffenbach, Chung, & Peterson, 1999; Gould, Greenleaf, Guinan, Dieffenbach, & McCann, 2001; Gould, Guinan, Greenleaf, Medbery, & Peterson, 1999; Gould, Guinan, Greenleaf, Medbery, Strickland, Lauer, Chung, & Peterson, 1998). Specifically, these investigators conducted several different studies that examined positive and negative factors influencing athlete and coach performance at the 1996 Atlanta and 1998 Nagano Olympic Games. In these studies, surveys as well as interviews were conducted with all U.S. athletes and coaches from the 1996 Atlanta and 1998 Nagano Olympic teams. Although the focus of this research was not on overtraining, overtraining was identified as a factor of consider-

ation that affected performance in Atlanta and Nagano.

Atlanta survey results, from 296 athletes representing 30 different sports, revealed that 84 (28%) of all U.S. Olympians reported that they were overtrained and that this had had a negative effect on their performance (Gould et al., 1998). Hence, when the athletes were asked about overtraining as one of a variety of almost 100 factors that influenced performance, a large number cited it as a negative performance influence. Similarly in open-ended responses, 35 of these Olympians identified overtraining and not getting enough rest as the number one coaching action that hurt their performance at the Games.

Nagano survey findings (Gould, Greenleaf, et al., 1999) revealed that 8 of the 83 U.S. Olympians, or approximately 10%, from 13 different sports reported that they were overtrained and that this had had negative effects on their performance. Also, in open-ended responses these same Olympians stated that they would taper, rest, not overtrain, travel less, and stay healthy if they could prepare again for the Olympics. Hence, these findings demonstrate that both summer and winter Olympic Games athletes consider overtraining a concern. They also identified a number of factors within overtraining, such as excessive traveling, lack of adequate rest, lack of proper taper, and a less-than-healthy lifestyle, as affecting performance.

To more specifically examine levels of overtraining in these athletes, table 2.1 summarizes the number of Atlanta athletes by sport who reported being overtrained, as well as the perceived impact of this overtraining on their performance. An inspection of this table reveals that the incidence of overtraining ranged from zero in judo and softball to 80% in synchronized swimming. Whereas some of these results are specific to particular coaches and contexts, generally, sports that require more physical training were characterized by higher levels of perceived overtraining. Moreover, the results show that overtraining is thought by athletes to be a major problem across a variety of sports.

Although the research by Gould and his colleagues is interesting and provides evidence for the need to study overtraining, its primary focus was not on overtraining. Other investigators, however, have conducted studies specifically designed to monitor overtraining and study the causes in athletes. For example, in studies of endurance

Table 2.1 Atlanta Olympian Frequency and Impact of Overtraining on Performance Responses

Sports	Yes (n)	No (n)	Yes (%)	Impact *M*	Impact *(SD)*
Athletics	13	41	24%	2.62	2.59
Baseball	1	7	13%	0.00	0.00
Canoe and kayak	5	6	45%	1.80	1.10
Cycling	4	4	50%	1.00	1.41
Diving	1	4	20%	0.00	0.00
Fencing	1	8	11%	2.00	0.00
Field hockey	14	5	74%	1.93	1.59
Gymnastics	3	6	33%	5.50	3.54
Rowing	16	13	55%	0.80	1.21
Shooting	1	16	6%	4.00	0.00
Soccer	1	13	7%	3.00	0.00
Swimming	4	20	17%	2.25	0.96
Synchronized swimming	4	1	80%	3.00	1.73
Handball	6	13	32%	2.50	1.23
Volleyball	5	8	38%	2.60	2.61
Wrestling	1	9	10%	4.00	0.00
Yachting	1	8	11%	2.00	0.00
Judo	0	8	00%	0.00	0.00
Softball	0	7	00%	0.00	0.00

Only data from sports that had five or more respondents are included. Impact ratings (1 = extremely negative effect; 3 = no effect; 5 = extremely positive effect).

athletes, especially in the sport of swimming, the yearly incidence of staleness ranged from 7% to 21% with an average of 10% of the athletes reporting symptoms (Hooper, Mackinnon, & Hanrahan, 1997; O'Connor, Morgan, Raglin, Barksdale, & Kalin, 1989; Raglin & Morgan, 1994). Morgan and his colleagues (1987, 1988), studying staleness in distance runners, also reported significant levels of overtraining. Specifically, these investigators found that 64% of males and 60% of females reported experiencing a minimum of one episode of staleness during their running careers. The overtraining percentage of nonelite runners, who recorded significantly less training mileage, was lower, but still noteworthy at 33%. Thus, overtraining is a significant problem for athletes.

Whereas most of the previous overtraining research focused on physical overtraining, Kellmann and Günther (2000) recently extended this research by focusing not only on physical training loads, but also on psychological stress levels and recovery activities in elite athletes. In this study the researchers examined changes in stress and recovery of 11 German rowers preparing for the 1996 Atlanta Summer Olympic Games. In order to explore the dose-response relationship between training volume and recovery-stress states as perceived by the athletes, the researchers asked

11 rowers to complete the Recovery-Stress Questionnaire for Athletes (Kellmann & Kallus, 2000, 2001) on four occasions leading up to the Olympics. In addition, the 8 rowers actually competing at the Olympics responded on a fifth occasion, two days before their Olympic preliminary races. Results revealed that significant components of somatic stress scales such as *Lack of Energy, Somatic Complaints,* and *Fitness/Injury* and recovery factors such as *Fitness/Being in Shape* paralleled the average lengths of daily training sessions. Moreover, significant changes in team conflicts and pressures as well as social relaxation were noted and reflected changes in interpersonal dynamics in the team. Together, then, these findings showed that training volume corresponded to stress levels in the athletes as did team dynamics. Also, recovery factors were found to be related to these factors and performance. These findings provide a detailed example of how elite athletes are influenced by training and recovery practices, demonstrating the importance of better understanding these topics.

Although certainly frequently noted in elite sport, overtraining is also a problem at other levels of participation. For example, Raglin and Wilson (2000) suggested that young athletes experience overtraining, the resulting staleness, and negative performance effects in youth sports, particularly when their training loads are comparable to those of elite adult athletes. In a well-conducted, cross-cultural study, Raglin, Sawamura, Alexiou, Hassmén, and Kenttä (2000) demonstrated this phenomenon. Specifically, 231 youth swimmers with a mean age of 14.8 years from Greece, Japan, Sweden, and the United States were administered surveys that assessed training volumes, mood states, and staleness. Staleness was defined as having a loss of performance for at least two weeks that did not result from injury or illness. Looking across all participants, it was found that 35% of the 231 young swimmers reported having been stale, with 45% of Greek, 34% of Japanese, 21% of Swedish, and 24% of U.S. athletes reporting staleness. The average length of staleness reported was 3.6 weeks, and stale swimmers reported greater mood disturbance than their healthy counterparts. Overall, then, staleness was found to be common in the young athletes studied, and although some differences were apparent, evidence of staleness was found in all four countries. It was also concluded that rates of staleness among young athletes were similar to those found among adult endurance athletes.

Finally, although statistical studies of the frequency of overtraining and factors related to it are important, they do not convey the devastating effects overtraining can have on athletes and their performance. For example, Gould, Guinan, et al. (1999) discussed a case study of an Atlanta Olympic Games team that unwittingly overtrained and suffered devastating performance effects. Specifically, being defending world champions, this team was highly favored to win a gold medal at the Games, but failed to medal. The primary negative performance influencing factor identified by both the athletes and coaches was overtraining, including quantity, intensity, and lack of an appropriate taper. As noted by one athlete, "we tried to get the edge by pushing the edge." Another stated, "some of the stuff we were doing was out of hand" in describing their pre-Games training load. One of the coaches also noted the problem, saying, "either I put a little too much overload in or we didn't get the taper right." The team focused so much on training hard and getting an edge over their opponents that they went too far and physically overtrained. Interestingly, the overtraining resulted from the inability of the athletes and coaches to recognize signs of overtraining and their failure to communicate training and recovery concerns with each other. The result was a dismal Olympic campaign and the failure to earn any medals.

Burnout in Athletes

Evidence emphasizing the importance of better understanding overtraining and underrecovery comes not only from overtraining research, but also from the related area of athlete burnout. To reiterate, burnout is defined as a psychological, physical, and emotional withdrawal from a formerly enjoyable and motivating activity resulting from prolonged or chronic stress (Smith, 1986). It results in a decline in sport participation by an athlete as a result of chronic excess stress.

In one attempt to explain athlete burnout, Silva (1990) suggested that athletic training physically and psychologically stresses the performer and can have both positive and negative effects. The desired impact of training is positive adaptation, the goal most athletes and coaches seek to achieve when overloading the body in training bouts. However, too much training and inadequate recovery can have a negative impact. Silva proposed that negative adaptation leads to negative training responses with athletes progressing from overtraining to staleness and ultimately to burnout (if the training stress is not reduced).

Physical Factors

In an initial attempt to study burnout, Silva (1990) conducted a survey of 68 elite collegiate athletes from a variety of sports. His results revealed that 7% of those athletes indicated that they had experienced burnout sometime during their university athletic experience. Moreover, causes of burnout cited included exhaustion, apathy, extreme fatigue, boredom, lack of recovery time from competitive sport, and severe practice conditions. Although Silva's results showed that burnout did occur in athletes and identified likely sources of burnout, no explanation of how the participants defined burnout was given, nor how burnout was distinct from staleness and overtraining. The sample size was also very small and represented only two universities.

Another early study of athlete burnout was conducted by Cohn (1990). In this qualitative investigation, 10 high school golfers (mean age = 16.4 years) were interviewed for the purpose of learning more about the stress and burnout they experienced. All 10 reported being burned out sometime during their careers with burnout being defined as "a negative reaction to physical or psychological stress leading to withdrawal from the activity" (p. 98). The mean length of time that they discontinued their golf was 10 days, ranging from a low of 5 days to a high of 14 days. Too much practice or playing time, lack of enjoyment, no new goals, going into a slump, and pressure from self and others were identified as causes of burnout. Unfortunately, since no distinctions were made among overtraining, staleness, and burnout in this study, there is no way to know what exactly these participants were experiencing. The results do show, however, that nonendurance-sport athletes also experience overtraining, underrecovery, and burnout.

Finally, in a recent study, Raedeke (1997) examined motivational factors that influenced burnout in 236 age-group swimmers who swam 40,000 meters per week. Various submeasures of burnout were employed and included emotional and physical exhaustion, devaluation, and reduced accomplishment, as well as a total burnout score. Although not presented in his original article, Raedeke's data can be used to estimate the extent of burnout experienced by young athletes (Gould & Dieffenbach, in press). Specifically, when those swimmers who scored 2 standard deviations above the mean on these various burnout subcategory scores and exhibited an overall burnout score of 4 (highest score possible) are grouped, approximately 3% to 5% of the athletes experienced some emotional and physical exhaustion, 3% to 5% of the athletes experienced devaluation, and 1% to 2% of the athletes experienced reduced accomplishment. Thus, between 1% and 5% of these 236 swimmers experienced some form of burnout. Hence, a small percentage of younger, nonelite athletes are experiencing burnout often as a result of hard physical training (some of the highest numbers in the study were for the *Emotional and Physical Exhaustion* subscale).

Social and Psychological Factors

When most of us think of overtraining and burnout, exhaustion from excessive physical training loads comes to mind. This is certainly justified based on the studies reviewed thus far. Burnout, overtraining, and underrecovery, however, are not solely caused by physical factors. Social and psychological factors have been shown to play an important role as well.

In 1992, for example, Coakley reported preliminary findings examining athlete burnout based on informal interviews with 15 young athletes between the ages of 15 and 18 years who had burned out of predominantly individual sports. Pressure and stress were mentioned by the participants as primary reasons for discontinuing participation. Moreover, it was reported that this pressure was typically tied to a lack of control over their lives (e.g., practice and competitions kept them from doing things with friends). The results also showed that sport participation was closely tied to the young athletes' self-definition, supporting the idea that burnout occurs when athletes do not have well-rounded self-identities, but instead define themselves solely through sport. Unfortunately, these results must be viewed cautiously because the results were not reported in enough detail to judge their scientific merit. They do, however, offer an interesting perspective on burnout and lead to the formation of an explanatory model of burnout.

According to the model Coakley (1992) developed from this data, the causes of burnout in young athletes are tied to the social organization of high-performance sport and its effects on identity and control issues in young athletes. Specifically, in terms of the identity of the young athlete,

Coakley proposed that burnout occurs because the structure of high-performance sport (e.g., time demands) does not allow the young athlete to develop a normal, multifaceted identity (e.g., they have no time to spend with peers or in other nonsport activities). Instead, identity foreclosure occurs in which the young athlete's identity is solely focused on sport success. Consequently, in many cases (e.g., when injury or performance failure occurs), this sole identity focus on being an athlete causes stress that can ultimately lead to burnout.

Coakley (1992) also contended that in high-performance sport the social worlds of young athletes are organized in such a way that their control and decision making is inhibited. In particular, young athletes' social environments "are organized in ways that leave them powerless to control events and make decisions about the nature of their experiences and the direction of their own development" (Coakley, 1992, p. 282). This lack of control and power also leads to stress and ultimately burnout.

The Coakley model was developed as an alternative to the stress-based models of burnout and is based on the perspective that stress is an outcome or symptom of burnout rather than a cause. This model is important for the emphasis it places on the social environment of the young athlete. Based on this model, specific recommendations for preventing burnout include changing the social structure of high-performance sport for children, changing the manner in which the sport experience is integrated in children's lives, and structuring the relationships between significant others and child athletes in differing ways.

Studies Guided by Smith's Model

In one of the more comprehensive studies to date, Gould and his colleagues (Gould et al., 1996a; Gould, Tuffey, Udry, & Loehr, 1996b, 1997) conducted a three-part investigation of burnout in junior tennis athletes. Although not testing any one model of burnout, the study was guided by Smith's (1986) cognitive-affective stress model. Specifically, Smith (1986) proposed a stress-based interpretation of burnout in sport. According to this view, a demand is placed on the athlete (e.g., high volumes of physical practice and training, pressure to win by significant others). Second, that demand is not perceived equally by all participants; some athletes will cognitively appraise it as more threatening or overwhelming than others

will. Third, if the demand is perceived as threatening, a physiological response occurs (e.g., anxiety, fatigue). Finally, the physiological response leads to some type of coping and task behavior, such as decreased performance, interpersonal difficulties, or withdrawal from the activity.

Smith's model also proposed that all four stages of the burnout process are influenced by personality and motivational factors such as self-esteem and trait anxiety (see figure 2.1). Additionally, Smith (1986) considered the model circular and continuous, with the coping and task behavior stage feeding back to the situational demand and resources stage. Reciprocal relationships also exist among all four stages of the model.

Finally, Smith contended that although some individuals discontinue sport participation because of burnout, burnout is not the primary cause of sport withdrawal for most individuals (Smith, 1986). Rather, Smith hypothesized, based on Thibaut and Kelly's (1959) social exchange theory and current youth sports research, that individuals withdraw from sport when costs are perceived to outweigh benefits relative to alternative activities. For most athletes this means that they discontinue because of changing interests, conflicting time demands among activities, low perceived competence, and a lack of fun (Gould & Petlichkoff, 1987; Weiss & Chaumenton, 1992). Thus, burnout only occurs when the costs outweigh the rewards and when the costs are stress induced.

Using this model as a general guide, then, the first phase of the Gould et al. (1996a) study involved a retrospective survey that was administered to a national sample of 30 male and female junior tennis players identified by the U.S. Tennis Association as having burned out. Thirty-two comparison players of similar age, gender, and competitive experience were also identified. All players completed a battery of psychological tests, and a series of discriminant function and univariate t-tests were conducted to compare the two groups. Relative to the comparison players, the burned-out players had significantly higher burnout scores, had less input into their tennis training and tennis-related decisions, were more likely to play up in an older age division, practiced fewer days (which lessened their involvement), were higher in amotivation, were lower in external motivation, reported being more withdrawn, differed in perfectionism (especially relative to concern over mistakes, personal standards, parental criticism, parental expectations, and a higher need for organization), were less likely to use planning coping

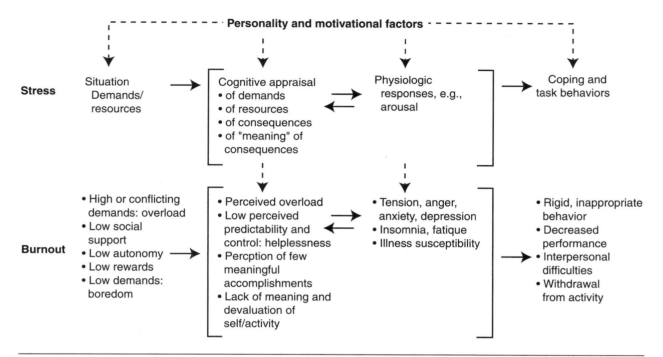

Figure 2.1 Smith's model shows the parallel relationships assumed to exist among situational, cognitive, physiological, and behavioral components of stress and burnout. Individual differences in motivation and personality are assumed to influence all of the components.

Reprinted, by permission, from R.E. Smith, 1986, "Toward a cognitive-affective model of athletic burnout," *Journal of Sport Psychology* 8: 40.

strategies, and were lower on positive interpretation and growth coping. The burned-out players did not differ from the comparison players relative to the number of hours trained. Both groups trained, on average, 2.3 hours per day. Hence, the results suggest that in this group of young athletes burnout was more psychologically than physically driven. The researchers also concluded that in addition to a variety of personal and situational factors, the personality disposition of perfectionism played a particularly important role in predicting burnout in junior tennis athletes.

The second part of the investigation (Gould et al., 1996b) involved extensive interviews with the 10 most burned out players identified in the quantitative part of the project. The interviews focused on signs and symptoms of burnout, how players dealt with their burned-out feelings, factors perceived to lead to burnout, suggestions for preventing burnout, involvement of significant others in tennis, and advice to others. Content analysis of the 10 interviews revealed two major categories of burned-out feelings—physical symptoms, which included injuries, illness, and/or being physically asymptomatic, and mental symptoms, which consisted of lacking energy/ motivation, negative feelings, feelings of isola-

tion, concentration problems, and high and low moods. Reasons for burning out included physical concerns, such as being sick and not being satisfied with performance, logistical concerns, such as time demands and too much travel, social interpersonal concerns, such as dissatisfaction with social life and negative parental influence, and (the largest category) psychological concerns, which included such things as unfulfilled and unrealistic expectations and pressure.

Burned-out athletes' recommendations for preventing and dealing with burnout included playing for one's own reasons, balancing tennis with other activities, such as school clubs or socializing with friends, stopping participation if playing tennis is not fun, focusing on making tennis fun, doing things to relax, and taking time off. The players recommended that parents recognize that some parental push is needed, but that it must be an optimal amount as too much contributes to burnout. Additionally, players suggested that parents reduce the focus on event and game outcomes, clarify their role in relationship with the coach, and solicit input from their junior player. Lastly, the results were examined in light of the burnout models of Silva (1990), Coakley (1992), and Smith (1986), with all three receiving some support.

Interestingly, all the players interviewed discussed how experiencing burnout negatively influenced their motivation and performance. As one participant indicated:

> *The biggest thing, though, was the lack of energy and lack of motivation, you know. I couldn't get myself to, you know, to give 100%. . . . I guess mentally and emotionally I'd feel really drained. (Gould et al., 1996b, p. 345)*

Other players put it this way:

> *Like, you know, I used to get sick a lot. I think a lot of it had do with the pressure because I couldn't handle stress very well and that is when I would get sick. (Gould et al., 1996b, p. 347)*

> *The grind of, you know, staying in a hotel and going there and having nothing to do for the rest of the day. And playing tennis just pretty much wore me out! So I guess pretty much for at least the five months prior to my quitting, I was very tired all the time. (Gould et al., 1996b, p. 347)*

In addition to these concerns, players talked about concentration problems, injuries, and numerous negative feelings that took a toll on both their performance and their enjoyment of the sport.

In the third part of the study Gould and colleagues (1997) highlighted individual differences in burnout by presenting the individual profiles of three players who represented different forms of burnout. The cases included (1) a player characterized by high levels of perfectionism and overtraining who burned out chiefly because of her personality orientation; (2) a player who experienced pressure from others and felt a strong need for a social life outside of tennis and burned out primarily because of social psychological factors; and (3) a player who was physically overtrained, failed to get enough sleep, and burned out because of physical factors. The researchers concluded that, based on these three cases and the earlier phases of the study, burnout might best be viewed within a stress-related strain model (see figure 2.2), with a "physically driven" strain resulting from physical overtraining and a "psychologically driven" strain composed of two additional substrains. One of the psychological substrains results from a young athlete having an "at risk" perfectionistic personality—a personality that predisposes them to burnout, even in nonpressure situations. The second psychological substrain focuses on burnout resulting from situational stress, such as coach or parent pressure to participate and perform. These two substrains are not totally independent of one another.

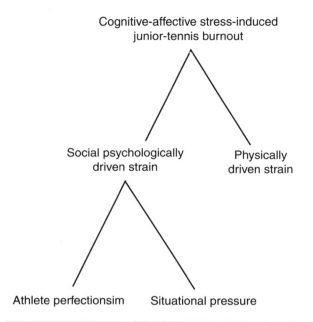

Figure 2.2 Burnout and burnout strains in athletes.

Adapted, by permission, from D. Gould, S. Tuffey, E. Udry, and J. Loehr, 1996, "Burnout in competitive junior tennis players: II. Qualitative analysis," *The Sport Psychologist* 10: 364.

Although the Gould et al. (1997) substrain notion is interesting, additional research is needed to verify its existence. Especially important is the need to examine whether various burnout strains and substrains differ across sports. These results do show, however, that burnout involves much more than excessive physical training demands and must be considered in light of social and psychological pressures as well.

Testing the Sport Commitment Model

In the most recent study of burnout in young athletes, Raedeke (1997) tested sport commitment model predictions in the previously discussed study of 236 age-group swimmers. Like Coakley's (1992) unidimensional identity development and external control model, the sport commitment model of burnout recognizes that stress is involved in the burnout process, but contends that other variables need to be examined if we are to better understand when and why burnout occurs. Raedeke (1997, p. 398), for example, contended that "everyone can experience stress, but not everyone who experiences stress burns out." Hence, sport commitment perspective theorists suggest that athletes burn out on sport because their reasons for being involved differ from those of athletes who do not burn out. Athletes who burn out do so because they are committed to sport for solely entrapment-related reasons (e.g., they feel that they "have to" maintain their involvement versus "want to" maintain their involvement).

Raedeke (1997) went on to indicate that athletes become entrapped in sport when they do not enjoy participation because of high perceived costs of involvement and low rewards (e.g., they must practice many hours and have few friends involved). However, they maintain their involvement because they feel they have too much invested in sport to discontinue (e.g., they have committed much time and effort to their training or their parents have invested much time, effort, and financial resources in their training). They also see a lack of alternative activities available in which to invest their efforts.

Raedeke's initial test of his model was designed to examine whether youth swimmers with motivation profiles representing sport entrapment, sport attraction, and low commitment, experience varying levels of burnout. As previously discussed, the teenage swimmers studied trained 40,000 meters a week and were extensively involved in swimming. The athletes all completed a 21-item athletic burnout scale, as well as assessments of the benefits and costs of swimming, swimming enjoyment, personal investment in swimming, alternative activity attraction, social constraints, swim identity, and perceived control. Cluster analysis was used to partition the swimmers into profile groups (e.g., enthusiastic, indifferent) based on their psychological characteristics. Swimmers who were characterized by an entrapment profile (i.e., they swam because they had to) exhibited significantly higher burnout scores than swimmers who were characterized by an attraction profile (i.e., they swam because they wanted to). Moreover, these swimmers were found to be entrapped because of their low perceived control (e.g., not having a say in what they do in swimming) and high social constraints (e.g., social norms and expectations that cause feelings of obligation to swim, such as parental pressure). Other entrapment sources, such as the attractiveness of alternative activities, received only scant support. The results are consistent with many of the sport commitment model predictions.

Summary

Looking across all the burnout models and investigations, then, it is clear that athlete burnout results from a complex interplay of situational factors and personal characteristics of the athlete. Numerous social and psychological factors beyond physical overtraining are involved. Hence, all these factors and their unique interactions must be considered when understanding burnout. It is also evident that even though the absolute numbers of athletes who experience excessive burnout are small, a significant minority of participants suffer from high levels of burnout.

Conclusions and Recommendations

Considering both the overtraining and athlete burnout research, several patterns are clear. First, athletes overtrain and burn out of sport, and although no exact numbers are available, many experts feel that the number of athletes doing so appears to be increasing. Overtraining, underrecovery, and burnout also affect athletes in a number of sports, at varied levels of competition, and of differing ages. It is also evident that researchers must look beyond mere physical training as a cause of overtraining and burnout, although physical training is certainly a major factor involved. Other factors such as psychological stress, inadequate rest, the type of recovery activity, travel, personality, and sociological issues must be examined in multifaceted models. Overtraining, underrecovery, and burnout, then, are issues that need to be further studied in sport psychology.

Although overtraining, underrecovery, and burnout are in need of further study, practitioners cannot wait for a full database to be developed before guiding practice. Practitioners must now be ready to help athletes cope with (and avoid) overtraining, design optimal recovery protocols, and effectively deal with burnout in sport based on the current state of knowledge. Fortunately, experienced athletes and coaches have conveyed a number of lessons for guiding practice in this area (Gould, Greenleaf, et al., 1999; Gould et al., 1996b). These include the following:

- Coaches and athletes should recognize that there is a fine line between training very hard and doing too much and overtraining. Studying exercise physiology and better understanding both the physical and social psychological factors influencing overtraining and burnout are critical.

- Coaches should realize that when an athlete is in top shape, he is very fragile and has an increased susceptibility to overtraining, staleness, and burnout. They should plan extensive recovery periods into training plans.

- When approaching critically important competitions like the Olympics or World Championships, coaches and athletes should recognize that although training hard and getting into top condition are essential, taking mental and physical breaks is equally important. Moreover, the type of break activity is an important consideration. Taking a break does little good if the athlete returns so fatigued or lethargic that she cannot function.

- Over time athletes and coaches should log the most effective ways to physically and psychologically regenerate.

- Coaches and athletes should realize that physical activity levels are only part of the overtraining process. Minimizing other stress factors, such as travel, leading up to important competitions is essential.

- Coaches should recognize that no single magic physical or psychological marker of training exists. The key is not only to use current available sport science tools (e.g., Recovery-Stress Questionnaire for Athletes; lactic acid assessments), but also to develop excellent athlete-coach communication patterns. Coaches must learn to recognize early signs of staleness, overtraining, and burnout in their athletes, and athletes must feel comfortable about speaking to their coaches about these issues (e.g., they must not be afraid the coach will feel they are mentally or physically weak if these symptoms are discussed).

- Athletes should understand their reasons for participating and be sure to play for themselves and not just to please others.

- The idea that intense training should not have any association with fun needs to be debunked. Hard physical training is often uncomfortable, but this does not mean fun cannot be included in workouts. Athletes and coaches should constantly be looking for ways to make the sport enjoyable and, in turn, less stressful and more satisfying.

- Although elite athletes cannot have the type of balance in their life that the more traditional 40-hour work week provides, they still must have some balance. Thus, they should have more in their lives than solely sport participation, whether it be family, school, part-time work, or hobbies.

- Significant others in athletes' lives (especially parents) must guard against becoming overinvolved in sport. Support, encouragement, and empathy are certainly needed, but must be offset by a healthy distancing from self-identification with results. The importance of repeatedly soliciting athlete input in decisions is critical.

- Coaches must continually cultivate personal involvement with their players and show interest in them not only as performers, but also as people. This will not only lower pressure placed on athletes, but will also encourage athletes to communicate more openly with their coaches.

- Coaches should develop good coach-athlete communication skills by fostering two-way communication with the player, soliciting and using athlete input on a regular basis, and striving to understand players' feelings.

References

Coakley, J. (1992). Burnout among adolescent athletes: A personal failure or a social problem? *Sociology of Sport Journal, 9,* 271-285.

Cohn, P.J. (1990). An exploratory study of sources of stress and burnout in youth golf. *The Sport Psychologist, 4,* 95-106.

Gould, D. (1996). Personal motivation gone awry: Burnout in competitive athletes. *Quest, 48,* 275-289.

Gould, D., & Dieffenbach, K. (in press). Psychological issues in youth sports: Competitive anxiety, overtraining, and burnout. In R. Malina & M. Clark (Eds.), *Youth sports in the 21st century: Organized sports in the lives of children and adolescents.* East Lansing, MI: Exercise Science Publishers.

Gould, D., Greenleaf, C., Dieffenbach, K., Chung, Y., & Peterson, K. (1999). *Positive and negative factors influencing U.S. Olympic athlete and coaches: Nagano Games assessment.* U.S. Olympic Committee Sport Science and Technology Final Grant Report. Colorado Springs.

Gould, D., Greenleaf, C., Guinan, D., Dieffenbach, K., & McCann, S. (2001). Pursuing performance excellence: Lessons learned from Olympic athletes and coaches. *Journal of Performance Excellence, 4,* 21-43.

Gould, D., Guinan, D., Greenleaf, C., Medbery, R., & Peterson, K. (1999). Factors affecting Olympic performance: Perceptions of athletes and coaches from more and less successful teams. *The Sport Psychologist, 13,* 371-395.

Gould, D., Guinan, D., Greenleaf, C., Medbery, R., Strickland, M., Lauer, L., Chung, Y., & Peterson, K. (1998). *Positive and negative factors influencing U.S. Olympic athletes and coaches: Atlanta Games assessment.* Final grant report submitted to the U.S. Olympic Committee Sport Science and Technology Division, Colorado Springs.

Gould, D., & Petlichkoff, L. (1987). Participation motivation and attrition in young athletes. In F. Smoll, R. Magill, & M. Ash (Eds.), *Children in sport* (pp. 161-178). Champaign, IL: Human Kinetics.

Gould, D., Tuffey, S., Udry, E., & Loehr, J. (1996a). Burnout in competitive junior tennis players: I. A quantitative psychological assessment. *The Sport Psychologist, 10,* 322-340.

Gould, D., Tuffey, S., Udry, E., & Loehr, J. (1996b). Burnout in competitive junior tennis players: II. Qualitative analysis. *The Sport Psychologist, 10,* 341-366.

Gould, D., Tuffey, S., Udry, E., & Loehr, J. (1997). Burnout in competitive junior tennis players: III. Individual differences in the burnout experience. *The Sport Psychologist, 11,* 257-276.

Hooper, S.L., Mackinnon, L.T., & Hanrahan, S. (1997). Mood state as an indication of staleness and recovery. *International Journal of Sport Psychology, 20,* 321-327.

Kellmann, M., & Günther, K. (2000). Changes in stress and recovery in elite rowers during preparation for the Olympic Games. *Medicine and Science in Sports & Exercise, 35,* 676-683.

Kellmann, M., & Kallus, K.W. (2000). *Der Erholungs-Belastungs-Fragebogen für Sportler; Handanweisung* [The Recovery-Stress Questionnaire for Athletes; Manual]. Frankfurt, Germany: Swets Test Services.

Kellmann, M., & Kallus, K.W. (2001). *Recovery-Stress Questionnaire for Athletes; User manual.* Champaign, IL: Human Kinetics.

Morgan, W.P., Brown, D.R., Raglin, J.S., O'Connor, P.J., & Ellickson, K.A. (1987). Psychological monitoring of overtraining and staleness. *British Journal of Sports Medicine, 21,* 107-114.

Morgan, W.P., Costill, D.L., Flynn, M.G., Raglin, J.S., & O'Connor, P.J. (1988). Mood disturbances following increased training in swimmers. *Medicine and Science in Sports and Exercise, 23,* 408-414.

O'Connor, P.J., Morgan, W.P., Raglin, J.S., Barksdale, C.N., & Kalin, N.H. (1989). Mood state and salivary cortisol levels following overtraining in female swimmers. *Psychoneuroendocrinology, 14,* 303-310.

Raedeke, T.D. (1997). Is athlete burnout more than just stress? A sport commitment perspective. *Journal of Sport and Exercise Psychology, 19,* 396-417.

Raglin, J.S., & Morgan, W.P. (1994). Development of a scale to use in monitoring training-induced distress in athletes. *International Journal of Sports Medicine, 15,* 84-88.

Raglin, J., Sawamura, S., Alexiou, S., Hassmén, P., & Kenttä, G. (2000). Training practices and staleness in 13-18 year old swimmers: A cross-cultural study. *Pediatric Exercise Science, 12,* 61-70.

Raglin, J.S., & Wilson, G.S. (2000). Overtraining in athletes. In Y.L. Hanin (Ed.), *Emotions in sport* (pp. 191-207). Champaign, IL: Human Kinetics.

Silva, J.M. (1990). An analysis of the training stress syndrome in competitive athletics. *The Journal of Applied Sport Psychology, 2,* 5-20.

Smith, R. (1986). Toward a cognitive-affective model of athletic burnout. *Journal of Sport Psychology, 8,* 36-50.

Thibaut, J.W., & Kelly, H.H. (1959). *The social psychology of groups.* New York: Wiley.

USOC (1998). Overtraining: The challenge of prediction. The second annual U.S. Olympic Committee/American College of Sports Medicine Consensus Statement. *Olympic Coach, 8*(4), 4-8.

Weiss, M.R., & Chaumenton, N. (1992). Motivational orientations in sport. In T.S. Horn (Ed.), *Advances in sport psychology* (pp. 61-90). Champaign, IL: Human Kinetics.

Kellmann, M. (2002). Psychological assessment of underrecovery. In M.
Kellmann (Ed.), *Enhancing recovery: Preventing underperformance in athletes* (pp. 37-55). Champaign, IL: Human Kinetics.

3

Psychological Assessment of Underrecovery

Michael Kellmann

A December 2000 MEDLINE and PSYCHLIT literature search for the terms *stress and sport* and
recovery and sport highlighted the imbalance in
the knowledge we have of these two processes.
Whereas a lot of research about the relationship
between stress and sport exists in the areas of
sport medicine, general psychology, and sport
psychology, the recovery research remains almost untouched. Currently, research has been
focused on detecting activities that reduce stress
rather than on the systematic enhancement of
recovery. Therefore, only little knowledge about
systematic recovery enhancement and the assessment of recovery exists.

Continuing the literature search for *recovery
and sport,* psychological and medical publications
dealing with recovery from sport injuries are found.
Papers focusing on active and passive recovery
after physical exercise follow as well. However,
almost all papers deal solely with the physical
issue of recovery, which is not sufficient to fully
cover the complex process of recovery. In particular, in the state of overtraining, physiological
changes and decrements of performance occur in
conjunction with psychic changes ranging from
disturbed sleep to depressed behavior. Consequently, it is necessary to assess recovery from a
multidimensional perspective in order to understand this complex process (Kellmann, 2000;
Kellmann & Günther, 2000; Kellmann & Kallus,
1999, 2000, 2001).

Athletes can only avoid overtraining and
achieve optimal performance when they are able
to recover and optimally balance training stress
and subsequent recovery. As a result of underrecovery, athletes may experience psychological
and physical consequences such as overtraining
and burnout. To achieve peak performance, athletes have to be able to recover quickly during
competition. When intensity and volume are increased during training, the subjective assessment of athletes turns out to be very important
because a long-term imbalance of stress (including training, competition, and nontraining stress
factors) and recovery can lead to a state of overtraining (Budgett, 1998; Foster, 1998; Hooper,
Mackinnon, & Hanrahan, 1997; Kenttä & Hassmén,
1998; Kuipers, 1998; Lehmann et al., 1997;
Lehmann, Foster, Gastmann, Keizer, & Steinacker,
1999; Lehmann, Foster, & Keul, 1993; USOC/ACSM,
1999; see Kellmann, this volume, chapter 1).

Stress and recovery should be monitored continuously during the training process (e.g.,
Berglund & Säfström, 1994; Hooper, Mackinnon,
& Howard, 1999; Kellmann & Günther, 2000;
Kellmann, Altenburg, Lormes, & Steinacker, 2001).
Smith and Norris (this volume, chapter 5) list a
number of training errors that can lead to overtraining (e.g., neglecting recovery, increasing
training demands too rapidly for the athlete to
adequately adapt, or extremely biased training
direction such as very high volume or very high-

intensity work). However, overtraining is due not only to training errors, but also to a high frequency of competitions that do not permit sufficient time for recovery. To avoid underrecovery—which has been identified as the precursor of overtraining—physiological and psychological recovery should be an integral part of the training plan (Hooper & Mackinnon, 1995; Kellmann, this volume, chapter 1).

Dealing with data assessment issues, Ulmer, Macsenaere, and Valasiadis (1999) reported difficulties measuring the level of exertion using objective tests. In this study 20 athletes had to run 400 meters with maximum effort and were tested five times within 19 minutes of the recovery period using a reaction and division test as an objective parameter. In addition, subjective degrees of mental and physical exhaustion were measured, and heart rate was assessed continuously. The results exhibited great variation (it resembled the course of the heart rate), whereas the objective parameters—namely, the time requirement for the reaction and division test—varied only slightly. Moreover, during recovery approximately 20% of the subjects showed even shorter reaction times. Since subjective scaling procedures seem to be more successful, test methods based on subjective tests have to be reconsidered.

The results of the Ulmer et al. study (1999) suggest that those assessing reactions to stress should consider method-specific reactions (or unexpected absences of reactions) in addition to individual-specific, stimulus-specific, and motivation-specific reactions. The authors concluded that standardized psychological methods turned out to be relatively stable, reliable, and sensitive—a result that is also reported in publications dealing with overtraining (e.g., Kenttä & Hassmén, 1998).

The objective when studying the effects of overtraining is to establish signs that predict negative processes. Physiological indicators, such as the presence of creatine kinase, represent shifts in training loads but are undependable for detecting early overtraining symptoms (Morgan, 1994; Raglin, 1993). Findings from physiological tests have been analyzed in an attempt to predict overtraining, but they are often inconsistent (e.g., Kuipers & Keizer, 1988). Distinguishing between normal and abnormal modifications in response to overtraining is complex because various physiological characteristics change when athletes shift from standard to intense training (Hooper, Mackinnon, Howard, Gordon, & Bachmann, 1995).

Kuipers (1998) asserted that no specific, simple, and reliable parameters are known for diagnosing overtraining at the earliest stage. However, studies to establish decisive factors of overtraining have demonstrated that psychological indicators seem to be more sensitive and consistent than physiological indicators (Kellmann, this volume, chapter 1; Kenttä & Hassmén, 1998; Raglin, 1993). The great advantage of psychometric instruments is the quick availability of information. Whereas common blood analyses and specific medical/physiological diagnostics may take hours or up to days (and even sometimes weeks), psychological data are available within minutes.

Psychometric Approaches

As pointed out in chapter 1 of this volume, interindividual differences in recovery potential, exercise capacity, nontraining stressors, and stress tolerance may explain the different degrees of vulnerability experienced by athletes under identical training conditions (Lehmann et al., 1993). In conclusion, it is necessary to evaluate athletes individually, monitoring them regularly and comparing the data longitudinally (Froehlich, 1993). In the following sections psychometric approaches currently used to monitor training will be discussed.

Sport psychological research of training/overtraining/underrecovery in North America deals mainly with the Profile of Mood States (POMS; McNair, Lorr, & Droppleman, 1971, 1992) and Borg's Rating of Perceived Exertion (RPE; Borg, 1975, 1998). In Germany in recent years a standardized scale of self-condition (Eigenzustandsskala; Nitsch, 1976) was also used in overtraining research (Urhausen, Gabriel, Weiler, & Kindermann, 1998; Urhausen & Kindermann, 2001). Kenttä and Hassmén (1998; this volume, chapter 4) recently introduced the method of Total Quality Recovery, which has been structured closely around the concept of RPE in order to emphasize the interrelationship between training and recovery. This new approach is an effective way of addressing the problem of assessing recovery and underrecovery.

The fact that the POMS and the RPE have been the instruments of choice for the psychological assessment of recovery in sport does not necessarily mean that they are properly designed for this purpose. Until recently no appropriate instrument existed to assess the complex processes of recovery and stress. This has been remedied by the Recovery-Stress Questionnaire for Athletes

(Kellmann & Kallus, 2000, 2001), which assesses stress and recovery simultaneously and consequently provides a differentiated picture of the current recovery-stress state (see Kellmann, this volume, chapter 1). This multilevel approach also includes the Recovery-Cue, which can serve as a recovery protocol (Kellmann, Botterill, & Wilson, 1999).

An alternative individualized approach introduced by Hanin (1997, 2000) suggests that each individual has a zone of optimal function. Performance efficiency is maximized when the level of one's subjective emotional experience falls within this zone. In other words, the Individual Zones of Optimal Functioning (IZOF) model provides an individualized framework and tools to describe, predict, and explain why and how individually optimal and dysfunctional states can affect athletic performance. An important extension of the IZOF model is that idiosyncratic emotion markers of these optimal and dysfunctional performance states are proposed as specific criteria of the optimal (sufficient) recovery process. It is also recommended in each case to individually identify optimal recovery strategies used by athletes. Since this model is discussed in detail in chapter 11 of this volume, where Hanin attempts to apply the IZOF model to an understanding of performance and recovery states in competitive sports, it will not be discussed further in this chapter.

In addition to the methods listed previously, an integrative, inexpensive, but effective method of monitoring training is the use of a training log.

Training Logs

Most athletes keep records of their daily training, including morning resting heart rate, distance or duration of training, exercise heart rate (where appropriate), and the type of activity. A careful review of the training log can offer valuable clues to overtraining (McKenzie, 1999). In addition to training details, athletes may record subjective ratings of fatigue, stress, sleep, and muscle soreness on a scale of 1 to 7 from very, very low, or good, (1) to very, very high, or bad, (7) (Hooper et al., 1995). Athletes may also track training enjoyment, irritability, and health together with causes of stress and unhappiness, incidence of illness, injuries, or menstruation (Hooper & Mackinnon, 1995).

Table 3.1 shows the training log of a female modern pentathlon athlete for a week of regular practice. Her individual entries range from a de-scription of training, to detailed information about physiological assessments (e.g., heart rate), to the subjective rating of feelings during and after practice, as well as social interactions and the improvement of her injury (shinsplints).

Training logs can range from prepared sheets, in which athletes mark their activities in standardized categories, to nonstandardized logs. A training log documents training and helps the athlete and/or coach evaluate it retrospectively, especially when performance development is unsatisfactory. It may also help the athlete and coach program appropriate training loads during intense training. Athletes using training logs would benefit from the regular use of one of the questionnaires discussed in the following sections. These can add to the systematic assessment of recovery begun in the training log.

Rating of Perceived Exertion

Borg's Rating of Perceived Exertion (Borg, 1975, 1998) is used in sport research to measure the level of perceived exertion of an individual. Noble and Robertson (1996) showed that the RPE was useful in various research areas in sport and exercise settings. Morgan (1994) pointed out that the RPE is usually accurate in estimating the intensity of an exercise stimulus. Ratings of perceived exertion are accurate indicators of training adaptation in exercise programs involving cardiac and hypertensive patients as well as clinically normal patients (Noble & Robertson, 1996).

Perceived exertion has also been studied in the context of overtraining. The direct relationship between training load and perceived exertion has been well established in numerous studies (for an overview, see Borg, 1998; Noble & Noble, 1998; Noble & Robertson, 1996). For example, a study by O'Connor, Morgan, and Raglin (1991) used the RPE scale on swimmers during their standardized training (at 90% of $\dot{V}O_2$max). The RPE results demonstrate that the perception of physical effort during a brief bout of submaximal exercise is sensitive to short-term increases in training volume. Urhausen et al. (1998) found significantly higher ratings of subjective exertion after 10 minutes of stress in overtrained participants. Snyder (1998) and Snyder, Jeukendrup, Hesselink, Kuipers, and Foster (1993) reported that changes in the ratio of RPE and blood lactate were found to be a reliable predictor of overreaching/overtraining. Foster (1998) recently reported a simple modification of the RPE in which athletes were asked to

Table 3.1 Training Log of a Female Modern Pentathlon Athlete

Day	Date	Week 6: Training camp/Poland	
Mon	02/08	Fence: Felt shinsplints during fencing, then I stopped; have pain in my upper thigh-muscle stiffness.	20'
		I set pressure points by myself (shinsplints), 1 · ultrasound	2 h
		Sauna and salt bath, massage (legs and back = 60')	
		Completion of the Recovery-Cue	1 h
Tue	02/09	Ride	1 h
		1 · ultrasound	
		Swim: 8 · 50 freestyle rhythm, 200 kick (25 back/25 but), 200 free	
		8 · 50 free, GA2, P 15", Ø 36/37"; pulse 160; 100 easy	
		4 · 100 free, GA2, P 30", Ø 1:18/16, pulse 156; 200 easy	
		16 · 25 free, GA2, P 10", Ø 18", pulse 168; 300 easy	2.6 km
		Run: 35' easy run Pᴀᴠɢ 151, Pᴍᴀx 163, shinsplints OK	7 km
		Shoot: 10 white, 10 normal, 10 hole, 10 estimate, aim:	
		4 · 46 with 30 shoots, 47/42/45/46/44/47	1:20 h
Wed	02/10	Lesson: Coach Iri	30'
		Group fencing: 19 bouts, 1 · 5 hits	
		Swim: 900 m easy	0.9 km
		Run: 37 min extensive run (Pᴀᴠɢ 159, Pᴍᴀx 170), 4 accelerations	
		(80-100 m) + walking, stretching	7 km
		Massage (back), foot bath, and laser left leg (shinsplints):	70'
Thur	02/11	Shoot: 20' gym, 30' technical exercises	
		30' ladder of success (shooting program)	1:30 h
		Swim: 8 · 25 free rhythm, 200 kick (free/but), 4 · 25 free kick max,	
		100 easy, 800 m free rhythm, 100 easy, 600 m pull	
		(paddles + pullboy); 100 easy; 8 · 50 free, P.15"; 200 easy	2.8 km
		Sauna, salt bath (90 min)	
		Laser (15'), shinsplints quite good	1:45 h
Fri	02/12	Ride: 20 min dressage, 40 min jumping	1 h
		Fence: lesson, Iri	30'
		Group fencing: 1 · 1 hits, 2 rounds, 16 people—everything seems a bit tough today.	
		Run: 48' easy run, Pᴀᴠɢ 149, Pᴍᴀx 168, short stretching	8 km
		Strength: Stabilization front and back (15') + stretching (15')	~ 30'
		Evening at Marek's house! Was nice and we had a lot of fun!	
Sat	02/13	Shoot: Training competition: 20 shoots, 41/47/45/49 = 182	1 h
		Swim: 4 · 100 m, 8 · 25 free kick max,	
		4 · 100 free pull + pullboy (2 + 4 paddles), 100 easy,	
		8 · 50 free start: 1', Ø 37"-34"; 200 m easy	
		16 · 25 free; rest: 10" (counting strokes, higher frequency!)	
		300 easy	2.4 km
		Run: 65' ext run (Pᴀᴠɢ 148, Pᴍᴀx 162), got lost, was running in	
		really deep snow!	11 km
		Sauna, laser, shinsplints very good! massage	2:15 h
Sun	02/14	Fence: Just fencing (30'), group lesson (20')	50'
		Ride: Short jumping course	1 h
		Shinsplints really good, almost no swelling left!	

Run: 25 km	Swim: 8.7 km	Shoot: 3 · 3:50 h	Ride: 3 ·	Fence: 3 · Group Fencing	3 · lesson

Run = running; shoot = shooting; fence = fencing; swim = swimming; ride = riding; but = butterfly; free = freestyle; back = backstroke; max = maximum; ext = extensive; P_{AVG} = pulse average; P_{MAX} = pulse maximum; min = minutes; 20' = 20 minutes; km = kilometer; GA2 = basic endurance 2 (special speed); 20" = 20 seconds; Ø = average; · = times rate the global intensity of the entire training. Twenty-five athletes (mostly speed skaters) recorded their training using a method that integrates the exercise session RPE and the duration (including warm-up, cool-down, and recovery intervals) of the training session. Athletes who exceeded individually identifiable training thresholds (mostly related to the strain of training) had a higher percentage of illness.

Despite significant research findings, most people use the RPE mainly because it is very economical to use and easy to complete. However, from the perspective of a biopsychological stress model (Janke & Wolffgramm, 1995), recovery and stress should be treated using a multilevel approach dealing with physiological, emotional, cognitive, behavioral, performance, and social aspects of the problem by considering these aspects both separately and together. Janke and Wolffgramm's (1995) approach matches Hanin's perspective (1997, 2000), which includes seven basic components of total human functioning that provide a relatively complete description of a performance state: cognitive, emotional, motivational, bodily-somatic, motor-behavioral, performance, and communicative. The one-item construction of the RPE cannot assess multidimensional aspects of recovery and stress. The POMS, with its multidimensional approach, takes more dimensions into account.

Profile of Mood States

Sport psychology research has dealt with the relationship between overtraining and emotional state and mood. Mood states are comparable to emotional states, but they are more persistent, less dynamic, and less specific than emotions (Carver & Scheier, 1990). However, they are more transient and fluctuating than personality characteristics. Mood states, emotions, and stress should be measured at different levels, which again encompass physiological, subjective-verbal, behavioral, cognitive, and social aspects. Within emotion research, facial expression, stature, and posture are indicators of emotional states as well (Kellmann & Kallus, 1999).

Research on emotional states is based mostly on the Profile of Mood States (McNair et al., 1971, 1992). The POMS is a self-assessment for mood and affective states. It is a 65-item Likert-format questionnaire that is rated on a scale of 1 ("not at all") to 4 ("extremely"). Shorter versions have also been discussed in the literature (for an overview, see LeUnes & Burger, 2000).

The POMS provides a measure of total mood disturbances and six mood states (*Tension, Depression, Anger, Vigor, Fatigue,* and *Confusion*). Total mood disturbances are determined by subtracting the *Vigor* score from the sum of the five negative scores. For case studies using the POMS to monitor training, see Kenttä and Hassmén, this volume, chapter 4.

A special issue of the *Journal of Applied Sport Psychology* (March 2000) discussed perspectives in mood in sport and exercise. Papers focusing on the POMS provided a good overview of the current POMS research in exercise settings (Beedie, Terry, & Lane, 2000; Berger & Motl, 2000; Lane & Terry, 2000; LeUnes, 2000; LeUnes & Burger, 2000; Prapavessis, 2000; Terry, 2000; Terry & Lane, 2000).

A 1987 publication by Morgan, Brown, Raglin, O'Connor, and Ellickson describes mood fluctuations reported by swimmers throughout their season. Initially, the athletes exhibited the iceberg profile (Morgan, 1985; Morgan & Costill, 1996). This profile suggests that athletes are in a mentally healthy state as a result of their positive athletic accomplishments. During overtraining, mood disturbances significantly increased and were accompanied by a profile reflecting diminished mental health. After the training intensity was significantly reduced, the swimmers again exhibited the original iceberg profile. A dose-response relation between mood disturbances and training intensity is prevalent (Raglin, 1993). There is a correspondence between such feelings as tension, fatigue, anger, depression, loss of vigor, and well-being (mood disturbances) and increased high levels of training. When training volume and/or intensity is reduced, desired mood states are dominant again (Berger et al., 1999; Morgan et al., 1987; Morgan, Costill, Flynn, Raglin, & O'Connor, 1988). This dose-response relationship between training and mood disturbance is well documented in different sports, such as swimming (Morgan et al., 1987), speed skating (Guttmann, Pollock, Foster, & Schmidt, 1984), wrestling (Morgan et al., 1987), rowing (Kellmann & Günther, 2000; Raglin, Morgan, & Luchsinger, 1990), and running (Wittig, Houmard, & Costill, 1989).

Recently, Berger et al. (1999) also found the dose-response relationship in cycling. The authors examined changes in mood and performance in response to high-intensity, short-duration overtraining and a subsequent taper. Eight cyclists completed the POMS and a simulated 4 km pursuit performance test throughout a six-week period including a baseline week, three weeks of overtraining (primarily high-intensity training), and a two-week taper. Total mood disturbance scores displayed a quadratic polynomial effect throughout the three weeks of overtraining, with highest scores in the second week. The average scores were lower during the taper than at baseline and lower at taper than at overtraining. Whereas performance improved during the three weeks of short-duration overtraining, and additional improvements were observed during taper, no significant correlation was reported for total mood disturbance and performance.

Advantages and Disadvantages of the POMS

Berger and Motl (2000) discussed the following advantages and disadvantages of the POMS in exercise settings.

- It is useful in detecting mood fluctuations in exercise.
- The six scales seem to measure mood subcomponents that are differentially responsive to diverse characteristics of exercise settings.
- Normative data for specific groups, including adults and frequently studied college students, is helpful for statistical interpretation of the POMS score.
- Data assessment is easy.
- It is highly reliable (for an overview, see LeUnes & Burger, 2000).
- An early identification of overtrained athletes is often listed in the literature.

The last point was questioned in a paper by Martin, Andersen, and Gates (2000), which described a study in which overtrained athletes were not identified. The authors studied 11 cyclists during a six-week, high-intensity interval training and a one-week taper. Whereas cycling performance changed over the weekly performance assessment, neither the high-intensity interval training nor the one-week taper significantly affected total mood or specific mood states. The individual assessment using the POMS scales to determine if athletes were overtrained did not work in this study. Therefore, the authors questioned the usefulness of the POMS to distinguish between periods of productive and counterproductive high-intensity training at the individual level.

Assuming that the POMS can identify overtrained athletes at an early stage, the question then arises as to what kind of intervention should take place. Because the items are in adjective form (e.g., *Tense, Annoyed, Bitter),* the POMS does not provide information about the cause of mood. Therefore, no direct recommendations for interventions can be drawn from the data assessed.

Furthermore, Berger and Motl (2000) noted the disadvantage that the POMS was initially developed for use with clinical populations (see also McNair et al., 1992) in order to have an economical method of identifying and assessing transient, fluctuating affective states. Berger and Motl (2000) continued that five of the six scales measured the negative mood characteristics of tension, depression, anger, fatigue, and confusion. They argued that a decrease in a negative mood state may not necessarily indicate mood benefits. This argument fits into the discussion of Kellmann and Kallus (2001), who pointed out that recovery cannot be merely characterized as lack or reduction of stress, but also as a proactive individualized process to replenish psychological and physiological resources. In addition, although low *Vigor* and high *Fatigue* scores on the POMS do reflect a need for recovery, it is not clear which specific recovery strategy is needed. Consequently, the POMS only vaguely reflects recovery processes and does not lead to the application of appropriate recovery strategies.

Recovery-Stress Questionnaire for Athletes

Kallus (1995) created the Recovery-Stress Questionnaire in order to obtain distinct answers to the question "How are you?" Taking a person's current state into account, Kallus searched for possible ways to anticipate peoples' responses to stress. This concept was founded on the assumption that someone in need of a vacation and someone presently in top psychological and physical fitness will respond differently to demands. Special measuring scales were added to provide a sport-specific version of the Recovery-Stress Questionnaire that could gauge stress and recovery in athletes.

The Recovery-Stress Questionnaire for Athletes (RESTQ-Sport, Kellmann & Kallus, 2000, 2001) measures the recovery-stress states of athletes. The recovery-stress state indicates the extent to which persons are physically and/or mentally stressed, whether or not they are capable of using individual strategies for recovery, as well as which strategies are used. The theory behind the questionnaire is that an accretion of stress in life, coupled with weak recovery potential, will cause a variation of the psychophysical general state. The specific characteristics of the RESTQ-Sport measure, in a direct and systematic manner, the frequency of appraised events, states, and activities together with stress and recovery processes. A scale measures the extent to which the respondent took part in different activities within the *past three days/nights*. A Likert-type scale is used with values ranging from 0 ("never") to 6 ("always") indicating how often the respondent participated in various activities during the past three days/nights. The questionnaire requires that respondents precisely appraise subjective events and focus on the frequency of behavior by using such statements as *I had a good time with friends,* instead of *I met some friends*. Specific interventions can be suggested based on these items.

The RESTQ-Sport consists of 12 general stress and recovery scales as well as 7 sport-specific stress and recovery scales (see table 3.2). The first seven scales deal with different aspects of *General Stress, Emotional Stress,* and *Social Stress* as well as resulting consequences. The scales *Conflicts/Pressure, Fatigue,* and *Lack of Energy* are concerned with performance aspects, whereas *Physical Complaints* addresses the physiological aspects of stress. *Success* is the only resulting recovery-oriented scale concerned with performance in general but not in a sport-specific context. *Social Recovery, Physical Recovery,* and *General Well-Being* are the basic scales of the recovery area with an additional scale assessing *Sleep Quality.*

The sport-specific scale *Disturbed Breaks* is sensitive to deficiencies of recovery and interrupted recovery during periods of rest (e.g., halftimes, time-outs). *Burnout/Emotional Exhaustion* is characterized by the component of wanting to give up or lack of persistence. This relates to any disappointments in the context of sport that might lead to quitting the sport. *Fitness/Injury* consists of any statements dealing with injuries, vulnerability to injuries, and an impairment of physical strength. *Fitness/Being in Shape* assesses subjective feelings about performance ability and competence, one's perceived fitness, and vitality. *Burnout/Personal Accomplishment* primarily asks about appreciation and empathy within the team and the realization of personal goals in sports. *Self-Efficacy* measures the level of expectation and competence regarding an optimal performance preparation in practice. *Self-Regulation* refers to the availability and use of psychological skills when preparing for performance (e.g., goal setting, mental training, motivation).

Reliability and Validation of the RESTQ-Sport

Cronbach α for the RESTQ-Sport scales is quite acceptable. Table 3.2 lists Cronbach α for a Canadian sample. The RESTQ-Sport attempts to portray the recovery-stress condition in temporary states that are composed of emotional, physical, and behavioral features with determined persistence (Bradburn, 1969). Faced with momentary functional fluctuations, the recovery-stress state, in comparison to the actual condition, is steady. Kallus (1995) showed that the test-retest reliability of all general stress and recovery scales is quite high after 24 hours for an instrument that records variable states. The consistently high short-term stability, however, clearly shows the reliability of the procedure. The test-retest reliability lies above $r = .79$, which implies that intraindividual differences in the recovery-stress states can be well reproduced. Moreover, the high test-retest reliability shows that the results of the RESTQ-Sport are stable concerning minor short-term functionary fluctuations and short-term changes in recovery-stress states. Corresponding with the measurement intention of the RESTQ-Sport, Kellmann and Kallus (2000, 2001) showed that the test-retest reliability is relatively stable for three days and declines with increasing time periods. Stress and recovery, according to Intercorrelations and Principle Component Analysis of the scales, must be viewed to some extent as independent components. This permits data analysis based on individual scales and on the factors of stress and recovery (for a detailed description, see Kellmann & Kallus, 2000, 2001).

Various studies with German and American athletes revealed high correlations between RESTQ-Sport and POMS scales (Birrer, Seiler, Binggeli, & Vogel, 2001; Kellmann, 1999; Kellmann, Fritzenberg, & Beckmann, 2000; Kellmann & Günther, 2000). *Tension, Depression, Anger, Fatigue,* and *Confusion* negatively correlate with recovery-related scales, whereas for *Vigor,* a positive relationship can be found. The stress-related RESTQ-Sport scales show a positive correlation between stress and *Tension, Depression, Anger, Fatigue,* and *Confusion* but a negative correlation between stress and *Vigor.* Whereas these studies reflected just a one-time

Table 3.2 Scales of the Recovery-Stress Questionnaire for Athletes

Scale	Scale summary	Cronbach α
1	**General Stress** Subjects with high values describe themselves as being frequently mentally stressed, depressed, unbalanced, and listless.	.91
2	**Emotional Stress** Subjects with high values experience frequent irritation, aggression, anxiety, and inhibition.	.84
3	**Social Stress** High values match subjects with frequent arguments, fights, irritation concerning others, general upset, and lack of humor.	.90
4	**Conflicts/Pressure** High values are reached if in the preceding few days conflicts were unsettled, unpleasant things had to be done, goals could not be reached, and certain thoughts could not be dismissed.	.80
5	**Fatigue** Time pressure in job, training, school, and life; being constantly disturbed during important work; overfatigue; and lack of sleep characterize this area of stress.	.82
6	**Lack of Energy** This scale matches ineffective work behavior like inability to concentrate and lack of energy and decision making.	.83
7	**Physical Complaints** Physical indisposition and physical complaints related to the whole body are characterized by this scale.	.78
8	**Success** Success, pleasure at work, and creativity during the preceding few days are assessed in this area.	.78
9	**Social Recovery** High values are shown by athletes who have frequent pleasurable social contacts and change combined with relaxation and amusement.	.86
10	**Physical Recovery** Physical recovery, physical well-being, and fitness are characterized in this area.	.83
11	**General Well-Being** Besides frequent good moods and high well-being, general relaxation and contentment are also in this scale.	.93
12	**Sleep Quality** Enough and recovering sleep, an absence of sleeping disorders while falling asleep, and sleeping through the night characterize recovery sleep.	.86
13	**Disturbed Breaks** This scale deals with recovery deficits, interrupted recovery, and situational aspects that get in the way during periods of rest (e.g., teammates, coaches).	.83
14	**Burnout/Emotional Exhaustion** High scores are shown by athletes who feel burned out and want to quit their sport.	.86
15	**Fitness/Injury** High scores signal an acute injury or vulnerability to injuries.	.82

Scale	Scale summary	Cronbach α
16	**Fitness/Being in Shape**	
	Athletes with high scores describe themselves as fit, physically efficient, and vital.	.87
17	**Burnout/Personal Accomplishment**	
	High scores are reached by athletes who feel integrated into their team, communicate well with their teammates, and enjoy their sport.	.72
18	**Self-Efficacy**	
	This scale is characterized by how convinced athletes are that they have trained well and are optimally prepared.	.88
19	**Self-Regulation**	
	The use of mental skills by athletes to prepare, push, motivate, and set goals for themselves is assessed by this scale.	.83

Cronbach α are taken from a Canadian sample listed in table 6.2 (p. 38) of the Recovery-Stress Questionnaire for Athletes.

Adapted, by permission, from M. Kellmann and K.W. Kallus, 2001, *Recovery-Stress Questionnaire for Athletes: User manual* (Champaign, IL: Human Kinetics), 6-7.

assessment, Kellmann et al. (2001) examined 24 female and 30 male rowers of the German Junior National Rowing Team six times during a six-week training camp before and during the World Championships. The authors observed that changes in mood, creatine kinase (CK) levels, and ergometer performance reflected the alteration and success of training. Results of MANOVAs revealed significant increases of stress and decreases of recovery when training load expanded, and vice versa. Because of page constraints in that publication, only the correlations between the POMS and the RESTQ-Sport, the development of CK, and the RESTQ-Sport scales during the training camp could be reported. However, of additional interest are the simultaneous changes over time of the POMS and RESTQ-Sport scales.

The training load of the 1998 German Junior National Team reached 248 minutes per day (T2) in the high-load phase (it was as high as 175 minutes per day [T1] in the previous phase), and 218 minutes (T3), 203 minutes (T4), 147 minutes (T5), and 118 (T6) minutes per day after the high-load phase. This was also reflected in the physiological measure of CK.

Figure 3.1 shows changes in participants' scores for two scales from each of the two questionnaires, respectively. The RESTQ-Sport scales with the highest correlation to the POMS scales were chosen, based on the correlation pattern, to present the changes in the athletes' subjective states throughout the training camp (see Kellmann

et al., 2001). The highest correlation of *Emotional Stress* was found with POMS-*Anger* ($r = .72$); POMS-*Depression* also correlated the highest with *Emotional Stress* ($r = .71$). POMS-*Fatigue* correlated the highest with RESTQ-Sport-*Fatigue* ($r = .73$), and POMS-*Vigor* with *Being in Shape* ($r = .71$). For the purpose of this chapter, only the development of two scales throughout the training camp were chosen. Figure 3.1 shows the scale *Fatigue,* which is part of the RESTQ-Sport and the POMS. Throughout the training camp a MANOVA for repeated measurements revealed a significant time effect for RESTQ-Sport-*Fatigue* ($p < 0.01$), whereas no gender effect occurred (upper-left panel). Similar developments were found for POMS-*Fatigue* ($p < 0.001$; lower-left panel); however, the gender effect turned out to be significant ($p < 0.001$). The scores in the recovery-related scale *Being in Shape* (upper-right panel) increased after the lowest scores at T2 during the training camp (time effect $p < 0.001$, gender effect $p < 0.001$, no interaction). In contrast, the development of POMS-*Vigor* was not significant (lower-right panel); however, a gender effect occurred ($p < 0.05$). Similar to *Being in Shape,* the lowest scores were measured at T2, and the increase of physical fitness was not reflected in the POMS-*Vigor.*

These results of the study by Kellmann et al. (2001) suggest that the RESTQ-Sport and the POMS seem to be sensitive to events in the lives of athletes that affect recovery-stress state and mood, respectively. Since the training load was

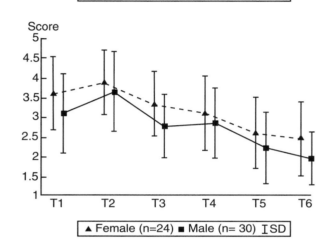

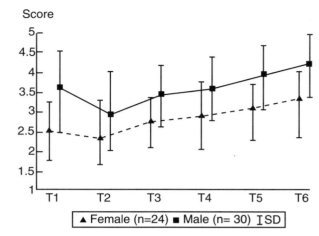

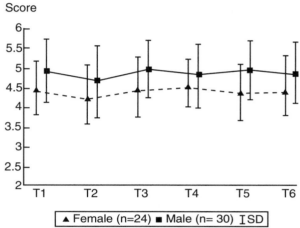

Figure 3.1 Means and standard deviations *(SD)* of the RESTQ-Sport scales *Fatigue* (upper-left panel) and *Being in Shape* (upper-right panel) as well as for the POMS scales *Fatigue* (lower-left panel) and *Vigor* (lower-right panel) for female (*n* = 24) and male (*n* = 30) rowers.

Upper panels: Reprinted, by permission, from M. Kellmann, D. Altenburg, W. Lormes, & J.M. Steinacker, 2001, "Assessing stress and recovery during preparation for the world championships in rowing," *The Sport Psychologist* 15: 151-167.

comparable for males and females, the study suggests either that females have a higher willingness to say how they feel or that they perceive the same training load differently than males. However, if females perceive a similar training load differently, they may need more attention during the training monitoring process.

Several studies have verified that training can be effectively monitored using the RESTQ-Sport and the POMS (e.g., Kellmann & Günther, 2000; Morgan et al., 1987). Similarities were found regarding the dose-response relationship (training volume/recovery-stress state, mood) and the interrelation of the scales. The test-retest reliability even seems to be in a comparable range (Kellmann et al., 2001). As a result, the question was raised: What advantage does the RESTQ-Sport have?

In contrast to the POMS, the advantage of the RESTQ-Sport is its systematic multilevel approach (Janke & Wolffgramm, 1995), which helps users assess subjective stress and recovery concurrently. Whereas the POMS' iceberg profile mainly incorporates negative mood states and only deals with one positive state of mood aspect, the RESTQ-Sport shows a distinct view of the athlete's state. The RESTQ-Sport's up-to-date recovery-stress profile presents solid solutions to current problems (Kallus & Kellmann, 2000; Kellmann, Kallus, Günther, Lormes, & Steinacker, 1997).

Applications of the RESTQ-Sport

The RESTQ-Sport identifies the current recovery-stress states of athletes and provides a complete picture of the extent of stress they are actually experiencing. To adequately manage the training process and prevent overtraining, it is important to gain information about the athlete's state in the past few days. Moreover, information based on an athlete's subjective perception is helpful for the coaching staff because the coaches' and athletes' perceptions often differ. By using the RESTQ-Sport, athletes and coaches can be informed about the importance of some daily activities. It can demonstrate how these activities relate to stress/recovery, as well as their effects on athletic performance.

The RESTQ-Sport provides a convenient way to monitor individuals and/or groups during training camps (Hogg, 2000; Kellmann et al., 2001; Kellmann & Günther, 1999, 2000) and over an entire season (Ferger, 1998a, 1998b). When data assessment is carefully planned, the effects of a yearly improved training schedule can also be evaluated (Kellmann & Altenburg, 2000). It is not necessary to complete the RESTQ-Sport on the day of competition. Because of the sufficient temporary stability of the results, the assessment can take place up to 48 hours before competition, allowing enough time for coaches or sport psychologists to intervene and optimize the recovery-stress state. During performance plateaus (times when performance does not increase), the questionnaire may also be beneficial to athletes and coaches in determining whether the intensity of training should be increased or decreased.

The RESTQ-Sport offers a complete profile that can be used as a screening method for individual problems. In contrast to the POMS, which assesses the current mood state, the RESTQ-Sport provides concrete recommendations for intervention (Kellmann & Günther, 2000; Kellmann & Kallus, 1999; Kellmann et al., 1997). For example, Kellmann et al. (2001) illustrated that training can be modified based on the RESTQ-Sport results if the underlying reason is clearly communicated to the athletes. The analysis on the basis of single scales, and in selected cases on item levels, provides information about activities that can be optimized and used as active steering elements to modify behavior.

The following case illustrates the applied use of the RESTQ-Sport. The main purpose is to identify athletes whose recovery-stress states do not correspond with the training schedule during the training camp. Through early intervention, individual training can be adapted in order to help these athletes deal with training stress, thus avoiding underrecovery and preventing overtraining. The internal consistencies for some scales suggest some limitations for individual diagnosis based on single scales. Therefore, the complete

profile will be considered. It should be noted that low scores in the stress-related areas and high scores in the recovery-related areas are "positively" labeled, and vice versa. However, in this context terms such as *good, bad, positive,* or *negative* do not exist. Kellmann and Kallus (2001) emphasized that the RESTQ-Sport profile reflects just one short period in a person's life, which may change drastically within a few days. The recovery-stress state varies during training camps, cycles of competition, working weeks of a year, different phases of life, and as a result of specific stressful events and recovery activities.

Figure 3.2 contains two RESTQ-Sport profiles of an 18-year-old rower. It shows a recovery-stress state with low scores in the stress-related areas and high scores in the recovery-related areas. Focusing on her profile at time 2, elevated *Fatigue* scores and, more important, very low *Sleep Quality* scores are detected. Since this pattern also occurred at the first measurement, the sport psychologist approached her and discovered she had immense problems falling asleep at night. She had been suffering from this situation for years but had never sought treatment. After she learned the relaxation technique of Progressive Muscle Relaxation in 10 weekly sessions, she was able to apply the technique at night. After that period the RESTQ-Sport was completed for a third time. In that measurement almost all stress-related scales increased slightly, but *Fatigue* went down, and although some scores in the recovery-related scales dropped, *Sleep Quality* increased drastically. Kellmann and Kallus (2001) described more case studies and subsequent interventions.

The case illustrated in figure 3.3 came from an applied research project with 17 male and female German junior rowers (median age: 17 yr) who completed the RESTQ-Sport six times throughout an interval of 24 weeks during the course of the 2000 season. The figure shows different developments of selected recovery scales. These results confirm Kallus and Kellmann's (2000) assertion that various processes of recovery can be dissociated. The multilevel concept of recovery (Kallus, 1995; Kallus & Kellmann, 2000) explains the different trends for *Being in Shape, Personal Accomplishment, Self-Efficacy,* and *Sleep Quality.*

The RESTQ-Sport includes behavioral- and performance-related items, as well as those that address emotional, physical, and social aspects of stress and recovery. Whereas *Being in Shape* deals with the physical side of the individual, *Personal Accomplishment* focuses on the person's integration into the team, communication with

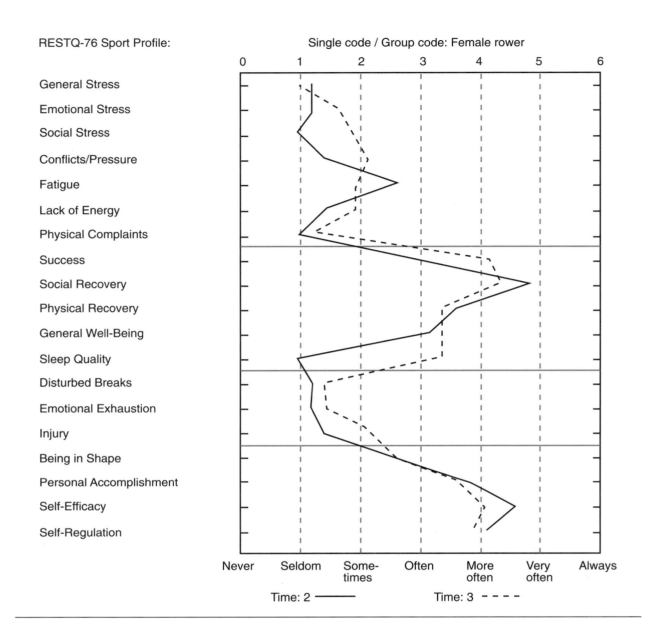

Figure 3.2 RESTQ-Sport profile for a female rower at week 5 (time 2) and at week 18 (time 4).

teammates, and enjoyment of the sport. *Self-Efficacy* assesses how convinced athletes are that they have trained well and are optimally prepared. Furthermore, *Sleep Quality* measures the quality and quantity of sleep and identifies sleeping disorders.

These results emphasize the importance of assessing recovery and stress on different levels (see also Steinacker et al., 1999). Keeping in mind that recovery is an individual process and applies to individual preferences (see Kellmann, this volume, chapter 1), athletes and their supporters should continuously monitor stress and recovery during the training process to determine the scale

that is most sensitive to the athlete's individual situation (e.g., Berglund & Säfström, 1994; Hooper et al., 1999; Kellmann & Günther, 2000; Kellmann et al., 2001).

Kellmann and Kallus (2001) summarized the advantages of the RESTQ-Sport as follows:

- Identifies athletes whose recovery-stress states during training camp do not correspond with changes in the training schedule. Training can be individually adapted (decreased or increased) based on that information.

- Provides a picture of athletes' conditions from a different point of view.

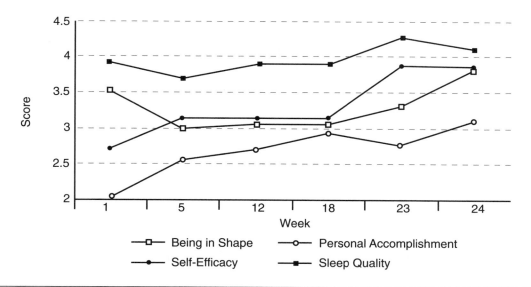

Figure 3.3 Comparison of the RESTQ-Sport scales *Being in Shape, Personal Accomplishment, Self-Efficacy,* and *Sleep Quality* (0 = never; 6 = always) in the course of the 2000 season of German Junior Rowers (mean of 17 rowers).

- Derives concrete solutions.
- Offers a systematic multilevel approach (simultaneous assessment of stress and recovery).
- Is economical.
- Is relevant, especially when there is no personal contact over an extended period of time (due to vacation or injuries).
- Reflects the subjective perception of an athlete, which can differ from that of the coach.
- Informs about the importance of activities (related to stress/recovery and to performance).
- Monitors and evaluates the effects of training.
- Compares individuals/groups during the season, training camps, and over the course of many years.

Psychological assessment tools are economical in repeated measurement designs. Within a short and limited period of time athletes can usually find the time to complete questionnaires several times. However, if the goal is to monitor training continuously, for instance, on a weekly basis over a complete season, most instruments—including the RESTQ-Sport—are too lengthy for applied use.

Recovery-Cue

Knowing that time is always an issue for athletes and coaches, Kellmann, Botterill, and Wilson

(1999) developed the Recovery-Cue (see Kellmann, Patrick, Botterill, & Wilson, this volume, chapter 12). The Recovery-Cue is a recovery protocol consisting of seven items (see table 3.3). Three items were developed from Kenttä and Hassmén's (1998) focus on perceived exertion, perceived recovery, and recovery efforts, while four items represent the areas of the RESTQ-Sport identified as being crucial for recovery processes *(Physical Recovery, Sleep Quality, Social Recovery, Self-Regulation)*. Being aware of the problems with one-item assessments, the authors tried to develop an applied tool for athletes and coaches that could be completed during training, and which would provide immediate feedback.

When using the Recovery-Cue, athletes are instructed to complete the items on a fixed day (ideally at the same time before, during, or after the same training session). In addition, it is important to consider the time and day of completion when the recovery-stress state is assessed. If the coach or athletes want to receive information about the recovery effects of the past weekend, Monday should be the assessment day. In contrast, if the interest is on monitoring the impact of training, the items should be completed during or at the end of the week.

As already described, 17 male and female German junior rowers completed the RESTQ-Sport six times throughout an interval of 24 weeks during the course of the 2000 season. In addition, they filled out the Recovery-Cue weekly during the 24-week period. The assessment time was scheduled

Table 3.3	The Seven Items of the Recovery-Cue

1. How much effort was required to complete my workouts last week? (excessive effort—hardly any effort)

2. How recovered did I feel prior to the workouts last week? (still not recovered—feel energized and recharged)

3. How successful was I at rest and recovery activities last week? (not successful—successful)

4. How well did I recover physically last week? (never—always)

5. How satisfied and relaxed was I as I fell asleep in the last week? (never—always)

6. How much fun did I have last week? (never—always)

7. How convinced was I that I could achieve my goals during performance last week? (never—always)

for Monday afternoon at the beginning of practice. Figures 3.4 and 3.5 show the changes in the scores (mean of 17 rowers) for the seven Recovery-Cue items over the 24-week period. For better visibility, standard deviation is not included in the figures.

The changes in figure 3.4 are drawn for the items *How much effort was required to complete my workouts last week?, How recovered did I feel prior to the workouts last week?,* and *How successful was I at rest and recovery activities last week?* Big changes occurred over time, starting the first week after the Christmas break when the athletes had some days off or regenerative training as part of the training plan. The seasonal highpoint—namely, the German Junior Championships—took place at the end of the assessment in week 24. Between week 1 and week 24 the periodization of the training plan was well re-flected in the subjective ratings. In addition, not all items advanced in the same direction each time. Occasionally a lack of time for perceived exertion and perceived recovery occurred. Besides the German Championships, two other major competitions took place, in week 19 (Hamburg) and week 23 (Munich). For both competitions, the taper phases are also reflected in the ratings.

In figure 3.5, a higher variability occurs for the remaining items *How well did I recover physically last week?, How satisfied and relaxed was I as I fell asleep in the last week?, How much fun did I have last week?,* and *How convinced was I that I could achieve my goals during performance last week?* For example, in week 6 the physical recovery showed the lowest scores, but more important, the athletes had fun. Week 6 referred to a special

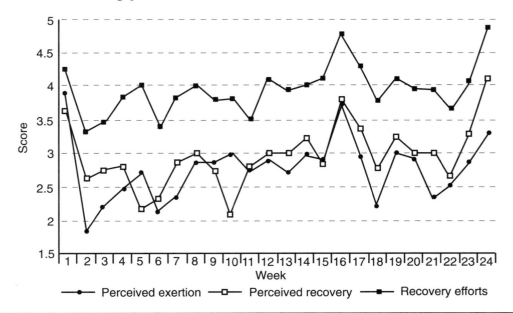

Figure 3.4 Comparison of recovery, effort, and recovery activities in the course of the 2000 season of German Junior Rowers (mean of 17 rowers). Week 19 = competition in Hamburg; week 23 = competition in Munich; week 24 = German Junior Championships.

training camp where the team went for a cross-country skiing trip. Cross-country skiing was quite an exhausting physical task, but obviously the athletes enjoyed themselves.

Figure 3.6 shows the protocol of a successful female modern pentathlon athlete (see also table 3.1, p. 40). Since the beginning of the year 2000, she completed the recovery protocol each Monday after the first training session. How stressful or how recovering the past week was could best be rated on how tight her muscles felt after the first running session. The subjective rating reflects the training schedule during the year, and the planned periodization turned out clearly. However, in personal communication with her, the data presented another aspect. Using this protocol she became more sensitized to the topic of

recovery and consciously reflected on whether the goal of the training schedule was appropriately reached in the past week. For example, she realized that after a "recovering week" she had not reached the aimed "recovery level," and consequently decided—in close consultation with her coach—to add a second easy week.

Information collected with the recovery protocol is also relevant for the coach, who receives information about the current recovery-stress state of the athlete (similar to a fever curve). Individual monitoring of the training is valuable information, especially if the subjective rating shows a time delay in the reactions. On that basis the coach has a good data foundation from which to decide how to intervene actively during the training process. In this case the athlete was able

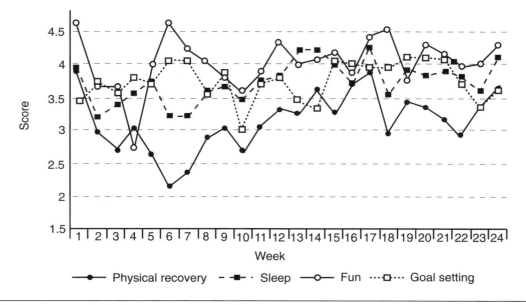

Figure 3.5 Comparison of physical recovery, sleep, fun, and goal setting in the course of the 2000 season of German Junior Rowers (mean of 17 rowers). Week 19 = competition in Hamburg; week 23 = competition in Munich; week 24 = German Junior Championships.

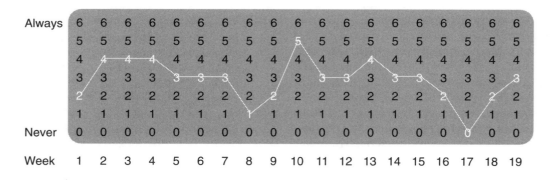

Figure 3.6 Individual rating for the recovery-protocol item *How well did I recover physically last week?*

to combine the Recovery-Cue with the training log, and in combination with the subjective ratings, training changes could be made for the next year.

Perspectives on the Psychological Assessment of Underrecovery

High-performance athletes regularly use questionnaires as a means of obtaining staff members' attention. Athletes often find it easier to mark a specific item on a piece of paper than to contact the coach, sport psychologist, or physician directly. From the applied perspective it is not important whether a problem really occurred, whether specific intervention has to take place, or whether the athlete "only" wants to talk or make direct contact. The key is that athletes need to feel assured that their concerns can be addressed and dealt with appropriately.

Some coaches and even sport psychologists are skeptical of using questionnaires for data assessment because they doubt the honesty of answers. Of course, cheating is easy on questionnaires, but athletes have to realize that the key to monitoring training is the "honesty principle." If the scoring of the instruments accurately reflects athletes' current conditions, they gain an increased awareness of the processes affecting their lives. By being honest in their questionnaires, athletes also accept responsibility when they realize that their recovery-stress profile was affected by their activities during the past three days.

When the appropriate monitoring tool is chosen, it often deals with areas not covered in a regular coach-athlete talk. Many coaches do not believe that "events outside of sports" are relevant to sport performance, or they think it may be too intimate to ask about athletes' private lives. Psychological assessment tools can thus start an educational process for athletes and coaches if the results are shared. However, this only works if explanations are provided as to why underrecovery is crucial and how questionnaires can be used to optimize training and performance.

In the applied work with the German Junior National Rowing Team the first round of data assessment opened with an introduction to the project. After information was given regarding the handling of data and when feedback would be provided to the athletes, questions from the athletes were answered. It is important for the athletes to know that they will receive feedback and will be informed about the results if desired. Up to 80% of the rowers asked for feedback after the World Championships and wanted to know how this information was used and how it connected with physiological and medical data. When athletes are told they will get feedback and are not just being used as subjects in a study, they are more committed to the process, especially when the data assessment takes place for research purposes rather then as training monitoring (Kellmann & Beckmann, in press). Open communication is important to get athletes involved voluntarily in the assessment of recovery.

As indicated by the Recovery-Cue, recovery should be measured on a longitudinal basis, which raises the scientific value and provides a better foundation for feedback. Although recovery should be integrated into the training and competition schedule, interdisciplinary cooperation is the key to a more effective diagnosis of the recovery-stress state of an individual. To optimize this process, the consultation of athletes should be done in close cooperation with coaches, sport physicians, and sport psychologists. Consequently, all physiological and psychological data, as well as training and performance data, should be used on an interdisciplinary basis (Froehlich, 1993; Kellmann & Altenburg, 2000; Kellmann et al., 1997; Kellmann & Kallus, 1999; Kenttä & Hassmén, 1998; Steinacker et al., 1999, 2000). This can be facilitated by the use of a staff training log (which unfortunately does not often exist), the assessment of subjective and objective physiological and psychological data, and the integration of an athlete's perspective. It is important that methods of the psychological assessment of recovery/underrecovery be part of the regular training routine—like lactate testing. The physiological parameter is discussed along with other physiological indicators in later chapters of this book.

References

Beedie, C.J., Terry, P.C., & Lane, A.M. (2000). The Profile of Mood States and athletic performance: Two meta-analyses. *Journal of Applied Sport Psychology, 12,* 49-68.

Berger, B.G., & Motl, R.W. (2000). Exercise and mood: A selective review and synthesis of research employing the Profile of Mood States. *Journal of Applied Sport Psychology, 12,* 69-92.

Berger, B.G., Motl, R.W., Butki, B.D., Martin, D.T., Wilkinson, J.G., & Owen, D.R. (1999). Mood and cycling performance in response to three weeks of high-intensity, short-duration overtraining, and a two-week taper. *The Sport Psychologist, 13,* 444-457.

Berglund, B., & Säfström, H. (1994). Psychological monitoring and modulation of training load of world-class canoeists. *Medicine and Science in Sports and Exercise, 26,* 1036-1040.

Birrer, D., Seiler, R., Binggeli, A., & Vogel, R. (2001). Kriterienvalidität des Erholungs-Belastungs-Fragebogens-Sport [Criteria validity of the Recovery-Stress Questionnaire for Athletes]. In R. Seiler, D. Birrer, J. Schmid, & S. Valkanover (Eds.), *Sportpsychologie: Anforderungen, Anwendungen, Auswirkungen* (pp. 161-163). Cologne, Germany: bps.

Borg, G. (1975). Perceived exertion as an indicator of somatic stress. *Scandinavian Journal of Rehabilitational Medicine, 2,* 92-98.

Borg, G. (1998). *Borg's Perceived Exertion and Pain Rating Scales.* Champaign, IL: Human Kinetics.

Bradburn, N.M. (1969). *The structure of physiological well-being.* Chicago: Aldine.

Budgett, R. (1998). Fatigue and underperformance in athletes: The overtraining syndrome. *British Journal of Sport and Medicine, 32,* 107-110.

Carver, C.S., & Scheier, M.F. (1990). Origins and functions of positive and negative affect: A control-process view. *Psychological Review, 97,* 19-35.

Ferger, K. (1998a). Saisonbegleitende Diagnose der individuellen Belastungs-Erholungsbilanz mit der athletenspezifischen Variante des EBF [Monitoring of the individual recovery-stress state using the Recovery-Stress Questionnaire for Athletes]. In D. Teipel, R. Kemper, & D. Heinemann (Eds.), *Sportpsychologische Diagnostik, Prognostik und Intervention* (pp. 131-133). Cologne, Germany: bps.

Ferger, K. (1998b). *Trainingseffekte im Fußball* [Training effects in soccer]. Hamburg, Germany: Feldhaus.

Foster, C. (1998). Monitoring training in athletes with reference to overtraining syndrome. *Medicine and Science in Sports and Exercise, 30,* 1164-1168.

Froehlich, J. (1993). Overtraining syndrome. In J. Heil (Ed.), *Psychology of sport injury* (pp. 59-70). Champaign, IL: Human Kinetics.

Guttmann, M.C., Pollock, M., Foster, C., & Schmidt, D. (1984). Training stress in Olympic speed skaters: A psychological perspective. *The Physician and Sportsmedicine, 12,* 45-57.

Hanin, Y.L. (1997). Emotions and athletic performance: Individual Zones of Optimal Functioning model. In R. Seiler (Ed.), *European Yearbook of Sports Psychology* (Vol. 1, pp. 29-72). St. Augustin, Germany: Academia.

Hanin, Y.L. (2000). Individual Zones of Optimal Functioning (IZOF) Model: Emotion-performance relationships in sport. In Y.L. Hanin (Ed.), *Emo-tions in sport* (pp. 65-89). Champaign, IL: Human Kinetics.

Hogg, J.M. (2000). *Canadian Women's World Cup Soccer 1999: Mental preparations. A report for the Canadian Soccer Association.* Edmonton, Alberta: University of Alberta.

Hooper, S.L., & Mackinnon, L.T. (1995). Monitoring overtraining in athletes. *Sports Medicine, 20,* 321-327.

Hooper, S.L., Mackinnon, L.T., & Hanrahan, S. (1997). Mood states as an indication of staleness and recovery. *International Journal Sport Psychology, 28,* 1-12.

Hooper, S.L., Mackinnon, L.T., & Howard, A. (1999). Physiological and psychometric variables for monitoring recovery during tapering for major competition. *Medicine and Science in Sports and Exercise, 31,* 1205-1210.

Hooper, S.L., Mackinnon, L.T., Howard, A., Gordon, R.D., & Bachmann, A.W. (1995). Markers for monitoring overtraining and recovery. *Medicine and Science in Sports and Exercise, 27,* 106-112.

Janke, W., & Wolffgramm, J. (1995). Biopsychologie von Streß und emotionalen Reaktionen: Ansätze interdisziplinärer Kooperation von Psychologie, Biologie und Medizin [Biopsychology of stress and emotional reactions: Starting points of an interdisciplinary cooperation of psychology, biology, and medicine]. In G. Debus, G. Erdmann, & K.W. Kallus (Eds.), *Biospsychologie von Streß und emotionalen Reaktionen* (pp. 293-349). Göttingen, Germany: Hogrefe.

Kallus, K.W. (1995). *Der Erholungs-Belastungs-Fragebogen* [The Recovery-Stress Questionnaire]. Frankfurt, Germany: Swets & Zeitlinger.

Kallus, K.W., & Kellmann, M. (2000). Burnout in athletes and coaches. In Y.L. Hanin (Ed.), *Emotions in sport* (pp. 209-230). Champaign, IL: Human Kinetics.

Kellmann, M. (1999). Die Beziehungen zwischen dem Erholungs-Belastungs-Fragebogen für Sportler und dem Profile of Mood States [The relationships between the Recovery-Stress Questionnaire for Athletes and the Profile of Mood States]. In D. Alfermann & O. Stoll (Eds.), *Motivation und Volition im Sport - Vom Planen zum Handeln* (pp. 208-212). Cologne, Germany: bps.

Kellmann, M. (2000). Psychologische Methoden der Erholungs-Beanspruchungs-Diagnostik [Psychological methods for the assessment of recovery and stress]. *Deutsche Zeitschrift für Sportmedizin, 51,* 253-258.

Kellmann, M., & Altenburg, D. (2000). Betreuung der Junioren-Nationalmannschaft des Deutschen Ruderverbandes [Consultation of the German Junior National Rowing Team]. In H. Allmer, W. Hartmann, & D. Kayser (Eds.), *Sportpsychologie in*

Bewegung—Forschung für die Praxis (pp. 67-80). Cologne, Germany: Sport und Buch Strauss.

Kellmann, M., Altenburg, D., Lormes, W., & Steinacker, J.M. (2001). Assessing stress and recovery during preparation for the World Championships in rowing. *The Sport Psychologist, 15,* 151-167.

Kellmann, M., & Beckmann, J. (in press). Research and intervention in sport psychology: New perspectives for an inherent conflict. *International Journal of Sport Psychology.*

Kellmann, M., Botterill, C., & Wilson, C. (1999). *Recovery-Cue.* Unpublished Recovery Assessment Instrument. Calgary: National Sport Centre.

Kellmann, M., Fritzenberg, M., & Beckmann, J. (2000). Erfassung von Belastung und Erholung im Behindertensport [Assessment of stress and recovery in sport with athletes with a physical handicap]. *Psychologie und Sport, 7,* 141-152.

Kellmann, M., & Günther, K.-D. (1999). Die Diagnose der Erholungs-Beanspruchungs-Bilanz während des WM-Trainingslagers des DRV [The Recovery-Stress-Balance Diagnosis during Competition Preparation]. In W. Fritsch (Ed.), *Rudern - informieren, reflektieren, innovieren* (pp. 287-293). Wiebelsheim, Germany: Limpert.

Kellmann, M., & Günther, K.-D. (2000). Changes in stress and recovery in elite rowers during preparation for the Olympic Games. *Medicine and Science in Sports and Exercise, 32,* 676-683.

Kellmann, M., & Kallus, K.W. (1999). Mood, recovery-stress state, and regeneration. In M. Lehmann, C. Foster, U. Gastmann, H. Keizer, & J.M. Steinacker (Eds.), *Overload, fatigue, performance incompetence, and regeneration in sport* (pp. 101-117). New York: Plenum.

Kellmann, M., & Kallus, K.W. (2000). *Der Erholungs-Belastungs-Fragebogen für Sportler; Handanweisung* [The Recovery-Stress Questionnaire for Athletes; manual]. Frankfurt, Germany: Swets Test Services.

Kellmann, M., & Kallus, K.W. (2001). *Recovery-Stress Questionnaire for Athletes: User manual.* Champaign, IL: Human Kinetics.

Kellmann, M., Kallus, K.W., Günther, K.-D., Lormes, W., & Steinacker, J.M. (1997). Psychologische Betreuung der Junioren-Nationalmannschaft des Deutschen Ruderverbandes [Psychological consultation of the German Junior National Rowing Team]. *Psychologie und Sport, 4,* 123-134.

Kenttä, G., & Hassmén, P. (1998). Overtraining and recovery. *Sports Medicine, 26,* 1-16.

Kuipers, H. (1998). Training and overtraining: An introduction. *Medicine and Science in Sports and Exercise, 30,* 1137-1139.

Kuipers, H., & Keizer, H.A. (1988). Overtraining in elite athletes: Review and directions for the future. *Sports Medicine, 6,* 79-92.

Lane, A.M., & Terry, P.C. (2000). The nature of mood: Development of a conceptual model with a focus on depression. *Journal of Applied Sport Psychology, 12,* 16-33.

Lehmann, M., Foster, C., Gastmann, U., Keizer, H.A., & Steinacker, J.M. (1999). Definition, types, symptoms, findings, underlying mechanisms, and frequency of overtraining and overtraining syndrome. In M. Lehmann, C. Foster, U. Gastmann, H. Keizer, & J.M. Steinacker (Eds.), *Overload, fatigue, performance incompetence, and regeneration in sport* (pp. 1-6). New York: Plenum.

Lehmann, M., Foster, C., & Keul, J. (1993). Overtraining in endurance athletes: A brief review. *Medicine and Science in Sports and Exercise, 25,* 854-861.

Lehmann, M., Lormes, W., Opitz-Gress, A., Steinacker, J.M., Netzer, N., Foster, C., & Gastmann, U. (1997). Training and overtraining: An overview and experimental results in endurance sports. *Journal of Sports Medicine and Physical Fitness, 37,* 7-17.

LeUnes, A. (2000). Updated bibliography on the Profile of Mood States in sport and exercise psychology research. *Journal of Applied Sport Psychology, 12,* 110-113.

LeUnes, A., & Burger, J. (2000). The Profile of Mood States research in sport and exercise psychology: Past, present and future. *Journal of Applied Sport Psychology, 12,* 5-15.

Martin, D.T., Andersen, M.B., & Gates, W. (2000). Using Profile of Mood States (POMS) to monitor high-intensity training in cyclists: Group versus case studies. *The Sport Psychologist, 14,* 138-156.

McKenzie, D.C. (1999). Markers of excessive exercise. *Canadian Journal of Applied Physiology, 24,* 66-73.

McNair, D., Lorr, M., & Droppleman, L.F. (1971). *Profile of Mood States manual.* San Diego: Educational and Industrial Testing Service.

McNair, D., Lorr, M., & Droppleman, L.F. (1992). *Profile of Mood States manual.* San Diego: Educational and Industrial Testing Service.

Morgan, W.P. (1985). Selected psychological factors limiting performance: A mental health model. In D.H. Clarke & H.M. Eckert (Eds.), *Limits of human performance* (pp. 70-80). Champaign, IL: Human Kinetics.

Morgan, W.P. (1994). Psychological components of effort sense. *Medicine and Science in Sports and Exercise, 26,* 1071-1077.

Morgan, W.P., Brown, D.R., Raglin, J.S., O'Connor, P.J., & Ellickson, K.A. (1987). Psychological monitoring of overtraining and staleness. *British Journal of Sport Medicine, 21,* 107-114.

Morgan, W.P., & Costill, D.L. (1996). Selected psychological characteristics and health behaviors of aging marathon runners: A longitudinal study. *International Journal of Sport Medicine, 17,* 305-312.

Morgan, W.P., Costill, D.L., Flynn, M.G., Raglin, J.S., & O'Connor, P. (1988). Mood disturbance following increased training in swimmers. *Medicine and Science in Sports and Exercise, 20,* 408-414.

Nitsch, J.R. (1976). Die Eigenzustandsskala (EZ-Skala) - Ein Verfahren zur hirarchisch-mehrdimensionalen Befindlichkeitsskalierung [The standardized scale of self-condition - An instrument for the hirachical multidimensional scaling of mood]. In J.R. Nitsch (Ed.), *Beanspruchung im Sport* (pp. 81-102). Wiebelsheim, Germany: Limpert.

Noble, B.J., & Noble, J.M. (1998). Perceived exertion: The measurement. In J.L. Duda (Ed.), *Advances in sport and exercise psychology measurement* (pp. 351-360). Morgantown, WV: Fitness Information Technology.

Noble, B.J., & Robertson, R.J. (1996). *Perceived exertion.* Champaign, IL: Human Kinetics.

O'Connor, P.J., Morgan, W.P., & Raglin, J.S. (1991). Psychobiologic effects of 3 d of increased training in female and male swimmers. *Medicine and Science in Sports and Exercise, 23,* 1055-1061.

Prapavessis, H. (2000). The POMS and sports performance: A review. *Journal of Applied Sport Psychology, 12,* 34-48.

Raglin, J.S. (1993). Overtraining and staleness: Psychometric monitoring of endurance athletes. In R.B. Singer, M. Murphey, & L.K. Tennant (Eds.), *Handbook of research on sport psychology* (pp. 840-850). New York: Macmillan.

Raglin, J.S., Morgan, W.P., & Luchsinger, A.E. (1990). Mood state and self-motivation in successful and unsuccessful women rowers. *Medicine and Science in Sports and Exercise, 22,* 849-853.

Snyder, A.C. (1998). Overtraining and glycogen depletion hypothesis. *Medicine and Science in Sport and Exercise, 7,* 1146-1150.

Snyder, A.C., Jeukendrup, A.E., Hesselink, M.K.C., Kuipers, H., & Foster, C. (1993). A physiological/psychological indicator of overreaching during intensive training. *International Journal of Sports Medicine, 14,* 29-32.

Steinacker, J.M., Kellmann, M., Böhm, B.O., Liu, Y., Opitz-Gress, A., Kallus, K.W., Lehmann, M., Altenburg, D., & Lormes, W. (1999). Clinical findings and parameters of stress and regeneration in rowers before World Championships. In M. Lehmann, C. Foster, U. Gastmann, H. Keizer, & J.M. Steinacker (Eds.), *Overload, fatigue, performance incompetence, and regeneration in sport* (pp. 71-80). New York: Plenum.

Steinacker, J.M., Lormes, W., Kellmann, M., Liu, Y., Reißnecker, S., Opitz-Gress, A., Baller, B., Günther, K., Petersen, K.G., Kallus, K.W., Lehmann, M., & Altenburg, D. (2000). Training of junior rowers before World Championships. Effects on performance, mood state and selected hormonal and metabolic responses. *Journal of Sports Medicine and Physical Fitness, 40,* 327-335.

Terry, P.C. (2000). Introduction to the special issues: Perspectives on mood sport and exercise. *Journal of Applied Sport Psychology, 12,* 1-4.

Terry, P.C., & Lane, A.M. (2000). Normative values for the Profile of Mood States for use with athletic samples. *Journal of Applied Sport Psychology, 12,* 93-109.

Ulmer, H.V., Macsenaere, M., & Valasiadis, A. (1999). Psychophysiologische Erholung nach einem 400 m-Lauf—Vergleich zweier Objektiver und zweier subjektiver Tests [Psychophysiological recovery after a 400-m run—A comparison between two objective and two subjective tests]. *Psychologie und Sport, 6,* 12-17.

Urhausen A., Gabriel, H.H., Weiler, B., & Kindermann, W. (1998). Ergometric and psychological findings during overtraining: A long-term follow-up study in endurance athletes. *International Journal of Sports Medicine, 19,* 114-20.

Urhausen, A., & Kindermann, W. (2001). Aktuelle Marker für die Diagnostik von Überlastungsschäden in der Trainingspraxis [Current markers for the diagnosis of overtraining syndrome in the practice of training]. *Deutsche Zeitschrift für Sportmedizin, 51,* 226-233.

USOC/ACSM (1999). *Human performance summit. Overtraining: The challenge of prevention: A consensus statement.* Retrieved April 6, 1999, from the www.acsm.org/sportmed/acsmusoc.htm

Wittig, A.F., Houmard, J.A., & Costill, D.L. (1989). Psychological effects during reduced training in distance runners. *International Journal of Sports Medicine, 10,* 97-100.

Kenttä, G., & Hassmén, P. (2002). Underrecovery and overtraining: A conceptual model. In M. Kellmann (Ed.), *Enhancing recovery: Preventing underperformance in athletes* (pp. 57-79). Champaign, IL: Human Kinetics.

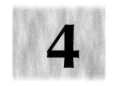

Underrecovery and Overtraining: A Conceptual Model

Göran Kenttä and Peter Hassmén

Oh tiredness,
where do you come from?
When you cover my body
with your blanket,
or wipe out my vision,
I crave for sleep.
Right then, right there.
I lie down on the ground,
close my eyes.

Leave everything.
Do not speak with me.
Do not ask me to speak.
Do not demand me to smile.
Let me be still.

Let me.
Allow me.
Forgive me.

Although great training loads can lead to performance development and success, they can also lead to performance deterioration and personal failure when recovery is insufficient. The lines to the left clearly illustrate the latter. The poem was written in frustration at the end of a five-year stretch during which intense training periods were interrupted by bouts of staleness brought on by negative overtraining and a serious lack of recovery. This young and talented canoeist's career ended in a severe case of burnout. She never realized her dream of participating in the Olympic Games. Perhaps the outcome could have been dramatically different if she had been assisted by a sensitive monitoring program that increased her self-awareness in her pursuit of excellence. In contrast, coaches and leaders frequently endorse attitudes such as "no pain, no gain" and "more is always better," which potentially foster "cultures of risk" instead of promoting self-awareness (Brustad & Ritter-Taylor, 1997).

How can aspiring elite athletes with little practical experience find the strength to challenge their coaches' great "wisdom"? We believe athletes can do so by educating themselves about the relationship between training and recovery. Coaches, too, for that matter, should understand this crucial relationship. Education is without a doubt an important tool in performance development, and close cooperation among sport scientists can further help to build the training process on a sound scientific base.

Training practices have indeed changed over the years, partly as a consequence of scientific progress. It is interesting to reflect on the changing perspectives of training over time. When world-famous middle- and long-distance runner Gunder Hägg reached his prime at the beginning of the 1940s, most athletes "just trained"—the more the better (Hägg, 1952). We will refer to this as the first developmental stage. The second stage introduced the art of periodization; that is, easy weeks were mixed with medium and heavy weeks according to a predetermined schedule. Still, very few athletes and coaches consciously acknowledged the importance of recovery within the process. In the third stage of the development of training, recovery in the form of rest from training was introduced as a vital part of the process.

Finally, in the fourth developmental stage, sport and exercise scientists realized that optimal performance required more than simply addressing physical training and rest. Athletes and their trainers must now strive to balance (1) the training and nontraining stress experienced, (2) the athlete's capacity to cope with this stress, and (3) all the recovery actions taken. Hence, the current consensus is that the individual is a living *psychosociophysiological* system (cf. Kenttä & Hassmén, 1998). Therefore, a monitoring system for training and recovery needs to consider psychosocial influences and interactions as well as physiological ones.

The aim of this chapter is to outline a monitoring system that builds on two user-friendly concepts that account for the training *and* the subsequent recovery processes. To enhance the implementation and application of this monitoring system, a conceptual model is presented that serves as a framework for the efficient use of the monitoring system. In order to address some practical implications, two authentic cases—that of a 17-year-old female racing canoeist and that of a 28-year-old male road racing cyclist—have been included.

A Monitoring System

The overall goal for monitoring training and recovery simultaneously is to yield optimal increases in performance. More specifically, when balancing the breakdown process (a natural result of training) and the following recovery process correctly, an overshoot in performance capacity occurs. This is frequently referred to as the *supercompensation principle* (e.g., Budgett, 1990;

Norris & Smith, this volume, chapter 7; Viru, 1984, 1994).

Despite accumulated research in the domain of sport science, a reliable method for accurately monitoring both training and recovery has been lacking for a long time. Such a method is badly needed because of the almost impossible task of initially distinguishing optimal training (which results in performance enhancement) from negative overtraining (which constitutes the first step toward staleness). This is most crucial during periods of heavy training when the outcome is still unknown (Kenttä & Hassmén, 1998; Koutedakis et al., 1999; Kuipers, 1998). The stock market can serve as a metaphor. Despite their best efforts, financial experts (comparable to coaches, athletes, and scientists in the world of sport) frequently fail to predict the actions of the stock market at predetermined dates (comparable to peak performances). Not surprisingly, Fry, Morton, and Keast (1992) stated that the training process is still "more art than a science" (p. 246). One important question is therefore: Can we increase our chances for predicting a positive training outcome (and peak performance at predetermined dates)? Our answer is yes. But in order to do so, we need to monitor carefully the complete process of training and recovery. Furthermore, we need to know what constitutes optimal training versus negative overtraining.

We suggest that a two-stage approach should be considered in order to develop a trustworthy monitoring system. First, we need to design a monitoring system that can be used easily by athletes and coaches in practical settings and that covers the full training process (i.e., includes both training and recovery). Several tools, such as structured training programs, training logs, and self-rating protocols, are integral parts in this work. Second, we need to define and set criteria for what constitutes optimal training as well as negative overtraining. Addressing important features of optimal and negative training, therefore, serves as a guideline for the monitoring system itself.

Optimal Training and Negative Overtraining Criteria

Optimal training primarily features the benefit of adaptation as opposed to maladaptation due to negative overtraining (Kuipers & Keizer, 1988; Lehmann, Foster, & Keul, 1993; Morgan, O'Connor, Sparling, & Pate, 1987). Essential components of optimal training include physical adaptation to the training performed and the possibility for competitive athletes to practice at the highest level of performance (optimal technique, speed, strength, aerobic power, and mental abilities). Furthermore, general well-being is maintained despite heavy training loads, and performance capacity increases in a steady fashion.

In contrast, pushing beyond optimal training will slowly diminish all positive effects. Depending on the degree and severity of negative overtraining, a number of less desirable outcomes will become obvious. For example, the potential for high-quality performance or technique training becomes limited, and training increasingly psychologically demanding. The immune system becomes negatively affected, resulting in more infections and the resultant absences from training. Uncertainty exists as to whether the body will adapt only to a previous level of performance or accomplish a supercompensation after recovery (Berglund & Säfström, 1994; Fry, Morton, & Keast, 1991; Kreider, Fry, & O'Toole, 1998).

A Complete Monitoring System

Although several methods have been developed to monitor and measure the training performed, methods aiming to monitor recovery are still scarce (Kellmann, this volume, chapter 3). A complete monitoring system is needed that will organize training practice and subsequent recovery in a conscious and systematic way. Such a system

needs to consider three phases: (1) stimulus, (2) perception of the stimulus, and (3) response to the stimulus (see figure 4.1).

Phase 1

Carefully tailoring the training program (i.e., stimulus) is the first important step in performance development. Frequently, athletes and coaches invest much effort in developing the "perfect" training program (Kellmann & Günther, 2000; Rowbottom, Keast, & Morton, 1998).

Arriving at a perfect program is insufficient, however, without considering two additional steps—the athlete's perception of the training performed (phase 2) and, perhaps most important and most neglected, the athlete's response to the stimulus (phase 3). All three phases must be addressed to ensure a complete monitoring system.

Phase 2

The second phase aims at understanding the magnitude of the stimulus. We are now referring to factors such as frequency, duration, work/rest ratio, but most important, actual intensity (Foster, Daniels, & Seiler, 1999). Even if the training program is meticulously detailed in terms of objective measures, the information content may still be insufficient to understand its effects on individual athletes. Objective variables, such as working heart rate, lactate thresholds, measured speed, and so on, are relatively easy to measure and unfortunately often thought of as the only

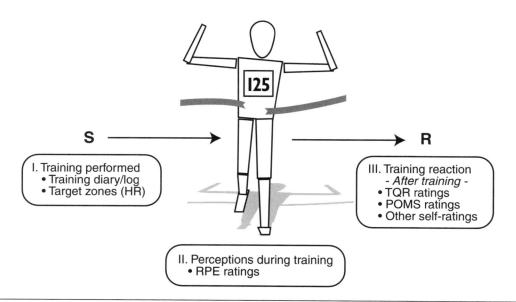

Figure 4.1 The training process containing stimulus (training), perception of the stimulus, and response to training.

necessary information about training load. Subjective variables, though more difficult to measure, can be combined with objective measures to offer a more complete picture of the true magnitude of training load exerted on the athlete (Kenttä & Hassmén, 1998). One purpose of this chapter is therefore to emphasize the importance, as well as the validity, of subjective self-reports in monitoring training and recovery. Furthermore, intraindividual (within the individual) approaches will be emphasized since development of optimal training regimens at the elite level must be highly individualistic endeavors (see Hanin, this volume, chapter 11).

But why do we have to question the athlete's "objective" training log for evaluating intensity? If the athlete is told to perform a standardized interval session, say at 80% of maximum intensity, and also notes this in the training log, isn't this knowledge sufficient? Consider a situation in which a number of elite athletes train together under the supervision of their head coach, and the similar but very different situation in which one of the athletes performs the "same" workout alone. Most likely, the two sessions will differ in intensity, despite the fact that the entries in the training log reveal no difference (cf. Ericsson, 1996).

Additionally, an extensive review regarding overtraining and staleness described how athletes of approximately equal capacity displayed heterogeneous responses to a standardized training stimulus (Raglin, 1993). This may explain why the same objective training load (i.e., same duration and intensity) can be perceived as optimal intensity for improving the performance capacity by one athlete (i.e., positive overtraining or overreaching), insufficient for another (who experiences a performance drop due to undertraining), and too heavy for a third athlete (who experiences a performance drop due to negative overtraining). Research has also shown that the same individual can perceive a given training load differently on two separate occasions depending on the training state (whether he is well rested or overreached) (Morgan, 1994; Raglin, Sawamura, Alexiou, Hassmén, & Kenttä, 2000) or on the current psychosocial stress load; see case 1 at the end of this chapter. Obviously, a strong need exists for more specific and appropriate assessments of training and recovery that are sensitive to individual differences. In addition, athletes' perceptions of the training load should be considered when evaluating the true impact of the training stimulus.

Phase 3

Finally, the last phase focuses on how athletes respond and adapt to the training performed, with particular emphasis on short-term responses. Annually or even monthly scheduled performance tests do not meet these criteria. And—importantly—due to the problem of successfully evaluating training load, we suggest a greater focus on response instead of stimulus—that is, shifting the focus somewhat from training load toward an ongoing evaluation of responses to the training performed. As long as training responses remain within a predetermined zone, major errors can be avoided. Short-term deviations from an anticipated response may only need some extra attention, whereas more long-term deviations will require substantial interventions. The latter may be a sign of poor adaptation leading to a performance plateau or decreased performance (i.e., maladaptation).

Tools of the Monitoring System

The most suitable tools for a complete monitoring system—Ratings of Perceived Exertion (RPE) and Total Quality Recovery (TQR) (Kenttä & Hassmén, 1998)—can each be viewed in terms of a global psychophysiological construct that focuses on the individual's own perceptions. The former relates to training, with the use of the RPE scale by Borg (1998); the latter, to recovery, with the use of the TQR scale by Kenttä (1996). These scales facilitate self-monitoring with a strong foundation in the athlete's perceptual and emotional experience. Self-monitoring, self-assessment, and didactic stress management generally serve the purpose of increasing the level of self-awareness in individuals. Self-understanding logically begins with self-observation (cf. Schaufeli & Enzmann, 1998). The concept of Total Quality Recovery is further separated into two elements, one focusing on perceptions of recovery as briefly noted previously and another focusing on stress management, or more specifically, recovery management.

Why Ratings of Perceived Exertion?

Research has shown that physical effort is best conceptualized as a complex psychobiological construct (cf. Borg, 1998). Numerous studies have verified that the RPE is accurate in estimating the intensity of exercise stimuli (Noble & Robertson, 1996). This demonstrates that the RPE can be valuable for prescribing exercise intensity as well as for monitoring purposes (Borg & Hassmén, 1999). RPE ratings can be given as local ratings (of working muscles, for example), central ratings (breathing, etc.), or overall ratings combining information from many parts of the body. See figure 4.2 for an explanatory model stemming from the work by Hassmén (1991).

Perceived exertion has also been studied in the context of overtraining. Morgan (1994) noted that, at given workloads, stale athletes increased their perceptions of effort measured by RPE. Changes in the ratio of RPE and blood lactate were found to be a reliable predictor of staleness (Snyder, 1998; Snyder, Jeukendrup, Hesselink, Kuipers, & Foster, 1993). Additionally, undesirable training outcomes were minimized when training load was successfully monitored using the RPE (Foster, 1998).

In summary, the RPE is user friendly, is easily performed on a regular basis, and has proved to be a highly reliable method for monitoring training. Furthermore, RPE ratings require athletes to observe and focus on psychophysiological cues in order to rate the perceived effort. Heart rate monitors, while being highly reliable, do not produce the same desirable effect of enhancing important cognitive functions and increasing the individual's self-awareness—at least not to the same degree. By using local and central RPE ratings, athletes and coaches may together contrast local working capacity (e.g., the specific endurance capacity in the legs during running) and central working capacity (e.g., the stroke

volume, which is critical for oxygen uptake). In other words, a runner may perceive that her running capacity is limited by the endurance capacity of her legs or the central capacity of her heart muscle to provide enough blood saturated with oxygen, thereby possibly identifying areas in greatest need of improvement. It seems reasonable to suggest that the integration of local and central cues into a global RPE is the best way to assess true individual training intensity. By being aware of "unexplainable" changes in RPE ratings during standardized training, athletes and coaches may also be able to detect early signs of staleness. We do recommend, however, that serious athletes use both a heart rate monitor and RPE ratings since the two sources together are superior to only one.

Why Total Quality Recovery?

According to the supercompensation principle, a more powerful training stimuli requires longer recovery. Logically, then, recovery should be monitored in close relationship with training load. The method of Total Quality Recovery (TQR) has therefore been structured closely around the concept of RPE in order to emphasize the interrelationship between training and recovery. A didactic advantage is also achieved by structuring the concept of recovery around the concept of perceived exertion (see figure 4.3). The initial purpose for developing the TQR was to prevent the occurrence of

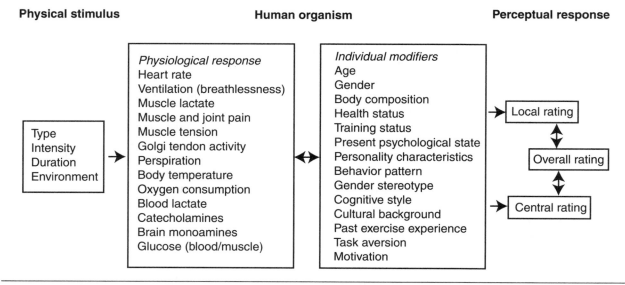

Figure 4.2 An explanatory model of the relationship between physical work and the physiological responses and psychological modifiers that affect the Ratings of Perceived Exertion.

The figure is based on a model suggested by Hassmén (1991).

Ratings of Perceived Exertion (RPE)	Total Quality Recovery (TQR)
6 No exertion at all	6 No recovery at all

7
   Extremely light
8
	7
	   Extremely poor recovery
	8

9 Very light	9 Very poor recovery
10	10
11 Light	11 Poor recovery
12	12
13 Somewhat hard	13 Reasonable recovery
14	14
15 Hard (heavy)	15 Good recovery
16	16
17 Very hard	17 Very good recovery
18	18
19 Extremely hard	19 Extremely good recovery
20 Maximal exertion	20 Maximal recovery

Figure 4.3. The RPE scale for training and the TQR scale.

RPE scale reprinted, by permission, from G. Borg, 1998, *Borg's Perceived Exertion and Pain Scales* (Champaign, IL: Human Kinetics), 47. © Gunnar Borg 1970, 1985, 1994, 1998. TQR scale from Kenttä, 1996.

staleness among racing canoeists (through pro-active recovery), thereby also optimizing the balance between training and recovery. In order to achieve this goal, and due to the lack of available instruments, it was necessary to develop a new method to measure psychophysiological recovery (Kenttä, 1996; Kenttä & Hassmén, 1998, 1999, 2000).

The TQR method is divided into two subdimensions, one focusing solely on the perception of recovery (TQR perceived scale) and the other on the recovery actions performed (TQR action scale). Specifically, they answer two questions: (1) How does it feel? and (2) What have you done?

The TQR perceived scale emphasizes the global perception of psychophysiological recovery. The correct instruction set is to ask the athlete before bedtime to rate his sense of recovery as an overall psychophysiological rating (i.e., physically and mentally) for the past 24 hours, including the previous night's sleep. This emphasizes the individual's subjective perception of recovery, which is qualitative in nature. It should therefore be used primarily to detect intraindividual changes.

The TQR action scale grades and monitors purposeful self-initiated recovery actions from four main categories (nutrition and hydration, sleep and rest, relaxation and emotional support, stretching and warm-down). A specially designed manual (Kenttä & Hassmén, 1999) explains how to earn recovery points, which are accumulated over 24 hours. The self-monitoring of TQR actions can be seen as a way to highly individualize recovery management. A successful implementation of the TQR concept thereby depends more than anything on each participant's learning process.

Athletes who use the TQR correctly can expect to experience a reduced risk of overuse injuries and infections, which in turn reduces the loss of possible training days. Furthermore, the TQR increases athletes' awareness of the possible need to accelerate the recovery process by active measures. The interrelationship between recovery actions and perceived recovery is graphically displayed in figure 4.4. Using TQR also clearly points to the close relationship between actual training load and adequate recovery. When training load increases, recovery actions also need to be upgraded. Finally, regular monitoring of recovery will indicate a state of underrecovery and thereby serve as an early staleness marker.

This approach can be contrasted to the more common approach in which coaches simply ask their athletes about recovery, stress, and sleeping habits. The main difference is that self-monitoring, even though implemented and supported by the coach, has a greater potential to promote the development of self-awareness, a sense of control, and an ability to proactively monitor adequate recovery.

Overview of TQR

The outcome of most methods applied in athletic settings depends heavily on the initial phase of implementation. Failing to deal with this phase comprehensively will result in the inefficient use of the monitoring system. Those overseeing the implementation must be careful to explain the overall purpose, the guidelines for assessing recovery actions, how to score, and perhaps most important for the athlete, how to interpret and use the scoring information. Giving appropriate attention to these matters during the initial implementation phase will assure the most efficient use of the recovery system for all participants.

Guidelines for Assessing Recovery Actions

The overall purpose of assessing recovery is to optimize performance development by balancing training and recovery and thereby simultaneously minimizing the risk of negative consequences of excessive training. Athletes using the TQR method collect recovery points (RPs) by performing predefined recovery actions over a 24-hour period. Recovery actions performed are preferably scored before bedtime each day as part of a standardized routine. All recovery actions performed during the day—including the last night's sleep—should be included. Evaluation is primarily focused on intraindividual changes. A total of 20 RPs is the maximum score and obviously most beneficial for overall recovery and subsequent adaptation potential.

The point on the TQR continuum at which adequate recovery becomes inadequate recovery is around TQR act 13. Swimmers and kayakers, for example, who were ready to perform optimally in a well-recovered state reported around TQR act 17, whereas the same athletes reported below TQR act 13 when they felt underrecovered. A low recovery score was often a consequence of time restriction and psychosocial stressors. In contrast, recovery was reportedly given more attention during training camps (Kenttä & Hassmén, 1999). This scenario is unfortunate since active recovery is even more crucial when athletes are under time pressure and when psychosocial stress is elevated. Arriving at a reasonable recovery score is usually a result of being somewhat good at dealing with each of the four recovery categories, namely, nutrition and hydration, sleep and rest, relaxation and emotional support, and stretching and warm-down. Nevertheless, since what constitutes a reasonable recovery score may differ both between athletes and for the same

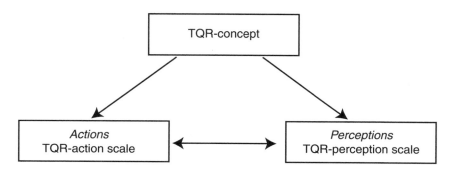

Figure 4.4 An overview of the TQR concept.

athlete over time, it is therefore important to examine every situation more specifically, especially if it results in persistent low ratings of perceived recovery.

Individual calculations (i.e., grading and scoring) of obtained RPs is made according to preset criteria in a standardized manual (see the following outline). These criteria serve as a foundation for scoring recovery actions as well as guidance for the process of acquiring RPs. After a supervised learning period, athletes are responsible for performing recovery actions as well as for grading them. By self-monitoring, athletes move toward enhanced self-awareness. Hence, each athlete judges her actions as adequate or inadequate in relation to her individual needs and the training performed. When she judges her actions as inadequate, the athlete is asked to evaluate the lack of recovery actions taken and express this as a percentage of full (adequate) recovery. For example, if she only ate half of a normal dinner, the full score would be reduced by 50%.

RPs have been allocated according to the degree of importance for the recovery process, but also in regard to practical limitations in the field setting. This was made after a comprehensive review of the recovery literature and consultation with experienced coaches and athletes. The first two recovery categories (nutrition and hydration, sleep and rest) can be seen as the most essential recovery actions. A lack of nutrition (carbohydrate intake) may have the most obvious short-term influence on recovery in terms of failing to restore energy (muscle glycogen) for the forthcoming training session. Failing to deal with the third and fourth categories (relaxation and emotional support; stretching and warm-down) may or may not have an immediate influence on recovery, but over time, severe consequences, such as feelings of chronic underrecovery and overuse injuries, may occur. In terms of striving for peak performance, however, every system needs to be fully recovered in order to maximize one's potential.

It should be noted that the distribution and calculation of RPs as explained in the manual (Kenttä & Hassmén, 1999) can be modified relatively easily to address sport-specific demands as well as individual needs. The version presented here was developed primarily to meet the demands of junior and senior endurance athletes. However, since the method is aimed at improving recovery at the individual level, modifications are encouraged as long as the same athlete always uses the method in the same way (as noted, intraindividual comparisons are the prime target).

How to Score Recovery Actions and Earn Recovery Points

This phase of implementing scoring and earning recovery points could preferably be integrated by adequate theoretical education about each category with emphasis on the importance of recovery and how recovery can be accelerated. Ultimately, athletes should theoretically understand the importance of recovery and practically know how to earn recovery points.

Nutrition and Hydration: 10 RPs (8 for Nutrition and 2 for Hydration)

Nutritional RPs are distributed as follows: excellence in breakfast—1 RP, lunch—2 RPs, dinner—2 RPs, snacks between meals and evening meal—1 RP, and fast carbohydrate refueling in conjunction with training—2 RPs. The recommendation for fast carbohydrate refueling is 1 gram of carbohydrates per kilogram of body weight immediately after training. Thereafter, every other hour up to six hours after training. The daily recommendation during heavy training is 8-10 grams of carbohydrates per kilogram of body weight (Coggan, 1997; Hawley, Schabort, Noakes, & Dennis, 1997; Ivy, 1991).

Excellence in nutrition has two different dimensions: qualitative and quantitative. The quantity demands emphasize the need to meet the individual's energy consumption with an adequate energy intake. Muscle glycogen storage will be drained during heavy training loads. Availability of glycogen determines the ability to maintain high-intensity training. It is therefore important to adjust to the energy demand and ingest carbohydrates to quickly restore muscle glycogen. Despite the need for "fast fuel," the necessity of other energy resources such as fat and protein should never be overlooked or underestimated, not even in the context of high-intensity training. A general recommendation of how energy intake should be distributed is 55-60 energy percent (E%) from carbohydrates, 20-30 E% from fat, and 10-15 E% from protein. Considering how the total energy intake is distributed from carbohydrates, fat, and protein is simply a way of demonstrating that the composition of energy sources matters. In other words, the energy intake is most efficient if it is distributed as noted.

The quality demands emphasize the need to eat sufficient amounts of vitamins and minerals. Iron in particular may need extra attention, especially for endurance athletes. An athlete with a well-balanced diet will seldom need to use expensive dietary supplements. However, this has to be decided on an individual basis (Costill et al., 1988; Morgan, Costill, & Flynn, 1988).

Drinking adequate amounts of water to maintain fluid balance in relation to current weather and training conditions allows athletes to accumulate the final 2 RPs. Note, however, that it is almost impossible to give any absolute recommendations regarding quantity of hydration since interactions among training type, environmental factors, and personal factors greatly affect the daily requirements. Athletes are therefore encouraged to use the "urine-color test" together with a measurement of body weight immediately before and after each training session. When urine has very little or no color, it indicates adequate fluid balance. Dark-colored urine indicates a lack of adequate hydration, although vitamin supplementation and certain foods will color urine as well.

In summary: Eat adequate amounts of a well-balanced diet in terms of energy sources and micronutrients (i.e., iron and certain vitamins). Drink appropriate amounts of fluid. Be aware of the importance of timing. Remember that appetite and thirst are insufficient indicators.

Sleep and Rest: 4 RPs

A full night of high-quality sleep adds up to 3 RPs, and an extra point is attainable with at least one period of "microrest" (i.e., similar to the "siesta" in Southern Europe or a "power nap" in other countries) during the day. Rating the degree of satisfaction should be based on a global individual perception. A combination of hours and perceived quality is emphasized instead of focusing exclusively on the number of hours. This pinpoints the fact that the amount of time needed for adequate sleep may vary from time to time. Eight hours of sleep is normally sufficient for an adult. However, the need for sleep and microrest becomes elevated during periods of heavy training or during an exhausting everyday life situation (Taylor, Rogers, & Driver, 1997).

Overtraining syndrome can in many cases be viewed as an error in the training program due to underrecovery and lack of rest days (cf. Kreider, Fry, & O'Toole, 1998). It is therefore important to include rest in the daily routine. But how many athletes actually dare to rest confidently and with a clean conscience? To encourage preplanned rest, we reserved some RPs for time off from training only. Hence, a preplanned day off from training equals 4 RPs, and a half-day off allows 2 RPs. This of course excludes unplanned rest forced by illness or injury. Giving bonus points for inactivity and time away from strenuous physical activity emphasizes the fact that rest should be part of a well-designed training program. A full day of rest each week is strongly suggested. These bonus points counterbalance the points achieved in conjunction with training.

In summary: Sleep comfortably for an adequate number of hours at the right time, and try to include microrest, especially during heavy periods of training. Moreover, make sure to take a day off each week.

Relaxation and Emotional Support: 3 RPs

When a state of full mental and muscular relaxation is reached as soon as possible after each training session, another 2 RPs are obtained. This state is reached through the use of relaxation techniques and is performed to decrease "afterburn time" (defined as the period of increased metabolism that occurs after exercise). Relaxation is also important for quickly eliminating above-normal muscle tone (i.e., tension). Decreased afterburn time and lowered muscle tone are strongly related to increased time for recovery and restoration between training sessions.

Active relaxation is preferably integrated with regular stretching. A stretching session can initially focus on muscular relaxation. Later in the session, when a feeling of comfort and muscle relaxation is achieved, the focus can shift toward mental relaxation. We like to call this technique of integrating muscular and mental relaxation into regular stretching "cyber-stretching."

The mental and muscular relaxation achieved after exercise should be distinguished from a mentally relaxed state that is generally desirable on a daily basis. A generally relaxed mental state is the opposite of being full of worries and negative emotions and being overwhelmed with psychosocial stress. Athletes should strive to reduce their vulnerability to unnecessary psychosocial stress and seek social support from significant others. They should concentrate on positive, relaxed thoughts and attitudes throughout the day. The third RP in this category is obtainable if the athlete can maximize the potential for psychosocial recovery, primarily by being able to maintain a mentally relaxed state throughout the day (Wilks, 1991).

Thoughts and mood states have the potential to influence recovery positively or negatively. In fact, cognitive behavioral techniques for stress prevention are based on the assumption of a relationship among thoughts (cognitions), emotions (feelings), and actions (behavior). Therefore, changing thoughts will change the appraisal of the situation, which in turn reduces negative feelings and finally eliminates undesirable behavior (Schaufeli & Enzmann, 1998). Negative feelings stem from stressful environments, which can result in anxiety and arousal levels that remain at high levels throughout the day. This will drain psychosocial energy resources and inhibit recovery. Additionally, elevations in nontraining stressors and limitations in recovery will negatively influence the recovery-stress state (see Kellmann & Kallus, 2001; Kellmann, this volume, chapters 1 and 3).

In summary: Work with a combination of muscular and mental relaxation techniques after physical training. Strive to maintain a mentally relaxed state throughout the day.

Stretching and Warm-Down: 3 RPs

Properly performed warm-down periods after each training session provides 2 RPs. Stretching all exercised muscle groups results in 1 RP. Warming up before a training session or a competition is normally viewed as an unquestionable part of preparation. Most athletes and coaches admit, however, that warming up before a competition or training session is prioritized to a higher degree than warming down afterwards.

The higher the degree of exercise intensity, the more important it is to perform stretching as well as warming down. When exercise intensity increases above a certain point, a large volume of lactic acid starts to accumulate in the muscles as a by-product from many forms of high-intensity anaerobic training, especially when exceeding a working duration of 10 to 15 seconds. The purpose of both warming down and stretching is to accelerate the elimination of rest products with an increased blood flow (Evjenth & Hamberg, 1985; McLellan, Cheung, & Jacobs, 1991).

Finally, instead of taking a full day off from training, a light training session (i.e., low volume, low intensity) followed by stretching can be performed with the single purpose of enhancing recovery. This type of recovery session will also allow for the maximum of 3 RPs from this category. Commonly, this type of training routine is referred to as active rest or active recovery. Exercising at moderate intensities will accelerate recovery more than passive rest (Ahmaidi et al., 1996; Wilmore & Costill, 1988). Easy training sessions are preferably conducted in a noncompetitive environment, maybe by engaging in a different sport without measuring performance (e.g., swimming for runners). In this sense, light training serves as a therapeutic tool. This benefits both psychological and physical recovery (Budgett, 1990).

In summary: Emphasize an accelerated recovery by reserving some time for warm-down and stretching. Make sure to use the benefits of an active recovery training session when appropriate.

How to Use the Scoring Information

A general recommendation is to constantly remind athletes that high levels of training load as well as increased training load must be followed by *matched* adequate recovery. This relationship between actual training load and actual recovery becomes obvious when simultaneously monitoring RPE and TQR as part of the daily training routine. Previous studies have shown that limited recovery, as compared to adequate recovery, distinguishes athletes who were unable to tolerate a given training load from those who did tolerate the training load (Costill et al., 1988).

Consequently, our recommendation is that both TQR ratings (especially TQR actions) should match the actual training stress (RPE) in order to ensure adequate recovery. A decrease in training load will momentarily lessen the recovery requirements, but it is always necessary to secure a sufficient base level even during periods of easy training. We recommend that athletes never go below TQR act 13 (reasonable recovery). Recovery scores below 13 will limit the recovery potential and subsequently the adaptation potential to a given training load. A chronic state of low recovery ratings will also place the athlete at greater risk of developing overtraining syndrome as a consequence of persistently being underrecovered.

The TQR action and perceived scales can also serve as markers of underrecovery. A decrease in perceived recovery has been suggested as a valid staleness marker (Kuipers, 1996; Kuipers & Keizer, 1988). Athletes may experience a feeling of poor recovery during heavy training despite doing everything possible to enhance recovery (TQR-perceived < TQR-action). In other words, a state of underrecovery is indicated when the majority of recovery action points have been obtained, but perceived recovery is still rated significantly lower. In this case, rest or reduced training is required since all available efforts to optimize recovery already have been made. For this reason, variations of perceived recovery and comparisons of the TQR action and perceived scales may indicate a state of underrecovery.

Finally, it is important to take care to select the most appropriate recovery actions. The best way to treat stress is by matching the treatment with the specific source and symptoms experienced. This suggests that somatic and cognitive stress should be treated by matched interventions. It is thus important to consider the origin of the perceived stress (i.e., training vs. nontraining stressors) in order to select recovery actions for the area of greatest need. It seems logical that a high level of stress caused by a family conflict needs other recovery interventions than the stress of glycogen depletion caused by a 25 km run. Matched recovery therefore always considers the source and the magnitude of the stress load. The most efficient recovery interventions are properly directed and sufficient in amount.

In summary, the TQR action scale promotes active recovery in and outside of sports.

Conceptual Model

So far, we have suggested a monitoring system covering the full process of training and recovery and addressed the difficulty of successfully balancing training and recovery actions in real-life situations. However, despite our effort to present a reliable method, it is safe to conclude that more knowledge is needed. Statements such as: "Unfortunately, relatively little is known about the quantitative relationship between training characteristics and physiological adaptation to that training" (Kuipers, 1998, p. 86) will continue to be highly valid. Regardless of knowledge level, performance development will continue to be a complex function involving a multitude of variables that are very hard to control for simultaneously. We nevertheless hope our method will be used as a guideline (or as a "training philosophy") rather than as a mathematical formula.

According to our view, optimal training can be seen as an ongoing *psychosociophysiological* balancing act. The ability to perform this act well is undoubtedly crucial for long-term performance development and short-term peak performances.

It is also imperative that the individual athlete take full responsibility for the training process. A coach can—and should in many cases—be deeply involved in planning the training program as well as overseeing the training performed. Nevertheless, only the individual athlete knows exactly in which way the training affects her body and mind and how she perceives recovery actions. The added influence of nontraining stressors occurring in the athlete's everyday life outside the training arena only lends more credibility to this statement.

To address the full context of optimal training and underperformance, we recently developed a conceptual model (Kentta & Hassmén, 1998). The purpose was to increase our understanding of the full complexity involved in monitoring training and recovery, and to differentiate between cause and consequence. Applying a *holistic* perspective to training and recovery will change the condition for planning, monitoring, and evaluation. To begin with, it may be frustrating to include and consider the individual's whole life situation. However, denying the fact that nontraining factors greatly influence the training process is neither the best nor the most constructive solution. In fact, performance development and optimal training depend heavily on the ability to integrate and react to as many relevant variables as possible. In other words, a holistic perspective can be described as the core feature of intelligent training, something that will help us use, and improve our understanding of, the previously described monitoring system.

The conceptual model starts out by making a clear distinction between *cause* (process) and *consequence* (result). Second, the process is described in terms of three major subsystems (physiological, psychological, and social), each containing three elements: specific *stress,* specific *capacity,* and specific *recovery.* These interdependent elements from the various subsystems accumulate into an actual magnitude of total stress, the present overall capacity to cope with this stress, and finally, the actual total recovery. Third, some negative consequences (i.e., markers or warning signals) associated with an unbalanced training process are described in the model (see figure 4.5).

The configuration of the process as described in the model depends on a function of nine elements falling into three categories: (1) physiological, psychological, and social *stress;* (2) physiological, psychological, and social *capacity;* and (3) physiological, psychological, and social *recovery.* These variables are both additive and interactive in nature. This further emphasizes the need

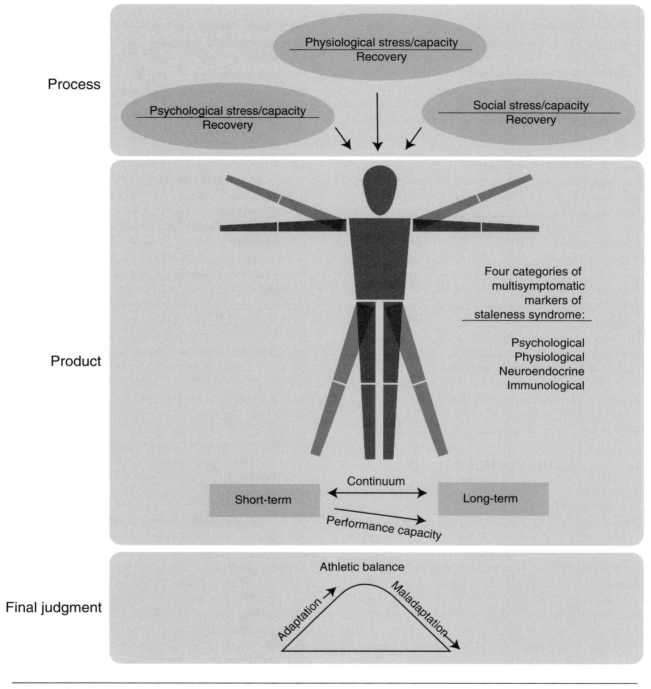

Process

Physiological stress/capacity
Recovery

Psychological stress/capacity
Recovery

Social stress/capacity
Recovery

Product

Four categories of
multisymptomatic
markers of
staleness syndrome:

Psychological
Physiological
Neuroendocrine
Immunological

Continuum

Short-term

Long-term

Performance capacity

Final judgment

Athletic balance

Adaptation

Maladaptation

Figure 4.5 Overtraining and recovery: a conceptual model.

Based on Kanttä and Hassmén, 1998.

for a holistic approach instead of focusing solely on single variables (e.g., training load) and wrongly assuming them to be independent of context. The ultimate goal of monitoring is to give each element the appropriate degree of individual attention while simultaneously watching and guiding all others.

Configuration of Total Stress Load

An examination of the total stress experienced suggests that athletes may encounter stress from three basic sources, which are physiological, psychological, and social in origin. Physiological stress—or more specifically, physical training stress (i.e., aerobic training, anaerobic training, weight training, etc.)—is usually described in the literature as the predominant cause of underperformance associated with staleness and burnout (Morgan, Brown, Raglin, O'Connor, & Ellickson, 1987; Morgan, Costill, & Flynn, 1988; Silva, 1990). However, nontraining stressors have more recently gained a wider acknowledgment in regard to overtraining and burnout among athletes (Gould, Udrey, Tuffey, & Loehr, 1996; Urhausen, Gabriel, Weiler, & Kindermann, 1998). This seems logical because different stressors accumulate into the same melting pot. For example, a small increase in total stress as a result of elevations of social stress might suddenly and unexpectedly elicit staleness (Budgett, 1990).

Increased knowledge about nontraining stressors will help athletes and their supporters adjust the physical training load in relation to variations in total stress experienced. It is also important to gain more knowledge about the extent to which nontraining stressors, and their origins, contribute to the overtraining syndrome. Social stress may arise from interactions with parents, family members, friends, coaches, team leaders, teammates, team officials, competitors, and colleagues. Psychological stress may arise from internal stressors, such as academic or performance situations in which the athlete perceives an imbalance between personal demands and performance capacity, especially when failing to meet these expectations (Kenttä & Hassmén, 1998, 2000).

Overall Capacity, or Stress Tolerance

Physical capacity can be divided into energy-producing capacities (ability to perform aerobic and anaerobic work) and neuromuscular capacities (general and specific strength and motor skills)

(see, for example, Hawley, Myburgh, Noakes, & Dennis, 1997; Kuipers, 1998; Morton, 1997). *Psychological* capacity divides into several subcategories such as self-confidence, attentional capacity, arousal control, motivational level, goal orientation, attitude control, positive mental health, and visualization capacity. Finally, *social* capacity can be described in terms of an existing social network and the ability to create, handle, and maintain relationships with others.

The aim of physical training is to disrupt the organism's homeostasis, that is, to create a stimulus that exceeds the individual's current ability, which then leads to adaptation and performance enhancement. During recovery, the organism is trying to reestablish the previous state of homeostasis. If the period of recovery is long enough, the organism will adapt to a higher level of performance (i.e., in line with the supercompensation principle previously described). This means that the organism will build up its own *capacity to handle more stress* for an equivalent homeostatic imbalance (Fry, Morton, & Keast, 1992). This of course also explains why an aerobically fit athlete tolerates a greater volume of endurance training as compared to a less aerobically fit athlete.

Research has shown that people with normal levels of anxiety, as compared to people with elevated anxiety levels, perceive and rate the intensity of a given stressor as being lower (Morgan, 1994). Clinical research is currently investigating the possibility of modifying the negative influence of mental stress on the immune system by meditation. A recent report suggests that the long-term practice of mediation may influence the immune system positively (Solberg, Halvorsen, & Holen, 2000). It appears that specific training of each subcapacity will be necessary to improve that subcapacity, and thereby help the individual reach the full potential of the overall capacity. By developing the overall stress capacity, the athlete will improve the ability to handle both training and nontraining stressors, thereby increasing the potential for adaptation. Additionally, each subcapacity is not only critical in relation to the total stress tolerance. They also explain a major proportion of global performance capacity (Carron & Hausenblas, 1998; Durand-Bush, Salmela, & Green-Demers, 2001; Kuipers, 1998; Martens, Vealy, & Burton, 1990; Moran, 1996; Morton, 1997; Roberts, 1992; Rushall, 1989).

Actual Total Recovery: Structuring the Recovery Process

World-class tennis player Pete Sampras stated in an interview that "Recovery is a huge factor now" (Clarey, 1998, p. 23), meaning that the key to successful performance is not so much harder training but better recovery actions. The question is, as previously discussed: How can recovery be integrated systematically into regular training practice? A diversity of recovery methods have been suggested throughout the sports literature: proactive rest, passive rest, active rest, flotation tanks, reading, listening to music, fluid and nutrition, and dietary supplements. Others include sleep, microsleep, cool-down, stretching, hydrotherapy, saunas, a variety of massage techniques, and hyperbaric oxygen therapy (i.e., increasing the availability of oxygen to the body). Eastern techniques are also suggested, such as acupuncture, accupressure, yoga, qigong, tai-chi, and meditation. In addition, some suggest physiotherapy; psychotherapy; counseling; relaxation techniques, such as progressive muscle relaxation, autogenic training, imagery, and breathing exercises; emotional support; social support; and daily "uplifting activities" (Calder, 1996; Marion, 1995; Orlick, 1999; Weinberg & Gould, 1999).

However, most suggestions given are general and incomplete without stating either a specific purpose or how it can be implemented and monitored in the context of training, and more specifically, in relation to training load. So clearly, the question still remains: How do we select appropriate recovery actions that are matched systematically with training load, and how do we measure and monitor recovery? Initially, the purpose of the recovery actions needs to be determined (e.g., prevention, rehabilitation, or simply an enhanced recovery rate).

If the focus is on prevention and enhancement of recovery, adequate recovery must consider the type and magnitude of stress and the individual's capacity (i.e., stress tolerance). We previously described in detail how the following four recovery categories could be used to establish an overall *psychosociophysiological* recovery.

1. Nutrition and hydration
2. Sleep and rest
3. Relaxation and emotional support
4. Stretching and active rest

Physiological recovery seems to get most of the attention (categories 1, 2, and 4), as compared to psychological and social recovery (category 3). This proportion may be appropriate for many endurance sports. In contrast, sports with low physical demands but high demands on technique and long-term concentration may require a greater focus on psychosocial recovery. For example, Swedish golfer Jesper Parnevik (among the top 10 golfers in the world in 1999-2000) described in a recent interview how a chronically high level of psychosocial stress drained his recovery potential. This finally evolved into a state of underperformance and chronic fatigue accompanied by medical disorders. This example emphasizes the fact that recovery actions must be matched with the original source. Consequently, it can be stated that each individual's recovery demands need to be met with a well-balanced mix of *psychosociophysiological* recovery.

Markers of the Overtraining Syndrome and Underrecovery

A large number of symptoms associated with the overtraining syndrome are listed in the literature. Fry et al. (1991) divided the variety of symptoms into four relatively homogeneous categories, namely, (1) psychological, (2) physiological, (3) biochemical, and (4) immunological. The value of these symptoms as early warning signs or simply being confirmatory in nature has been discussed among researchers (Hooper & Mackinnon, 1995; Morgan, 1994). Generally, symptoms are milder at the initial stage (overreaching) and will require less recovery as compared with a stale state when more severe symptoms exist. While underperformance is furthermore regarded as the hallmark of staleness, no consensus has been reached regarding the degree to which performance will drop at different overtraining stages (Hooper & Mackinnon, 1995; O'Connor, 1998; Raglin, 1993). A decrease in physiological markers such as $\dot{V}O_2$max, max lactate, and max heart rate obviously explain and confirm decreased performance. But athletes, coaches, and sport scientists are, for obvious reasons, more interested in finding a valid early warning signal that can prevent undesired underperformance (Hedelin, Kenttä, Wiklund, Bjerle, & Henriksson-Larsén, 2000). In fact, some researchers have argued that psychological testing is most effective in detecting staleness at an early stage (Kellmann & Günther, 2000; O'Connor, 1998; Shephard & Sheck, 1994).

O'Connor (1998) listed four advantages of using psychological markers to monitor the overtraining process: (1) Psychological changes are more reliable and mood shifts display a dose-response relationship with training load. (2) Some mood states are sensitive to the training load (e.g., fatigue), whereas others are more sensitive to staleness (e.g., depression). (3) Variations in mood measures often covary with physiological markers. (4) Titration of training load based on monitoring mood responses appears to have potential for preventing the overtraining syndrome. Not surprisingly, and in light of O'Connor's suggestions, the POMS (McNair, Lorr, & Droppleman, 1992) inventory has been used extensively within the overtraining literature. In the following sections, two real-life cases will exemplify how the POMS inventory can be used either for monitoring the additive effects of psychosocial stress (in the canoeist example), which may contribute to the development of staleness, or for monitoring recovery from a stale state (in the cyclist example).

Case Studies

Case 1 describes the impact of heavy schoolwork (i.e., a predominantly psychosocial stressor) on recovery and athletic training in a 17-year-old elite canoeist. Case 2 focuses on the recovery process of a 28-year-old racing cyclist who, due to both training- and nontraining-related stressors, became stale. The first scenario exemplifies how an increase in nontraining-related stressors can make the training load seem much heavier than it seems when the psychosocial stress level is lower. The second scenario shows that recovery from staleness is a tedious process that requires much time and patience.

Case 1: A 17-Year-Old Female Racing Canoeist

The primary interest in this case is the relationship between a standardized one-week training regimen and POMS *Vigor* and *Fatigue* scores, as modified by varying degrees of schoolwork. This young female canoeist had won several individual medals at junior national championships and had an extensive training background.

Method: Initially, researchers, in cooperation with the athlete and coach, chose two weeks that were expected to differ regarding schoolwork. The first week in December was anticipated to consist of heavy schoolwork (end of semester), and the second week in March, only light schoolwork. Both the athlete and the coach agreed to standardize and control for all other possible stressors besides schoolwork and to keep the physical training load equal during the two weeks. A similar baseline at the beginning of each week was also strongly emphasized. During both weeks, the athlete followed a physical training program considered to be heavy. At the end of the seven-day training period (Monday to Sunday), the athlete was rewarded with a full day of rest. The POMS was administrated almost every day from Monday to Monday. The scale of TQR as described before, ranging from 6 to 20, was used to assess recovery actions and the athlete's perception of overall psychosocio-physiological recovery. The POMS and recovery ratings were made at 7 P.M. each evening. Training load was rated after each workout, with the help of the 6-20 RPE scale (Borg, 1970, 1998).

Results: The athlete's training log was collected together with a diary of brief notes. The athlete trained for a total of 14 hours on 12 separate occasions during each week. The training performed followed the preplanned training schedule during both weeks. Most of the training was of high intensity; it was rated as "Hard" on the scale (i.e., RPE 15). Two short notes from the diary at the end of each week may characterize the difference between the weeks: Monday, December 8: "Dead tired, just wanted to sleep." Monday, March 9: "Generally this week felt more relaxed compared to the week in December." The perception of the overall psychosociophysiological recovery was rated poorer at the end of the "heavy" school week as compared with the "easy" school week (i.e., TQR was rated as 13 on Saturday and Sunday evenings during the heavy week, in contrast to 17 and 16 during the easy week). A visual inspection of the profiles displayed in figure 4.6 is also enlightening.

The two profiles initially display the same slight downward trend for both weeks with only small fluctuations. However, a somewhat strong maladaptive reaction seems to occur between Friday and Saturday in the heavy week, whereas only a small change is detected in the easy week. In addition, the athlete responded more favorably to recovery on the Monday after the easy week as opposed to the Monday after the heavy week.

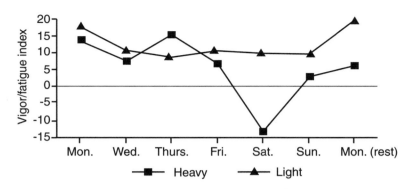

Figure 4.6 Ratios between *Vigor* and *Fatigue* for the heavy and light school weeks, respectively, for a 17-year-old female racing canoeist.

Case 2: A 28-Year-Old Male Racing Cyclist

This experienced racing cyclist had reached a severe state of staleness, probably to a great extent due to a tough training regimen in combination with poor recovery. He was a 28-year-old male with an annual training load during the previous years of about 850 hours. This training load had been managed before, but additional stressors during the last year had started to take their toll.

Method: During the first session the cyclist was asked to recall and describe in detail the previous 18 months leading up to staleness. The cyclist also completed the POMS inventory. The goal was then to monitor the process of rehabilitation until a healthy state was reached. This led to a monitoring period of two months with four measurements, initially every second week and with the last measurement four weeks after the previous one. Each POMS result was evaluated immediately, and feedback was given to the athlete. Comments focused on positive aspects of active recovery and on ensuring a low-volume, low-intensity, noncompetitive exercise regimen performed strictly for therapeutic benefits.

Results: When describing the previous 18 months leading up to staleness, the athlete identified both training and nontraining stressors. The annual training load had indeed been 850 hours, and he was aiming to increase this to 950 hours during the coming year. Nontraining stressors had started to influence the athlete at the end of the previous year.

For example, his girlfriend had moved to another city due to job opportunities. Forced to live on only one salary, he had had to move into a smaller apartment. This allegedly increased his stress level and was perceived as negative, something which in turn made him feel even more stressed. After the first competition of the year he had felt "dead tired." He also perceived a severe loss of motivation, and for the first time ever, viewed his sport as "boring." On top of this, his girlfriend had a short fling with another man. This was, according to the cyclist, a consequence of the girlfriend's unhappiness with the long-distance relationship. The cyclist therefore felt a pressing need to move to the same city as his girlfriend. The stress associated with a possible move, and the need to find a new job with new routines in a new city, was also taxing. As a consequence, the athlete's performance kept worsening, but he tried to keep training according to his plans anyway. The struggle to keep up was finally lost in July, when he sank into a deep depression. At the first session with the athlete, his *Fatigue* score widely outnumbered his *Vigor* score (see figure 4.7). Gradually, during the process of recovery, the *Vigor* scores increased and the *Fatigue* scores decreased.

In figure 4.8, the initial stale POMS profile is shown together with the healthy profile observed at the end of the two months. The athlete clearly started out stale; the profile resembles an inverted iceberg profile. After the two-month period, the healthier iceberg profile (e.g., Morgan, 1985) emerged.

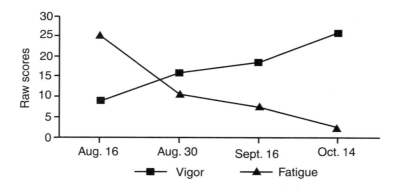

Figure 4.7   POMS *Vigor* and *Fatigue* scores during a 28-year-old male racing cyclist's recovery from staleness.

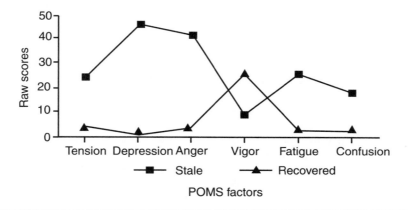

Figure 4.8   Cyclist's initial (stale) POMS profile and the profile obtained after rehabilitation.

Discussion of Cases 1 and 2

Nontraining stressors were present in both of the described cases. The different school weeks made a significant change in how the 17-year-old canoeist felt in relation to *Vigor* and *Fatigue,* despite the fact that the training load was equal during those weeks. The 28-year-old cyclist had reached a state of staleness that, to a certain extent at least, could be blamed on the psychosocial stressors occurring in his life. Consequently, one can infer from these cases that nontraining stressors can indeed be responsible for stress reactions otherwise only associated with the physical training load. With a rapid increase in nontraining stressors, the cumulative level of stress may increase to a level at which a person experiences a lack of recovery, which eventually may lead to staleness and ultimately burnout. Obviously, more research is needed in order to establish to what extent psychosocial stress interacts with training-induced stress in the development of the overtraining syndrome.

We nevertheless suggest that every coach who uses periodization (alternating tough training periods with easier ones) for the athletes in training also pay close attention to nontraining-related stressors. Evidence suggests that staleness can develop even during moderate levels of physical training, provided that high levels of psychosocial stress coexist. In fact, Gould et al. (1996) reported a larger number of psychosocially driven burnout cases among tennis players as compared to physically driven burnout cases (Gould & Dieffenbach, this volume, chapter 2).

The length of rehabilitation needed for full recovery is most likely a complex function of several variables (Lehmann, Foster, Gastmann, Keizer, & Steinacker, 1999), including the severity of the initial state; the recovery actions undertaken; the individual's capacity to recover; social support; and the professional assistance of a nutritionist, sport psychologist, or other relevant personnel. It is clearly not an easy task to predict the adequate length of recovery for any given person. Hence, monitoring of mood states suggests a possible method to determine the length for adequate recovery from accumulated fatigue as well as overreached or stale states.

A Strategic Formula for Optimizing Adaptation

It is possible to derive a formula for maximizing adaptive training from the previously presented model. This formula consists of three strategies:

1. Optimizing Total Quality Recovery by applying the matching principle, that is, considering the *source* and magnitude of stress when aiming for the most efficient recovery interventions.

2. Eliminating or minimizing psychological and social stressors.

3. Focusing training on improving all critical capacities, which will correspond not only to an increased stress tolerance in that specific capacity, but also to the overall stress tolerance. For example, enhanced self-efficacy or arousal control will primarily improve coping skills, but it will also benefit the total psychological capacity (stress tolerance) and, ultimately, the overall stress tolerance.

By and large, these strategies attempt to minimize unnecessary nontraining stressors, maximize recovery, and build up the individual's tolerance for stress. This will serve the purpose of using all available resources for one single purpose, namely, adaptation to the highest possible training load. The first two strategies will have immediate effects on the actual adaptation potential and can thereby be seen as short-term interventions, whereas the latter is more of a long-term intervention. Some capacities may improve within a short period, but others may require long-term practice. Building a good team spirit/atmosphere/cohesion,

for example, will require more of a long-term approach. However, a good team climate will reduce unnecessary psychosocial stress and at the same time contribute to social recovery. This will subsequently influence the athletes' ability to tolerate higher training loads than they would be able to tolerate in a nonsupportive team environment.

Furthermore, the model can provide a structure for studying and understanding cause and consequence in a large variety of important performance areas. Monitoring individual variations in total stress, total capacity, and total recovery over time may increase the understanding of why the same athlete responds differently to a given training stimulus under different conditions, why homogeneous groups of athletes display different responses to a given training stimulus, and why some athletes seem to be more vulnerable to staleness. The model may ultimately enhance the knowledge base regarding the characteristics of optimal training and negative overtraining.

Athletes undergoing elite training—balancing on the verge of staleness—constantly need to know whether it is OK to maintain the scheduled training intensity. Will continued training result in the desired adaptation? Alternatively, will early signs of negative overtraining develop? A comprehensive assessment and evaluation of all available cues from the *psychosociophysiological* process as well as possible negative consequences assessed by various early warning signs (i.e., markers of staleness and variation in performance capacity, see figure 4.5 on p. 68) may contribute to the most accurate answer achievable. To address this highly individual and critical question, it will be necessary to obtain individual baselines and measures of intraindividual changes.

Summary and Recommendations

In conclusion, we suggest that athletes and their supporters consider the following recommendations:

- Apply a *holistic* perspective to performance development and the training process.
- View training as an ongoing psychosociophysiological *balancing act*.
- Create a monitoring system that involves the *entire process* of training and recovery.
- *Tailor* the training load carefully with respect to individual states and differences.

- Treat the athlete as a *dynamic* psychosociophysiological system.
- Focus on the *content* of each training session, instead of merely chasing training hours.
- Focus on the individual's *perception* of training and recovery.
- Focus and carefully assess short-term *training responses.*
- Increase the *knowledge* and *awareness* of Total Quality Recovery for performance enhancement.
- Take *personal responsibility* for psychosociophysiological recovery, and make it happen.
- Emphasize *self-monitoring* as an important tool for developing self- and body awareness.
- Support *cognitive strategies* that enhance attention and sensitivity to bodily cues and signals.
- Increase the *collaboration,* and emphasize a *shared responsibility,* between coach and athlete in planning, performing, and evaluating training.
- Increase the knowledge and awareness of *nontraining stressors* occurring in everyday life, and their influence on the training process.
- Increase the awareness of *psychosocially* driven underperformance states.

References

Ahmaidi, S., Granier, P., Taoutaou, Z., Mercier, B., Dubouchaud, H., & Prefaut, C. (1996). Lactate kinetics during passive and active recovery in endurance and sprint athletes. *European Medicine and Science in Sports and Exercise, 28,* 450-456.

Berglund, B., & Säfström, H. (1994). Psychological monitoring and modulation of training load of world-class canoeists. *Medicine and Science in Sports and Exercise, 26,* 1036-1040.

Borg, G. (1970). Perceived exertion as an indicator of somatic stress. *Scandinavian Journal of Rehabilitation Medicine, 2,* 92-98.

Borg, G. (1998). *Borg's perceived exertion and pain scales.* Champaign, IL: Human Kinetics.

Borg, G., & Hassmén, P. (1999). Physical activity and perceived exertion: Basic knowledge with applications for the elderly. In P. Capodaglio & M.V. Narici (Eds.), *Physical activity in the elderly* (pp. 17-34). Pavia, Italy: Maugeri Foundation Books.

Brustad, R.J., & Ritter-Taylor, M. (1997). Applying social psychological perspectives to the sport psychology consulting process. *The Sport Psychologist, 11,* 107-119.

Budgett, R. (1990). Overtraining syndrome. *British Journal of Sports Medicine, 24,* 231-236.

Calder, A. (1996). Recovery training. In P. Reaburn & D. Jenkins (Eds.), *Training for speed and endurance* (pp. 97-119). Sydney: Allen & Unwin.

Carron, A.V., & Hausenblas, H.A. (1998). *Group dynamics in sport* (2nd ed.). Morgantown, WV: Fitness Info Tech.

Clarey, C. (1998, September 2). After the glory of victory, the agony of recovery. *The New Yorker,* p. 23.

Coggan, A.R. (1997). Plasma glucose metabolism during exercise: Effects of endurance training in humans. *Medicine and Science in Sport and Exercise, 5,* 620-627.

Costill, D.L., Flynn, M.G., Kriwan, J.P., Houmbard, J.A., Mitchell, J.B., Thomas, R., & Park, S.H. (1988). Effects of repeated days of intensified training on muscle glycogen and swimming performance. *Medicine and Science in Sport and Exercise, 20,* 249-254.

Durand-Bush, N., Salmela, J.H., & Green-Demers, I. (2001). The Ottawa Mental Skills Assessment Tool (OMSAT-3*). *The Sport Psychologist, 15,* 1-19.

Ericsson, A.K. (1996). *The road to excellence: The acquisition of expert performance in the arts and sciences, sports, and games.* Mahwah, NJ: Erlbaum.

Evjenth, O., & Hamberg, J. (1985). *Muscle stretching in manual therapy* (Vol. 1 & 2). Örebro, Sweden: Alfta Rehab förlag.

Foster, C. (1998). Monitoring training in athletes with reference to overtraining syndrome. *Medicine and Science in Sport and Exercise, 7,* 1164-1168.

Foster, C., Daniels, J.T., & Seiler, S. (1999). Perspectives on correct approaches to training. In M. Lehmann, C. Foster, U. Gastmann, H. Keizer, & J. Steinacker (Eds.), *Overload, performance incompetence, and regeneration in sport* (pp. 27-41). New York: Plenum.

Fry, R.W., Morton, A.R., & Keast, D. (1991). Overtraining in athletes: An update. *Sports Medicine, 12,* 32-65.

Fry, R.W., Morton, A.R., & Keast, D. (1992). Periodisation and the prevention of overtraining. *Canadian Journal of Sport and Science, 3,* 241-248.

Gould, D., Udry, E., Tuffey, S., & Loehr, J. (1996). Burnout in competitive junior tennis players: II. A qualitative analysis. *The Sport Psychologist, 10,* 341-366.

Hägg, G. (1952). *Gunder Häggs dagbok, en världsmästares erfarenheter och träningsråd* [Gunder Hägg's diary, a world champion's experiences and training advice]. Stockholm: Tryckeriaktiebolaget Tiden.

Hassmén, P. (1991). *Perceived exertion: Applications in sport and exercise.* Edsbruk, Sweden: Akademitryck AB (doctoral dissertation).

Hawley, J.A., Myburgh, K.H., Noakes, T.D., & Dennis, S.C. (1997). Training techniques to improve fatigue resistance and enhance endurance performance. *Journal of Sports Sciences, 15,* 325-333.

Hawley, J.A., Schabort, E.J., Noakes, T.D., & Dennis, S.C. (1997). Carbohydrate-loading and exercise performance: An update. *Sports Medicine, 24,* 73-81.

Hedelin, R., Kenttä, G., Wiklund, U., Bjerle, P., & Henriksson-Larsén, K. (2000). Short term overtraining: Effects on performance, circulatory responses, and heart rate variability. *Medicine and Science in Sports and Exercise, 32,* 1480-1484.

Hooper, S.L., & Mackinnon, L.T. (1995). Monitoring overtraining in athletes: Recommendations. *Sports Medicine, 20,* 321-327.

Ivy, J.L. (1991). Muscle glycogen synthesis before and after exercise. *Sports Medicine, 11,* 6-19.

Kellmann, M., & Günther, K.D. (2000). Changes in stress and recovery in elite rowers during preparation for the Olympic games. *Medicine and Science in Sport and Exercise, 32,* 676-683.

Kellmann, M., & Kallus, K.W. (2001). *Recovery-Stress Questionnaire for Athletes; User manual.* Champaign, IL: Human Kinetics.

Kenttä, G. (1996). *Överträningssyndrom: En psykofysiologisk process* [Overtraining syndrome: A psychophysiological process]. Unpublished master's thesis, Högskolan i Luleå, Luleå, Sweden.

Kenttä, G., & Hassmén, P. (1998). Overtraining and recovery: A conceptual model. *Sports Medicine, 26,* 1-16.

Kenttä, G., & Hassmén, P. (1999). *Träna smart: Undvik överträningssyndrom* [Train smart: Avoid overtraining syndrome]. Stockholm: SISU Idrottsböcker.

Kenttä, G., & Hassmén, P. (2000). Non-training stressors and recovery from staleness. In B.A. Carlsson, U. Johnson, & F. Wetterstrand (Eds.), *Sport psychology conference in the new millennium* (pp. 217-221). Halmstad, Sweden: Halmstad University.

Koutedakis, Y., Myszkewycz, L., Soulas, D., Papapostolou, V., Sullivan, I., & Sharp, N.C.C. (1999). The effects of rest and subsequent training on selected physiological parameters in professional female classical dancers. *International Journal of Sports Medicine, 20,* 379-383.

Kreider, R.B., Fry, A.C., & O'Toole, M.L. (Eds.). (1998). *Overtraining in sport.* Champaign, IL: Human Kinetics.

Kuipers, H. (1996). How much is too much? Performance aspects of overtraining. *Research Quarterly for Exercise and Sport, 67,* 65-69.

Kuipers, H. (1998). Advances in the evaluation of sports training. In W.P. Morgan (Ed.), *Physical activity and mental health* (pp. 63-94). New York: Hemisphere.

Kuipers, H., & Keizer, H.A. (1988). Overtraining in elite athletes: Review and directions for the future. *Sports Medicine, 6,* 79-92.

Lehmann, M., Foster, C., Gastmann, U., Keizer, H., & Steinacker, J. (Eds.). (1999). *Overload, performance incompetence, and regeneration in sport.* New York: Plenum.

Lehmann, M., Foster, C., & Keul, J. (1993). Overtraining in endurance athletes: A brief review. *Medicine and Science in Sports and Exercise, 25,* 854-861.

Marion, A. (1995). Overtraining and sport performance. *Coaches Report, 2,* 12-19.

Martens, R., Vealey, R., & Burton, D. (1990). *Competitive anxiety in sport.* Champaign, IL: Human Kinetics.

McLellan, T.M., Cheung, K.S.Y., & Jacobs, I. (1991). Incremental test protocol, recovery mode and the individual anaerobic threshold. *International Journal of Sports Medicine, 2,* 190-195.

McNair, D.M., Lorr, M., & Droppleman, L.F. (1992). *EdITS manual for the Profile of Mood States* (revised 1992). San Diego: Educational and Industrial Testing Service.

Moran, A.P. (1996). *The psychology of concentration in sport performers: A cognitive analysis.* Exeter, UK: Taylor & Francis.

Morgan, W.P. (1985). Selected psychological factors limiting performance: A mental health model. In D.H. Clarke & H.M. Eckert (Eds.), *Limits of human performance* (pp. 70-80). Champaign, IL: Human Kinetics.

Morgan, W.P. (1994). Psychological components of effort sense. *Medicine and Science in Sports and Exercise, 26,* 1071-1077.

Morgan, W.P., Brown, D.R., Raglin, J.S., O'Connor, P.J., & Ellickson, K.A. (1987). Psychological monitoring of overtraining and staleness. *British Journal of Sports Medicine, 21,* 107-114.

Morgan, W.P., Costill, D.L., & Flynn, M.G. (1988). Mood disturbance following increased training in swimmers. *Medicine and Science in Sports and Exercise, 20,* 408-414.

Morgan, W.P., O'Conner, P.B., Sparling, P.B., & Pate, R.R. (1987). Psychologic characterization of the elite female distance runner. *International Journal of Sport Medicine, 8,* 124-131.

Morton, R.H. (1997). Modeling training and overtraining. *Journal of Sports Sciences, 15,* 335-340.

Noble, B., & Robertson, R. (1996). *Perceived exertion.* Champaign, IL: Human Kinetics.

O'Connor, P.J. (1998). Overtraining and staleness. In W.P. Morgan (Ed.), *Physical activity and mental health* (pp. 145-160). New York: Hemisphere.

Orlick, T. (1999). *Embracing your potential.* Champaign, IL: Human Kinetics.

Raglin, J.S. (1993). Overtraining and staleness: Psychometric monitoring of endurance athletes. In R.B. Singer, M. Murphey, & L.K. Tennant (Eds.), *Handbook of research on sport psychology* (pp. 840-850). New York: Macmillan.

Raglin, J.S., Sawamura, S., Alexiou, S., Hassmén, P., & Kenttä, G. (2000). Training practices and staleness in 13-18-year-old swimmers. A cross-cultural study. *Pediatric Exercise Science, 12,* 61-70.

Roberts, G.C. (1992). *Motivation in sport and exercise.* Champaign, IL: Human Kinetics.

Rowbottom, D.G., Keast, D., & Morton, A.R. (1998). Monitoring and preventing of overreaching and overtraining in endurance athletes. In R.B. Kreider, A.C. Fry, & M.L. O'Toole (Eds.), *Overtraining in sport* (pp. 47-66). Champaign, IL: Human Kinetics.

Rushall, B.S. (1989). Sport psychology: The key to sporting excellence. *International Journal of Sport Psychology, 20,* 165-190.

Schaufeli, W., & Enzmann, D. (1998). *The burnout companion to study and practice: A critical analysis.* Padstow, UK: Taylor & Francis.

Shephard, R.J., & Shek, P.N. (1994). Potential impact of physical activity and sport on the immune system—A brief review. *British Journal of Sports Medicine, 28,* 347-355.

Silva, J.S. (1990). An analysis of the training stress syndrome in competitive athletics. *Applied Sport Psychology, 2,* 5-20.

Snyder, A.C. (1998). Overtraining and glycogen depletion hypothesis. *Medicine and Science in Sport and Exercise, 7,* 1146-1150.

Snyder, A.C., Jeukendrup, A.E., Hesselink, M.K.C., Kuipers, H., & Foster, C. (1993). A physiological/psychological indicator of overreaching during intensive training. *International Journal of Sports Medicine, 14,* 29-32.

Solberg, E.E., Halvorsen, R., & Holen, A. (2000). Effect of meditation on immune cells. *Stress Medicine, 16,* 185-190.

Taylor, S.R., Rogers, G.G., & Driver, H.S. (1997). Effects of training volume on sleep, psychological, and selected physiological profiles of elite female swimmers. *Medicine and Science in Sport and Exercise, 5,* 688-693.

Urhausen, A., Gabriel, H.H.W., Weiler, B., & Kindermann, W. (1998). Ergometric and psychological findings during overtraining: A long-term follow-up study in endurance athletes. *International Journal of Sports Medicine, 19,* 114-120.

Viru, A. (1984). The mechanism of training effects: A hypothesis. *International Journal of Sport Medicine, 5,* 219-227.

Viru, A. (1994). Molecular cellular mechanism of training effects. *Journal of Sports Medicine and Physical Fitness, 34,* 309-322.

Weinberg, R., & Gould, D. (1999). *Foundations of sport and exercise psychology* (2nd ed.). Champaign, IL: Human Kinetics.

Wilks, B. (1991). Stress management for athletes. *Sports Medicine, 11,* 289-299.

Wilmore, J.H., & Costill, D.L. (1988). *Training for sport and activity: The physiological basis of the conditioning process.* Dubuque, IA: Wm. C. Brown.

Part II

Determinants of Underrecovery

Smith, D.J., & Norris, S.R. (2002). Training load and monitoring an athlete's tolerance for endurance training. In M. Kellmann (Ed.), *Enhancing recovery: Preventing underperformance in athletes* (pp. 81-101). Champaign, IL: Human Kinetics.

5

Training Load and Monitoring an Athlete's Tolerance for Endurance Training

David J. Smith and Stephen R. Norris

In the athletic world, coaches and athletes constantly push the window of positive training adaptation in order to gain an edge in performance. However, by increasing either the frequency, duration, or intensity of training, coaches and athletes risk creating excessive fatigue that may lead to functional impairment, which has been described as staleness or burnout (Hooper & Mackinnon, 1995; Koutedakis, Budgett, & Faulmann, 1990). During the training year, the athlete is in constant flux along a continuum of positive and negative responses, a continuum ranging from peak performance to, in extreme cases, an inability to perform or train at previously attainable levels.

The aim of training is to provide successive stressors that will displace the homeostasis of an athlete and provide a stimulus to initiate adaptation (Matveyev, 1981). Thus, the purpose of physical training is to disturb homeostasis and create fatigue through training loads that are greater than the load to which the body is normally accustomed. However, once an adaptation to one load has occurred, a greater load (progressive overload) must be applied at the appropriate time in order to gain performance improvements. Unfortunately, a nonlinear relationship exists between the amount of training and training effect. When initial fitness is low, improvements in performance will occur quickly. However, further improvements will take effect more slowly, with the athlete eventually reaching a plateau. Exces-

sive levels of fatigue, although purposely induced, may lead to performance incompetence in some situations. The difficulty for coaches is that no two athletes react the same way to training loads. Genetics, training, background, years of training, health, and tolerance to both physical and psychological stress influence an individual's response to a given training load.

In this chapter we describe the continuum of endurance from short- to long-duration performance and examine training load classification, a continuum of fatigue, modeling fitness and fatigue, and methods of quantifying and tracking training load. We also offer practical methods for monitoring tolerance to training.

Performance, Fatigue, and Endurance

A superior athletic performance is characterized by the ability to sustain either a maximal or submaximal intensity for a relatively longer period of time than other competitors. Whether the sport is running, swimming, canoeing, or a triathlon, the winner is able to sustain a higher average speed or power output than his fellow competitors. In 1925, A.V. Hill commented that an important and interesting problem for a young athlete is: How fast can I run some given distance? He suggested that the problem before us, physiologically speaking, is clearly: How long can a given effort be maintained?

Hill commented further to say that fatigue determines performance, and the type of fatigue changes as the distance increases.

Research has established that the primary factors influencing fatigue vary as the intensity and duration of performance are altered. Muscle fatigue has been defined as the inability of muscle to maintain the force required to achieve a given power output (Edwards, 1981). Fatigue that results from extreme effort, and fatigue that results from an effort of more moderate intensity that is continued over a long period of time (referred to as exhaustive fatigue) are both considered muscular (Hill, 1925). A third type of fatigue was described by Hill (1925) as due to wear and tear on the body as a whole: soreness, stiffness, nervous exhaustion, metabolic changes and disturbances, sleeplessness, and similar factors that may affect an individual long before the muscular system has given out. He commented further that the third type was so indefinite and complex that one could not hope at the time (1925) to determine it accurately or to measure it.

When the average speeds of running records for a given distance are plotted against time, a curvilinear relationship is observed. Running speed initially declines quickly up to a duration of approximately 2 minutes and is then followed by a relatively small decline in speeds for events lasting up to approximately 13 minutes for the 5,000-meter run. From that time to 60 minutes there is a relative plateau in speeds to the half-marathon distance. Based on these observations, Hill (1925) suggested that the curvilinear model of speed versus time could be roughly expressed as a series of essential linear compartments with systematically declining slopes. Thus, performance may be classified in the following manner:

- short-duration endurance (20-120 seconds);
- medium-duration endurance (2-13 minutes);
- long-duration endurance (13-60 minutes); and
- extended endurance (greater than 60 minutes) (see figure 5.1).

Consequently, different fatigue-inducing factors may limit performance.

Short-duration performance is primarily supported by ATP muscle concentration, the ATP-CP system, and anaerobic glycolysis (Bouchard, Taylor, Simoneau, & Dulac, 1991) in varying percentages according to the duration of the activity. The time frame of medium-duration endurance performance is between 2 and 13 minutes; this category of performance uses a combination of anaerobic glycolysis and the aerobic system. The boundary of 13 minutes for the beginning of long-duration endurance performance is a compromise between 11 minutes suggested by Harre (1982, p. 127) and 15 minutes suggested by Hawley, Myburgh, Noakes, and Dennis (1995) and may reflect the limit of the attainment of $\dot{V}O_2$max during constant load exhaustive exercise and the beginning of sub-$\dot{V}O_2$max exercise. Long-duration endurance performance depends primarily on the aerobic system and may be subdivided in categories of 13 to 30 minutes, 30 to 60 minutes, and greater than 60 minutes (extended endurance) since different metabolic, mental, and training requirements are needed for success in each subcategory. In activity between 13 and 60 minutes, the intensity is less than $\dot{V}O_2$max but greater than or similar to the anaerobic threshold, whereas in extended endurance activities, intensities below the anaerobic threshold are sustained.

Endurance in sport may be defined as the athlete's capacity to resist fatigue and is specific

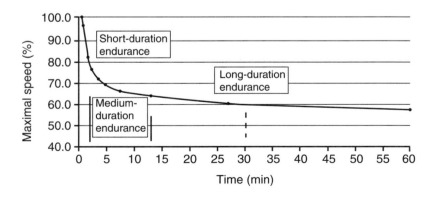

Figure 5.1   Decline in running speed as a percentage of maximal speed versus time.

to the duration of effort. It underpins the attainment of an optimum intensity throughout the time required by the competition; it leads to a high quality of movement and the ability to optimize technical and tactical problems during the entire competition and facilitates mastery of a large volume of hard work during training (Harre, 1982, p. 124). Endurance is thus not only a crucial and highly important factor in competitive performances for the majority of sports, but it is also a decisive factor for the athlete's performance in training and general capacity (Harre, 1982).

For those sports in which activity lasts up to approximately 45 seconds (short bursts, as in tennis or ice hockey), the energy systems required for maximal performance are principally anaerobic, a combination of the ATP-CP and anaerobic glycolytic systems. For longer durations, the aerobic system starts to gradually play a more important role and up to approximately 13 minutes of exhaustive activity, all three systems are used in varying proportions. A model of the energy system continuum and the contribution to various sport events is presented in figure 5.2.

Any sport will require some combination of basic or sport-specific endurance together with a component of strength and speed. The specifics will depend on the resistance to be overcome, the speed of muscle contraction, the duration of the activity, and whether the required performance is repetitive (intervals) or continuous in nature. In addition to short-duration or long-duration endurance training, the training overload required to improve strength and speed will also contribute to fatigue. Thus, since the tolerance to physical training or competition is multifaceted, a careful analysis of a sport is required in order to identify which component may be contributing to a performance decrement.

Continuum of Training Fatigue

Since the purpose of training is to displace the homeostasis of an athlete's functional systems (Matveyev, 1981), the natural consequence is some degree of fatigue. A continuum of fatigue exists from day-to-day training fatigue (Costill, 1986) to the fatigue generated from an excessive load (Viru, 1995), a load that may result in performance incompetence or lead to underperformance. With continued heavy training, primary symptoms of a training overload may develop into more complicated, more chronic symptoms (Noakes, 1991). In order to clarify the flow of the continuum from one level to the next (Fry, Morton, & Keast, 1991), a time frame of expected recovery is suggested (see table 5.1).

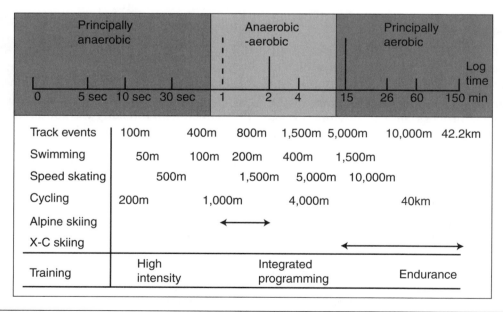

Figure 5.2 Model of the energy system continuum illustrating the time frames of various sport disciplines and the type of training undertaken for a specific event.

Table 5.1   Overview of Approximate Recovery Times Relative to the Imposed Training Load

Training loads (process)	Recovery from induced fatigue (outcome fatigue)
Acute training stress	Normal training fatigue; recovery in < 24 hr
Unaccustomed exercise	Overstrain; recovery in 3-5 days, peak soreness 24-48 hr
Training overload	Overload fatigue; recovery in 5-7 days with reduced training
Excessive training load	Short-term overtraining/overreaching; recovery in 10-14 days
	Long-term overtraining/underperformance; recovery in > 28 days

Classification of the Training Load

In order to assess an athlete's tolerance to training, a system of classifying the training loads must be developed. It has previously been stated that in order to achieve a training effect, an overload must be applied. However, an athlete who works out twice a day, six days a week will not be able to tolerate an overload every training session. In such cases a continuum of training load is needed. One classification system (Viru, 1995) evaluates the loads of a single session or microcycle of training (three to five days) in the following manner:

1. Excessive load—surpasses the functional capacity of the body and results in overtraining.
2. Trainable load—results in a specific training effect.
3. Maintenance load—is insufficient to stimulate net protein synthesis but is sufficient to avoid a detraining effect.
4. Recovery load—favors promotion of the recovery process after a previous excessive or trainable load.
5. Useless load—is below the intensity or value necessary to achieve any of the previous effects.

In addition to subjectively classifying the training load, an objective quantification of the volume and intensity of training should be documented. The volume of training, which has to increase continuously from year to year, and change in a cyclic pattern within yearly macrocycles, is a quantitative measure. It may be assessed in kilometers or miles covered per session, the total weight lifted in weight training, the number of movement repetitions in technical events, or the number of hours of training. The intensity of training, however, may be measured in relative or absolute terms: relative intensity reflects the intensity of load compared to the maximum ability of an athlete for a specified task per unit of time; absolute intensity is measured as maximal speed or weight lifted in a given time, or the maximum height or distance jumped or thrown. In racket or team sports absolute intensity may be measured by the frequency or pace of movement or the tempo of a game.

Another factor influencing tolerance to training is load density, which reflects the relationship among relative intensity, duration, and recovery time within or between training sessions. When technical work is a training objective, the recovery periods are constructed to ensure that the volume of training can be attained while maintaining the technical execution of the skill(s). As an athlete achieves improved tolerance, the training load may become denser in order to achieve a "trainable load." However, load density must be considered in the overall evaluation of training load since if recovery is inadequate within or between high-intensity workouts, what was considered a trainable load becomes an excessive load. At that point the difference between fitness and fatigue may become large leading to an underperformance situation. Coaches and athletes know that high-intensity loads produce a relatively rapid improvement in performance. However, the performance is not necessarily stable or reliable without moderate or high volumes of low-intensity training to support the fitness and load tolerance of the athlete.

The need to accurately assess and record training demands is an integral part of the practicalities of sport science intervention and involvement in the training of elite athletes. The retrospective evaluation and prospective development of the "training history" of an individual athlete is crucial in the assessment of her current and future needs, as well as her ability to withstand future training demands. It is important, therefore, to understand the "path" she has taken en route to her present trained state and competitive level, particularly since this may be extremely complex and highly individualistic due to the myriad of variables that contribute to her condition at any one moment in time. Furthermore, the direct and residual effects of "historical" training may well have longer-reaching consequences than the short-term training gains that are often the focus of athletes and coaches.

Figure 5.3 illustrates the concept of a growthlike evolution in the training history of athletes. The actual progression, or path, of an athlete's training history is open to great variation depending on many factors, such as activities engaged in, various coaching or sport system biases, and even athlete decision making. Attention is drawn to the fact that the actual combinations of intensity, volume, and time course are somewhat limitless and that the illustrated path (denoted by the zigzag line) is purely for illustrative purposes.

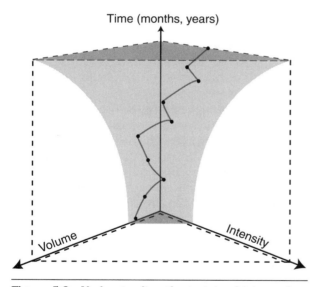

Time (months, years)

Volume

Intensity

Figure 5.3 Understanding the training history of an athlete and the pattern of this history en route to the current status.

Modeling Fitness and Fatigue

With the objective of improving performance and peaking at a significant competition, coaches and athletes have found that by applying the principles of repetition, summation, or duration, followed by a reduced training load, an enhanced performance can be achieved. However, the quantity and quality of the training overload and degree of recovery necessary to maximize the performance are unique to the individual and circumstances, and therefore difficult to characterize.

General training models have been suggested to assist coaches in planning and understanding the training process. Individual tolerances to training dictate that the general models should be individually adapted based on observed training and competition performance. One- and two-factor models have been suggested in organizing the training load–recovery sequence, since the process of adaptation is the result of the current interplay of work and recovery. The one-factor model is based on the theory of supercompensation, which states that the immediate training effect of a workout is the result of a depletion of certain biochemical substances followed by a supercompensation effect (Zatsiorsky, 1995). The classic example of this effect is glycogen depletion/supercompensation in preparation for long-distance running. In theory, a workout or training load results in a degree of fatigue or depletion, which is followed by a supercompensation or training effect (see figure 5.4). It is believed that if the rest intervals between consecutive workouts are of optimal duration, the next training session will coincide with the supercompensation phase, and the performance ability will increase (Zatsiorsky, 1995).

The supercompensation theory has been advanced to the microcycle level where several training sessions of high training loads are conducted with insufficient recovery time between each session (the principle of summation). After this microcycle a sufficient recovery period is introduced with the belief that a significant supercompensation in performance will follow and that the training load tolerance will be enhanced permitting even greater training loads (see figure 5.5).

Although this one-factor, supercompensation model is simple and convenient, the complexity of the biological adaptive process is more sophisticated than the demonstrable laboratory glycogen depletion/supercompensation procedure. Obvious differences exist in the protein synthesis sites and rates of adaptation between strength training and endurance training. Strength training increases the myofibrillar proteins in the overloaded muscles, while endurance training increases the activity of oxidative enzymes in

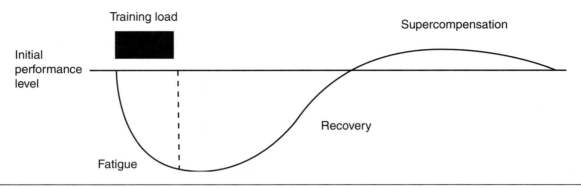

Figure 5.4 Theoretical model of the time course of athlete preparedness after a workout.

Adapted, by permission, from V.M. Zatsiorsky, 1995, Basic concepts of training theory. In *Science and practice of strength training,* edited by V.M. Zatsiorsky (Champaign, IL: Human Kinetics), 13.

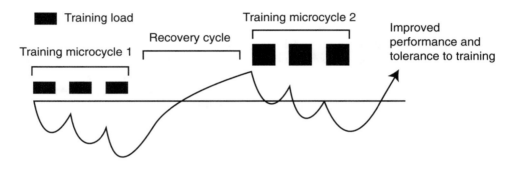

Figure 5.5 Theoretical model of the time course of athlete preparedness after a microcycle of training.

Adapted, by permission, from V.M. Zatsiorsky, 1995, Basic concepts of training theory. In *Science and practice of strength training,* edited by V.M. Zatsiorsky (Champaign, IL: Human Kinetics), 15.

mitochondria. The process of the training effect can be monitored through blood samples and muscle biopsies; however, the actual performance level can only be plotted theoretically since the other component confounding performance is the degree of fatigue produced by the training load. Consequently, this has led to the development of a two-factor model of training, which is based on fitness and fatigue components.

The two-factor model is based on the premise that repeated training loads affect performance and that, at any point in time, their difference (Fitness-Fatigue) should represent how well an athlete performs at that time (Banister, 1991). "Athlete preparedness," or readiness, is determined by the positive (fitness) and negative (fatigue) changes, with fitness gain from a training session suggested to be moderate in magnitude but long lasting, and fatigue hypothesized to be greater but relatively short in duration (Zatsiorsky, 1995). A fitness impulse and fatigue impulse generated from a training session can be calculated;

their decline is suggested to be predictable based on an exponential decay equation defined separately for each. On average, the fitness decay time constant may be taken as 45 days and that for fatigue as 15 days (Banister, 1991). Thus, if fatigue decays three times as quickly as fitness from any attained position at the end of a period of training, then fitness may now be revealed, as fatigue drops away faster than fitness does (Banister, 1991). Consequently, at any point in a training program or macrocycle

Predicted Performance = Fitness – Fatigue

as demonstrated in figure 5.6.

Again, the problem of this model is the generalized decay constants. Although the model portrays visually the effects of specific workouts, the principle of individualization confounds the generalization to a group of athletes unless empirical performance data allow athletes to be subgrouped on performance changes and recovery rates.

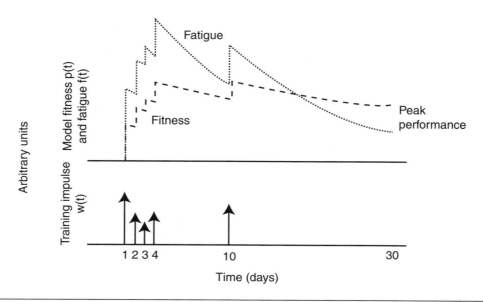

Figure 5.6 An example of the accumulation and decay of fitness and fatigue. The degree of training impulse influences the two factors.

Adapted, by permission, from E.W. Banister, 1991, Modeling elite athletic performance. In *Physiological testing of the high-performance athlete,* 2nd ed., edited by J.D. MacDougall, H.A. Wenger, and H.J. Green (Champaign, IL: Human Kinetics), 414.

Methods of Quantifying and Tracking Training Load

The aim of training is to maximize performance at a specified time while minimizing the risk of illness and fatigue in the period leading up to the competition (Morton, 1991). This necessitates an understanding of the training load that produces a given response and the identification of training situations that may precipitate underperformance or illness.

The heart rate response of an individual to training, stress, or sickness is a useful indicator of the body's reaction to a shift in homeostasis. Heart rate monitors allow the collection of heart rate data for long periods of time in both interval and continuous situations, and the response to a given absolute load allows identification of a training effect (decreased heart rate response) or a fatigue response (elevated heart rate response). A training effort (dose) is calculated as the product of duration of effort and the average functional elevation of the maximum heart rate range. This index, termed *training impulse* (TRIMP), was defined as

Duration × Training × Delta Heart Rate Ratio
(ΔHR Ratio)

where

$$\Delta \text{HR Ratio} = \frac{\text{HR}_{ex} - \text{HR}_{rest}}{\text{HR}_{max} - \text{HR}_{rest}}$$

Banister (1991) remarked that as a guard against giving a disproportionate importance to long-duration activity at a low heart rate compared with intense, short-duration activity, the delta HR ratio should be weighted in such a manner that reflects the intensity of effort. A multiplying factor *(y),* which is based on the classically described increase in blood lactate in male and female subjects, respectively, weights the delta HR ratio proportionately higher the higher its elevation during exercise. The multiplying factor is $0.64e^{1.92x}$ for males and $0.86e^{1.67x}$ for females, where e is the Napierian logarithm having a value of 2.712, and x is the delta HR ratio in exercise. This method of quantifying a training session illustrates the pattern of the training load. Moreover, this method, together with an assessment of standard test performances or competition efforts, allows coaches and athletes to assess the effectiveness of training sequences or microcycles.

One of the most widely used methods of evaluating physical effort is the Rating of Perceived Exertion (RPE) category scale developed by Gunnar Borg in 1970 (see also Kellmann, this volume, chapter 3). A modified category-ratio scale from 0 to 10 (CR10; Borg, 1982) provides a means of identifying each quantitative rating with a verbal expression. The scale ranges from 0 to 10 applying a wide range of intensities from "very, very weak"—set at 0.5—to "very, very heavy"—set at 10. In order to quantify training load, Foster et al. (1995) used the CR10 scale for session RPE, and training load was defined as the product of the rating of the global intensity of an entire training session and the duration of the session.

$$\text{Load} = \text{Session RPE} \times \text{Duration}$$

The "session RPE" was demonstrated to relate to the average percent heart rate reserve during the exercise session and to the percentage of a training session during which the heart rate was in blood-lactate-derived heart rate training zones (Foster et al., 1995).

In order to further quantify training load, other indices have been suggested as monitoring tools. It is recognized that inappropriate training sequence can lead to underperformance particularly when the training load on "easy" days is increased (Bruin, Kuipers, Keizer, & Vandervuisse, 1994). The increased training volume and increased intensity studies by Lehmann et al. (1992) demonstrated that during the increased training volume, study subjects developed some performance incompetence. However, with increased intensity and substantially more day-to-day variation in training, subjects demonstrated improved performance.

These observations led Lehmann, Foster, and Keul (1993) and Foster and Lehmann (1997) to suggest that some index of training variability together with training load might contribute to underperformance. They suggested that this index of training variability can be defined as the mean of the daily load divided by the standard deviation of that weekly load calculated over a period of a week, and can be labeled "training monotony" (Foster & Lehmann, 1997). Since high training load and high training monotony are both factors related to negative adaptations in training, Foster and Lehmann suggested that the product of training load and training monotony, what they called "training strain," may also relate to negative adaptations to training (Foster, 1998). Using these indices, Foster (1998) reported that when monitoring episodes of illness, a quantitative relationship was demonstrated between the various indices of training and the presence of negative adaptations to training. He observed that a high percentage of illnesses could be accounted for when individual athletes exceeded individually identifiable training thresholds, mostly related to the strain of training (Foster, 1998).

Practical Methods for Monitoring Tolerance to Training

When initiating a strategy to monitor an athlete's tolerance to training, we must develop a procedure that can be used to evaluate the degree of fatigue along the continuum from normal training response to long-term overtraining/underperformance. Since the risk of poor performance, injury, illness, and premature retirement are likely to be greatly increased with the overtraining syndrome, prevention is paramount. Some prevention methods are suggested in table 5.2 (Hooper & Mackinnon, 1995). Because the transition from adequate training to long-term overtraining is a gradual one, it is difficult to diagnose an overtraining syndrome in its earliest stage (Kuipers, 1998). Because diagnosis usually occurs prospectively in real-world sports, at present attempts to identify reliable, specific, and sensitive parameters have failed (Hooper, Mackinnon, Howard, Gordon, & Bachmann, 1995; Rowbottom, Keast, & Goodman, 1995). Researchers have had some success, however, in using decrements in performance or the inability to train at customary levels as markers of overtraining.

Some have suggested that the key to separating overreaching and underperformance from the normal training response of a training overload may lie in examining the structure of a training program. At the end of a training block, into which a designated recovery phase has been programmed, an assessment of recovery status should be undertaken. Poor training performance or indications of an imbalance between fitness and fatigue at the end of a designated recovery phase would indicate incomplete recovery; subsequent heavy training should not be initiated (Fry et al., 1991). However, overreaching is used by some coaches as a large stimulus for adaptation to promote a fitness peak prior to a major competition (Brown, Frederick, Falsetti, Burke, & Ryan, 1983). This results in decreased performance for a short period but, after extended recovery, results in an increased performance level (Kuipers & Keizer, 1988). If this tactic is used, the problem of timing the overreaching training phase is compounded by individual rates of recovery and the degree of nontraining stress

Table 5.2   Suggested Methods for Preventing Overtraining Syndrome

Identify susceptible athletes.

Minimize known causes, such as sudden increases in training or lack of adequate rest between seasons.

Individualize training in recognition that athletes have different backgrounds and tolerances.

Monitor athlete for early warning signs in known moderate-to-heavy training cycles.

Minimize poor nutrition.

Examine lifestyle and nontraining stressors.

Adapted, by permission, from S.L. Hooper and L.T. Mackinnon, 1995, "Monitoring overtraining in athletes," *Sports Medicine* 20: 323. © Adis International Ltd., Auckland, NZ.

factors. Consequently, knowledge of individual recovery rates and the identification of athletes susceptible to overreaching is critical for timing a peak performance (see Norris & Smith, this volume, chapter 7).

Step-by-Step Assessment

The process of individually monitoring and preventing overtraining should be conducted in steps, beginning with the inexpensive method of using a training log. Most athletes keep records of their daily training, including morning resting heart rate (MRHR), distance or duration of training, exercise heart rate (when appropriate), and the type of activity. A careful review of the training diary offers valuable clues to overtraining (McKenzie, 1999). Details of subjective ratings of fatigue, sleep patterns, and assessment of training responses can provide useful information regarding the athlete's response and adaptation to the workload.

Heart Rate

MRHR has been suggested to be a marker of training tolerance (Brown et al., 1983). Classically, a reduced MRHR is an indication of the effect of endurance training and improved cardiovascular fitness (Steinhaus, 1933). However, MRHRs that rise progressively during intensified training may reflect the early stages of fatigue leading to overtraining. A progressive rise of 10 b · min^{-1} above the lowest recorded level suggests that the training load may have exceeded the athlete's functional adaptive limit (Dressendorfer, Wade, & Scaff, 1985). However, before overreaching or any other state of fatigue can be suspected, other possible causes such as infection, emotional upset, insufficient or poor sleep, inadequate carbohydrate intake, and de-

hydration must be investigated (Hooper & Mackinnon, 1995).

In addition to MRHR, changes in submaximal heart rate and maximal heart rate have been examined. At the same submaximal power output, a decreased submaximal heart rate was observed with no change in maximal heart rate in response to an induced increase in training volume (Lehmann et al., 1991). No clear pattern of sensitivity to training load has emerged with these heart rate variables, although a decreased maximal heart rate and maximal performance was observed at the end of a two-week intensified training regimen (Jeukendrup, Hesselink, Snyder, Kuipers, & Keizer, 1992). The explanation for the reduced measures was local muscle fatigue in the legs. Since heart rate and oxygen uptake were lower, it was suggested that the capacity of the cardiorespiratory system was not the limiting factor and that peripheral fatigue resulted in the lower scores. The cyclists in this intensified training study attained an overreaching stage of fatigue that was also marked by an increase in sleeping heart rate but not in MRHR (Jeukendrup et al., 1992).

The Rusko orthostatic heart rate test (Rusko, Härkönen, & Pakarinem, 1994) shows promise as an indicator of training or nontraining stressors. The test requires an athlete to lie down for 10 minutes at the same time of day, and the resting heart rate for the last 2 minutes of the 10-minute resting period is recorded. Then, after the athlete stands up, the 15-second, 90-second, and 120-second heart rates are recorded. Athletes not on the verge of overreaching or long-term overtraining display constant heart rate responses at the specified recording times. However, severe change in the 120-second post-standing-up heart rate (e.g., > 10 b · min^{-1} above normal) may indicate the approach of fatigue and reduced performance.

Excessive training loads may initially induce changes in the nervous regulation of cardiovascular autonomic functions without changes in hormone concentrations.

Iron

A decrease in training or performance may occur as a result of iron deficiency, particularly in women (Gledhill, Warburton, & Jamnik, 1999), and should be used as a routine screen several times per year. The influence of hemoglobin concentration ([Hb]) on aerobic power ($\dot{V}O_2$max) and performance has been studied extensively (Freedson, 1981; Kanstrup & Ekblom, 1984; Woodson, Willis, & Lenfant, 1978); a suboptimal [Hb] clearly impairs aerobic performance (Gledhill et al., 1999). Sport anemia often occurs in endurance athletes due to plasma expansion without a concurrent increase in red blood cells (RBCs). This results in suboptimal [Hb] but with normal values for other indices of iron status, including ferritin and percentage transferrin saturation (Weight, 1993), and in the absence of any recognized disease process (Clement, 1981). True anemia, on the other hand, is characterized by at least two of the following criteria: serum ferritin < 20 mg/L; red blood cell protoporphyrin (RBCP) levels >1.8 mmol/L RBC; and percentage transferrin saturation (%sat) below 18%. In addition, when [Hb] falls below 12.0 g/100 ml in women and 14.0 g/100 ml in men, the athlete is considered iron deficient and anemic (Bothwell & Baynes, 1987).

The three stages of iron deficiency are outlined in table 5.3 as defined by Garza et al. (1997).

Low [Hb] and ferritin independent of sport anemia may be the result of poor nutrition (Clement & Sawchuk, 1984); excessive menstrual blood loss (Haymes & Lamanca, 1989); hematuria (Jones & Newhouse, 1997); and training (Candau, Busso, & Lacour, 1992; Roberts & Smith, 1992). Because of the importance of hemoglobin and iron to normal function, it is suggested that the monitoring of hematological status in athletes should be one of the first invasive screening procedures performed at the beginning of the training year.

Table 5.3   Classification of Iron-Deficiency States

Stage I: Storage iron depletion (prelatent iron deficiency)

Low serum ferritin levels	and	Normal total iron-binding capacity
		Normal percent transferrin saturation
		Normal serum iron concentration
		Normal hemoglobin

Stage II: Storage iron-deficient erythropoesis (latent iron deficiency)

Low serum ferritin levels	and	Increased total iron-binding capacity
		Decreased percent transferrin saturation
		Normal hemoglobin
	or	
Low serum ferritin levels	and	Decreased serum iron concentration
		Normal hemoglobin

Stage III: Iron-deficiency anemia (manifest iron deficiency)

Low serum ferritin levels	and	Increased total iron-binding capacity
		Decreased percent transferrin saturation
		Decreased serum iron concentration
		Low hemoglobin

Adapted, by permission, from A.B. Garza, I. Shrier, H.W. Kohl, P. Ford, M. Brown, and G.O. Matteson, 1997, "The clinical value of serum ferritin tests in endurance athletes," *Clinical Journal of Sport Medicine* 7 (1): 46-53.

Chatard, Mujika, Guy, and Lacour (1999) suggested an algorithm for guiding treatment decisions. Monitoring procedures should ensure that an inflammation response is not present at the time of sampling since inflammation increases ferritin production without increasing iron stores (Lipschitz, Cook, & Finch, 1974). Finally, adequate iron stores are important for altitude training or exposure.

Glycogen

It is well established that with prolonged continuous exercise, time to fatigue at a moderate submaximal intensity is related to preexercise muscle glycogen concentration (Bergström, Hermansen, Hultman, & Saltin, 1967). Recently, Balsom (1999) demonstrated that pregame muscle glycogen concentration influences the amount of high-intensity exercise performed during small-sided (four-on-a-side) games of soccer. The total amount of high-intensity exercise performed was significantly greater (~ 33%) following an exercise and diet regimen that included a high carbohydrate (CHO) diet. The author suggested that although high-intensity running is only a small percentage of the game (~ 3%), this type of exercise is extremely important when one considers the outcome of the game. Although some degree of caution should be taken when extrapolating the results to full-sided game situations in sports such as soccer, rugby, basketball, field hockey, and ice hockey, the findings suggest that to optimize performance a high carbohydrate (CHO) diet should be administered in preparation for intense training or competition (Balsom, 1999). This in-the-field study supports other laboratory studies demonstrating the effects of CHO consumption on performance during repeated short-duration exercise (Bangsbo, Nørregaard, Thorsøe, 1992; Nicholas, Williams, Lakomy, Philips, & Nowitz, 1995).

A further question relates to the influence of CHO stores on training tolerance and the ability to maintain customary levels of training. A classic study (Costill, Bowers, Branam, & Sparks, 1971) demonstrated that runners who trained intensely over three days and ate a low CHO diet (40% total calories) often experienced a day-to-day decrease in muscle glycogen. However, when these athletes consumed a high CHO diet (70% total calories), their muscle glycogen levels recovered almost completely within 22 hours of the training bouts. Thus, adequate ingestion of CHO is important to avoid the potential consequences of glycogen depletion on endurance performance and training.

In a longer training study, the effects of a 10-day period of approximately twice the normal training on male swimmers revealed that a third of the group (nonresponders) had difficulty completing the training load (Costill et al., 1988). They had significantly reduced muscle glycogen levels, and dietary analysis indicated that they consumed fewer calories and fewer CHO than those who handled the training load well. However, performance tests of muscular power, sprinting ability (approximately 11 seconds), and a maximal swim effort over 365 meters (approximately 270 seconds) revealed that the nonresponders were not affected by the increased training load and reduced muscle glycogen levels. The implication of this study is that training, as opposed to short-duration performance, was compromised as a result of the athletes' failure to ingest sufficient CHO to meet the energy demands of heavy training (Costill et al., 1988). This is a classic real-world situation showing that inadequate CHO intake, rather than too much training, can be the cause of acute training problems. The compromised training can be rectified quickly by taking a few days' rest and ingesting adequate calories and CHO.

Chronic glycogen depletion may lead to symptoms of overreaching, reduced customary training levels, and decreased muscle mass. Furthermore, low muscle glycogen levels can reduce the levels of branched-chain amino acids and lead to central fatigue (Newsholme, Parry-Billings, McAndrews, & Budgett, 1991). It is therefore important in the assessment of tolerance to training to determine if low glycogen levels are a factor of overreaching or underperformance.

Plasma Glutamine and Glutamate Concentrations

Glutamine is an amino acid found in relatively high amounts in muscle and plasma. Injury, infection, nutritional status, and exercise can all influence the plasma glutamine concentration ([Gm]). After an overnight fast the normal [Gm] range is between 500 and 750 mmol · L^{-1} (Walsh, Blannin, Robson, & Gleeson, 1998) depending on the measurement technique. Glutamine is associated with significant body functions, including the transfer of nitrogen between organs and the detoxification of ammonia (Newsholme & Leech, 1983), a possible regulator of protein synthesis and degradation (MacLennan, Brown, & Lennie, 1987). It is also used by cells of the immune system (Ardawi &

Newsholme, 1983). Significantly lower resting [Gm] has been reported in athletes diagnosed as over-reached or overtrained (Kingsbury, Kay, & Hjelm, 1998; Parry-Billings et al., 1992; Smith & Norris, 2000b) compared to healthy control athletes.

Parry-Billings et al. (1992) were the first to suggest a possible link between overtraining and lower [Gm]. Rowbottom et al. (1995) reported that only [Gm] deviated significantly from the normal range among a battery of standard blood parameters in overtrained athletes. We recently reported lower [Gm] in overtrained athletes but similar [Gm] was also observed in athletes who did not exhibit overtraining (Smith & Norris, 2000b). Consequently, we suggested that low [Gm] alone does not indicate overtraining but may instead suggest that the volume of training has exceeded the athlete's capacity to tolerate work. Several possibilities may be responsible for the decline in muscle [Gm], including increased levels of glucocorticoids (Falduto, Young, & Hickson, 1992; Muhlbacher, Kapadia, Colpoys, Smith, & Wilmore, 1984) or decreased nutritional intake of protein (Kingsbury et al., 1998). Increased protein intake has been suggested for endurance athletes particularly in heavy training (Lemon, 1991). With additional protein intake, [Gm] increased to above $500 \text{ mmol} \cdot \text{L}^{-1}$, and increased training was resumed in a group of athletes exhibiting low [Gm] (Kingsbury et al., 1998). However, Hiscock and Mackinnon (1998) reported a wide variation in [Gm] across sports, and there was no relationship between [Gm] and total dietary protein intake when expressed as $g \cdot day^{-1}$.

With respect to [Gm] reflecting tolerance for the volume of work, we observed high [Gm] in individual athletes with a background in long-duration aerobic work, particularly swimmers, cross-country skiers, and all-round speed skaters (Smith & Norris, 2000b). Relatively high [Gm] has also been reported for cyclists, and low [Gm] for power lifters (Hiscock & Mackinnon, 1998). In addition, we suggest that the timing of measurement is critical to interpretation since high [Gm] has been observed in a recovered-rested-early macrocycle training situation compared to relatively lower values during heavy training (Smith & Norris, 2000b).

Metabolic acidosis stimulates the rate of glutamine release from muscle, and this in turn is used by the kidney in acid-base balance (King, Goldstein, & Newsholme, 1983). Ammonia, produced by the hydrolysis of glutamine to glutamate, reacts with excess hydrogen ions (H^+) to form

ammonium ions, which are excreted in the urine. Significantly higher plasma glutamate concentrations [Ga] have been reported in overtrained athletes compared to controls (Parry-Billings et al., 1992) and nonovertrained athletes in heavy training (Smith & Norris, 2000b). We observed that high-intensity training was associated with high [Ga], which leads us to the hypothesis that [Ga] may increase significantly when recovery from intensity training is impaired through either repeated high-intensity training or lack of adequate recovery time. Based on these observations we proposed an athlete tolerance to training model, in which the blood [Gm]/[Ga] ratio may be used as an overall indicator of training tolerance (Smith & Norris, 2000b).

In a rested or early-season condition, the [Gm]/[Ga] ratio is relatively high, but with increased training load, a pattern of a decrease in [Gm] and an increase in [Ga] occurs. As training volume and intensity increase during a training cycle, athletes react depending on their individual tolerances (Lehmann et al., 1993). Normal rested or low-training status is represented by a [Gm] of 585 ± 54 $\text{mmol} \cdot \text{L}^{-1}$ and a [Ga] of $101 \pm 16 \text{ mmol} \cdot \text{L}^{-1}$. When athletes are in heavy training and are managing the training load, values for [Gm] are $522 \pm 53 \text{ mmol} \cdot$ L^{-1}, whereas those for [Ga] are $128 \pm 19 \text{ mmol} \cdot \text{L}^{-1}$. These values are represented in figure 5.7.

We acknowledge that there are always "gray areas" between managing the training load and overreaching, but this model may assist sport scientists and coaches in monitoring athletes that they know are prone to underperformance. The classification of tolerance to training is presented in table 5.4.

The measure presented here should not be used as a single robust measure of overreaching or overtraining. Underperformance and an inability to sustain relative high-intensity exercise may still occur within the normal [Gm]/[Ga] ratio range, with muscle soreness and tenderness reported by the athlete. However, since training load, infection, and nutrition may all influence [Gm], and chronic high-intensity training is associated with high [Ga], these markers may be useful in monitoring an athlete's tolerance to training.

Immune Function

A common perception among elite athletes and their coaches is that prolonged and intense exercise lowers resistance to upper respiratory tract infections (URTIs; Neiman, 1997, 1998). URTIs are

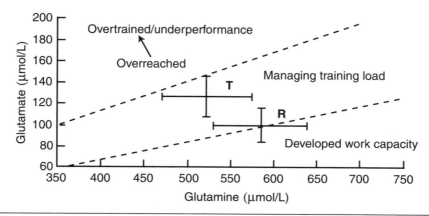

Figure 5.7 Athlete training tolerance model: **R** represents mean (± *SD*) plasma glutamine and glutamate values under rested or low-training volume conditions and **T** represents values during high-volume and intensity training. The managing training load area is bordered by an upper boundary line equal to a [Gm]/[Ga] ratio of 3.58 μmol · L⁻¹ and a lower boundary line equal to 5.88 μmol · L⁻¹.

Table 5.4   [Gm]/[Ga] Ratio (μmol · L⁻¹) As a Classification of Athlete Training Tolerance

[Gm]/[Ga] ratios	Condition	Characteristics
> 5.88	Developed work capacity	Athletes with years of training background. Blood sample obtained during early season when training volume is low to moderate or in a tapered condition.
3.58–5.88	Managing training load	Athletes are managing training stressors and are performing to expected levels.
< 3.58	Overreached	Complaint of fatigue and below-par expected training levels or performance. Recovery to > 3.58 occurs within two weeks with reduced training load.
	Overtrained	[Gm]/[Ga] ratio does not recover to > 3.58 with rest or low-intensity aerobic exercise within four weeks; decreased training and competition performance.

the most common infections in trained athletes (Peters, 1997), and one of the most common symptoms of overtraining is an increased susceptibility to infection. Although an athlete's health and well-being may suffer from the symptoms typically associated with URTIs, performance may not be compromised unless moderate or more severe problems are encountered (Pyne et al., 2001). Symptoms of URTI may include sore throat, runny nose, mild fatigue, and headache.

Host defense at mucosal surfaces is largely mediated by the family of secretory immunoglobulins (Ig) (Mackinnon, 1996). The predominant antibody is immunoglobulin-A (IgA), which acts to prevent viral replication and inhibit viral and bacterial attachment to the mucosal epithelium of the mouth, throat, and upper respiratory tract (Mackinnon, 1996). Salivary IgA has been suggested as a promising indicator of overtraining (McKenzie, 1999) or as a marker for identifying those athletes more prone to URTI (Pyne & Gleeson, 1998; Shephard & Shek, 1998).

The effects of acute exercise on salivary IgA vary among sports and appear to depend on the level of fitness of the subjects, the experimental design (Gleeson, 2000a), and the phase of training under investigation. In general, postexercise salivary IgA levels are lower than preexercise levels as reported for elite cross-country skiers (Tomasi, Trudeau, Czerwinski, & Erredge, 1982), swimmers

(Gleeson et al., 1999; Tharp & Barnes, 1990), cyclists (Mackinnon, Chick, van As, & Tomasi, 1989), rowers (Nehlsen-Cannarella et al., 2000), and kayakers (Mackinnon, Ginn, & Seymour, 1993). Recovery to preexercise levels usually occurs within 24 hours but may remain depressed for longer periods after high-intensity exercise (Gleeson, 2000b). However, it has been suggested that the magnitude of change in immunity that occurs after each bout of prolonged exercise has more clinical significance than the training-induced alterations in resting immunity (Neiman, 1997; Shephard & Shek, 1995). During this theoretical "open window" of altered immunity, viruses and bacteria may gain a foothold, increasing the risk of infection (Neiman, 2000).

A recent 12-month study of athletes at the University of Freiburg (Germany) suggests that increased training in hours per week is related to an increased rate of URTIs. Furthermore, endurance athletes appear to be at a considerably higher risk of developing infections than athletes performing power sports or a mixed type of sport (König, Grathwohl, Weinstock, Northoff, & Berg, 2000). Additionally, athletes reporting daily stress, lack of nutritional awareness, or sleep deprivation had significantly more infections than athletes adhering to a healthier lifestyle (König et al., 2000).

In a two-week study of the effects of multiple training sessions on an elite kayaker, pretraining salivary IgA concentrations failed to recover to the initial IgA concentration of the day, prior to subsequent sessions (Gleeson, Ginn, & Francis, 2000). Furthermore, very intense early morning training sessions resulted in an 80% decrease in IgA prior to the second training session. Thus, recovery rates to pretraining block levels appear to be significantly influenced by the intensity and number of daily sessions. When monitoring has occurred over a microcycle(s) of training, there is less consensus. A recent study of elite swimmers reported no significant differences in median salivary IgA concentration between May and August over a training macrocycle prior to a major competition (Pyne et al., 2001). A previous study by the same group showed a significant decrease over a seven-month training period (Gleeson et al., 1995). In a study of Russian athletes several key findings were reported: the levels of salivary Ig showed a sudden decrease during periods of maximum intensity training and a significant increase in the incidence of URTIs during the maximum intensity period (Levando, Suzdal'nitskii, Pershin, & Zykov, 1988).

The significance of lower salivary IgA levels and incidences of URTIs is the effect on training and competitive performance. A study examining the relationship between swimming performance and incidences of URTIs reported no statistical difference in performance between ill and healthy swimmers. However, in real-world performance terms, the data suggested that swimmers with URTIs could experience performance decrement compared with their counterparts who remained free from illness (Pyne et al., 2001).

Individual responses, real-world differences in training design, and testing regularity all influence the degree of immunosuppression, but it is highly likely that repeated high-intensity training will cause immunosuppression and have long-term effects on the recovery rate from the suppression (Gleeson, 2000a).

Hormonal Markers of Training Tolerance

The determination of hormone concentrations for monitoring training and potentially identifying overtraining has been a focus of sport science over the last 15 years. Endogenous hormones are essentially involved in exercise-induced acute or chronic adaptations and influence the regeneration phase through modulation of anabolic and catabolic processes after exercise (Urhausen, Gabriel, & Kindermann, 1995). A study by Adlercreutz et al. (1986) suggested that overtraining must be related to decreased testosterone levels, or at least to a pronounced decrease in the testosterone/cortisol ratio. Results of a study of long-distance runners who had undertaken one week of intensive training in comparison to a control group that trained normally suggested that the testosterone/cortisol ratio was more useful for monitoring the intensity of training than for monitoring overtraining. However, despite the numerous training studies, no essential changes in levels in resting testosterone or cortisol during overtraining, or correlations with performance, have been established that satisfy the sport science community. Urhausen and Kindermann (2000) suggested that the ratio seems to indicate the physiological strain of training from a hormonal perspective, but in most cases it does not diagnose overtraining or underperformance.

Resting cortisol levels have also been used to monitor the status of athletes and have been recommended for the determination of overtraining. The literature is equivocal, however, with some investigations finding no change in resting cortisol concentration during overtraining (Flynn et al., 1994; Schnabel, Kindermann, Schmitt, Biro, & Stegmann, 1982) and others reporting an increase (Barron, Noakes, Levy, Smith, & Millar, 1985; Kraemer et al., 1989; Stray-Gundersen, Videman, & Snell, 1986).

Nocturnal urinary catecholamine excretion (NUCE) has been investigated as a tool for diagnosing short-term overreaching. In a study designed to induce overtraining, eight experienced distance runners increased their training volume significantly over a four-week period (Lehmann et al., 1991). After the four weeks, the runners' NUCE fell to 28-30% of baseline values, and their urinary noradrenaline excretion was correlated with a complaint index, such as muscular stiffness, fatigue, or exhaustion ($r = 0.91$). Similar decreased NUCE has been observed in soccer players (Lehmann et al., 1992; Naessens, Chandler, Kibler, & Driessens, 2000) and cyclists (Gastmann & Lehmann, 1999). Under fatigue conditions, NUCE is seen as an indicator of intrinsic sympathetic activity, with a decrease considered a sign of an overexertion exhaustion of the sympathetic system (Lehmann et al., 1992). With reduced training, normalization of NUCE occurs (Gastmann & Lehmann, 1999).

Training Sequencing and Load Tolerance

The next phase of athlete assessment for the avoidance of long-term overtraining/underperformance requires that adequate rest or recovery training be planned and implemented within a training program. Planned training will assist in the administration of correct loads and adequate regeneration periods to avoid excessive fatigue (Fry et al., 1991). Periodization is a well-established concept (Bompa, 1983; Krüger, 1973; Matveyev, 1981) and appreciably diminishes the danger of monotony and mental saturation through built-in variation in spite of a high training frequency (Harre, 1982). A training monotony index was recently suggested, and a low index, indicative of training monotony, was found to be associated with incidence of illness (Foster, 1998). However, currently no definitive guidelines of training work for all athletes in all individual endurance disciplines (Foster, Daniels, & Seiler, 1999). This is due to the principle of individualization and the individual variability in recovery potential, exercise capacity, nontraining stress factors, and stress tolerance that may explain the different vulnerabilities of athletes who train under

identical training stress conditions (Lehmann et al., 1993). Monitoring processes tend to emphasize the individual athlete's response to training. The inability to cope with a training load may not be the fault of the athlete; instead it may be related to an inappropriate structure of training.

Authors, as reviewed by Foster, Daniels, and Sieler (1999), have suggested a variety of training strategies for avoiding recurrent fatigue or underperformance, including the following:

- The total volume of low-intensity, background training should serve as a platform for progressively higher-intensity "specific" training (Seiler, 1997).

- High-intensity loads produce a relatively rapid improvement in performance, but the improved performance standard is less stable and needs to be consolidated by a great deal of work at a lower intensity (Harre, 1982).

- Most of the noninterval training should be at fairly low intensities below the aerobic threshold (Seiler, 1997).

- Middle intensities (above aerobic threshold) should be avoided as they do little more than tire athletes (Seiler, 1997).

- Athletes should alternate hard and easy training (Noakes, 1991) or build a program around two high-intensity interval sessions per week (Seiler, 1997) or at a maximum three (Daniels, 1998).

- Athletes should train easily enough on easy days in order to be able to train hard enough on hard days (Seiler, 1997).

- Athletes should not train hard and race hard at the same time (Lydiard & Gilmore, 1962).

- More variation in the day-to-day training load is likely to result in more effective adaptation to training (Foster et al., 1999).

- The adaptive response to the addition of specific training is quantitatively dependent on the total volume of training performed during the build-up period (Foster et al., 1999).

- Athletes and coaches should understand the holism of training (Noakes, 1991).

Holism of Training and the Global Aspects of Performance

Noakes (1991) suggested that training holism encompasses two ideas: (1) training itself must be balanced and varied and (2) nontraining time has a major influence on training itself. It is important therefore that all factors outside the realm of the training session be evaluated as to their possible negative influence on total fatigue. The factors include diet, sleep, other physical effort of the day, and work stress (Noakes, 1991). In order to create optimum development of the standard of performance, it is essential to recognize the reasons for overloading as early as possible and to eliminate them. This requires close cooperation among the coach, athlete, and sports physician (Harre, 1982, p. 69; see also Norris & Smith, this volume, chapter 7). Nontraining stress may include a way of life harmful to training and environmental factors that create physical and psychological stress and health problems. The coach must be aware of what the athlete takes on and coordinate training with the athlete's educational and professional responsibilities (Harre, 1982, p. 69).

The preparation of an athlete for Olympic or World Championship success may require many years of training. The dynamics of the athlete's sporting achievements over many years may be presented in the general form as a parabolic curve (Matveyev, 1981, p. 293). Most agree that in the first years of high-level sport, athletes improve at a rapid rate. Then the pace gradually slows until finally there is a tendency for a decrease in performance. However, as the athlete endeavors to make small improvements, he emphasizes the mastery and stabilization of competitive performance. Over the many years of training, a tolerance to training manifests itself in an ability to execute the necessary skills, tactics, endurance, power, and psychological preparedness within a small margin of variance from best performances. The ability to achieve stability of international performance requires the optimization of five parameters of performance, originally described by Matveyev (1981) as criteria for sporting form.

> Sporting form is characterized by a complex of physiological, health, and psychological indices. Sporting form is a harmonious unity of all components of the athlete's optimum readiness: physical, psychological, health, technical, and tactical. (Matveyev, 1981, p. 260)

In order for an athlete to realize best performance, all aspects should be near or at optimal level during a given time frame. If any one component is below par, top sporting form will not be attained (Matveyev, 1981).

Smith and Norris (2000a, 2000b) developed a model of the five components of sporting form and characterized a competitive performance as a "global performance" on a continuum from optimal to underperformance. Since tolerance to training impacts all components of the global performance, they have incorporated and developed further the "reasons for overloading (underperformance)" presented by Harre (1982, p. 70) into the overall model presented in figure 5.8.

We suggest that each component (physiology, biomechanics, psychology, tactics, and health/lifestyle) can be evaluated at any point in time (although especially around competitive events) on a scale from optimal to underrested/underperformance/poor or sick. Furthermore, the competition sequence or frequency and training macro, meso, micro design determine the outcome optimization/underperformance. Everything has to come together for the athlete to realize her full potential.

Summary

The process of monitoring an athlete's tolerance to training should be systematic and long-term. Readiness for competition requires, at any point on the parabolic curve of performance, the harmonious unity of physiological, biomechanical, technical, tactical, and medical components (Matveyev, 1981). Underperformance, on the other hand, occurs as the result of the accumulation of training and nontraining stress; performance abilities are influenced by factors such as training, lifestyle, health, and environment (Norris & Smith, this volume, chapter 7) and the sequence of competition and training.

The monitoring process should include the following:

- Sport analysis—evaluation of the sport relative to long-, medium-, or short-duration endurance and the requirements of speed and strength.

- Load demands of sport—assessment of the different types of training that are frequently used within a sport. Evaluation of training volume, intensity, and general and specific type of training.

- Competition sequencing and selection—evaluation of the competitive calendar and an assessment of appropriate competitive opportunities.

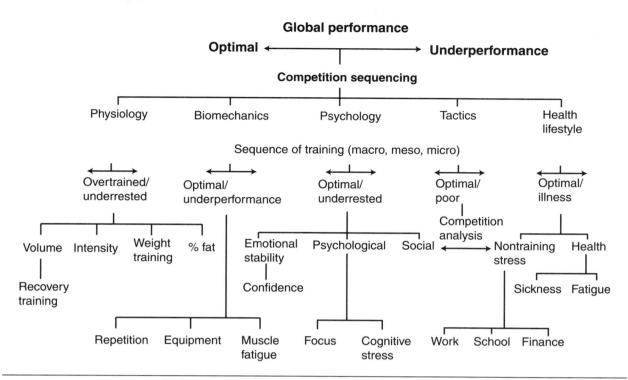

Figure 5.8 A model of five components of performance that impact the global performance of an athlete.

Reprinted, by permission, from D.J. Smith and S.R. Norris, 2000, "Building a sport science program," *Coaches Report* 6 (4): 19-21.

- Athlete performance maturation—assessment of yearly performance relative to the parabolic curve of performance.

- Health evaluation—yearly or more frequent evaluation of basic health parameters such as hemoglobin, ferritin, and other standard parameters.

- Nutrition assessment—appropriate education and dietary analysis when applicable.

- Training log—maintain a diary of training details and include subjective ratings of sleep, stress, fatigue, and muscle soreness.

- Avoidance of glycogen depletion—glycogen depletion is an avoidable condition if attention is paid to diet and the sequence and training load. The consequence of depletion is underperformance.

- Individualization—genetics, training background and years of training, health tolerance to physical stress, and psychological stress determine the individual response to a given training load.

Clearly, evaluations of any kind undertaken in a random fashion will not yield coherent assessments that will lead to understanding. Carefully

determined entry and exit assessments relative to a training block or cycle are important for monitoring the effectiveness of a training program (Smith & Norris, 2000a, p. 21).

References

Adlercrentz, H., Harkonen, K., Kuoppasalmi, K., Naveri, H., Huthamieri, H., Tikkanen, H., Remes, K., Dessypms, A., & Karvonen, J. (1986). Effect of training on plasma anabolic and catabolic steroid hormones and their response during physical exercise. *International Journal of Sports Medicine,* 7(Suppl. 1), 27-28.

Ardawi, M.S.M., & Newsholme, E.A. (1983). Glutamine metabolism in lymphocytes of the rat. *Biochemical Journal, 212,* 835-842.

Balsom, P.D. (1999). Carbohydrate intake and multiple sprint sports: With special reference to football (soccer). *International Journal of Sports Medicine, 40,* 48-52.

Bangsbo, J., Nørregaard, L., & Thorsøe, F. (1992). The effect of carbohydrate diet on intermittent exercise performance. *International Journal of Sports Medicine, 13,* 152-157.

Banister, E.W. (1991). Modeling elite athletic performance. In J.D. MacDougall, H.A. Wenger, & H.J. Green (Eds.), *Physiological testing of the high-performance athlete* (2nd ed., pp. 403-424). Champaign, IL: Human Kinetics.

Barron, J.L., Noakes, T.D., Levy, W., Smith, C., & Millar, R.P. (1985). Hypothalamic dysfunction in overtrained athletes. *Journal of Clinical Endocrinology and Metabolism, 60,* 803-806.

Bergström, J., Hermansen, L., Hultman, E., & Saltin, B. (1967). Diet, muscle glycogen, and physical performance. *Acta Physiologica Scandia, 71,* 140-150.

Bompa, T.O. (1983). *Theory and methodology of training.* Dubuque, IA: Kendall/Hunt.

Borg, G. (1982). Psychophysical bases of perceived exertion. *Medicine and Science in Sports and Exercise, 14,* 377-381.

Bothwell, T.H., & Baynes, R.D. (1987). Iron deficiency and anaemia—Nutritional and clinical aspects. *South African Journal of Continuing Medical Education, 5,* 1524-1529.

Bouchard, C., Taylor, A. W., Simoneau, J.-A., & Dulac, S. (1991). Testing anaerobic power and capacity. In J.D. MacDougall, H.A. Wenger, & H.J. Green (Eds.), *Physiological testing of the high-performance athlete* (2nd ed., pp. 175-221). Champaign, IL: Human Kinetics.

Brown, R.L., Frederick, E.C., Falsetti, H.L., Burke, E.R., & Ryan, A.J. (1983). Overtraining of athletes: A round table. *Physician and Sportsmedicine, 11*(6), 92-110.

Bruin, G., Kuipers, H., Keizer, A., & Vandervuisse, G. J. (1994). Adaptation and overtraining in horses subjected to increasing training loads. *Journal of Applied Physiology, 76,* 1908-1913.

Candau, R., Busso, T., & Lacour, J. R. (1992). Effects of training on iron status in cross-country skiers. *European Journal of Applied Physiology, 64,* 497-502.

Chatard, J.-C., Mujika, I., Guy, C., & Lacour, J.-R. (1999). Anaemia and iron deficiency in athletes. *Sports Medicine, 27*(4), 229-240.

Clement, D.B. (1981). Anemia and iron deficiency in athletes. *Sport Science Periodical on Research and Technology in Sport, Nutrition 0-2,* 1-4.

Clement, D.B., & Sawchuk, L.L. (1984). Iron status and sports performance. *Sports Medicine, 1,* 65-74.

Cook, J.D. (1982). Clinical evaluation of iron deficiency. *Seminars in Hematology, 19,* 6-18.

Costill, D.L. (1986). *Inside running—Basics of sports physiology.* Indianapolis: Benchmark Press.

Costill, D.L., Bowers, G., Branam, G., & Sparks, K. (1971). Muscle glycogen utilization during prolonged exercise on successive days. *Journal of Applied Physiology, 31,* 834-838.

Costill, D.L., Flynn, M.G., Kirwan, J.P., Houmard, J.A., Mitchell, J.B., Thomas, R., & Park, S.H. (1988). Effects of repeated days of intensified training on muscle glycogen and swimming performance. *Medicine and Science in Sports and Exercise, 20,* 249-254.

Daniels, J. (1998). *Daniels' running formula.* Champaign, IL: Human Kinetics.

Dressendorfer, R.H., Wade, C.E., & Scaff, J.H. (1985). Increased morning heart rate in runners: A valid sign of overtraining? *Physician and Sportsmedicine, 13*(8), 77-86.

Edwards, R.T.H. (1981). Human muscle function and fatigue. In R. Porter & J. Whelan (Eds.), *Ciba Foundation Symposium, 82* (pp. 1-18). London: Pitman Medical.

Falduto, M.T., Young, A.P., & Hickson, R.C. (1992). Exercise inhibits glucocorticoid-induced glutamine synthetase expression in red skeletal muscles. *American Journal of Physiology: Cell Physiology, 262,* C214-C220.

Flynn, M.G., Pizza, F.X., Boone, J.B., Jr., Andres, F.F., Michaud, T.A., & Rodriguez-Zayas, J.R. (1994). Indices of training stress during competitive running and swimming seasons. *International Journal of Sports Medicine, 15,* 21-26.

Foster, C. (1998). Monitoring training in athletes with reference to indices of overtraining syndrome. *Medicine and Science in Sports and Exercise, 30,* 1164-1168.

Foster, C., Daniels, J.T., & Seiler, S. (1999). Perspectives on correct approaches to training. In M. Lehmann, C. Foster, U. Gastmann, H. Keizer, & J.M. Steinacker (Eds.), *Overload, performance, incompetence, and regeneration in sport* (pp. 27-41). New York: Kluwer Academic/Plenum.

Foster, C., Hector, L., Welsh, R., Schrager, M., Green, M.A., & Snyder, A.C. (1995). Effects of specific versus cross training on running performance. *European Journal of Applied Physiology, 70,* 367-372.

Foster, C., & Lehmann, M. (1997). Overtraining syndrome. In G.N. Guten (Ed.), *Running injuries* (pp. 173-188). Philadelphia: W.B. Saunders.

Freedson, P.S. (1981). The influence of hemoglobin concentration on exercise cardiac output. *International Journal of Sports Medicine, 2,* 81-86.

Fry, R.W., Morton, A.W., & Keast, D. (1991). Overtraining in athletes: An update. *Sports Medicine, 12,* 32-65.

Garza, A.B., Shrier, I., Kohl, H.W., Ford, P., Brown, M., & Matteson, G.O. (1997). The clinical value of serum ferritin tests in endurance athletes. *Clinical Journal of Sport Medicine, 7*(1), 46-53.

Gastmann, U.A.L., & Lehmann, M.J. (1999). Monitoring overload and regeneration in cyclists. In M. Lehmann, C. Foster, U. Gastmann, H. Keizer, & J.M. Steinacker (Eds.), *Overload, performance incompetence, and regeneration in sport* (pp. 131-137). New York: Kluwer Academic/Plenum.

Gledhill, N., Warburton, D., & Jamnik, V. (1999). Haemoglobin, blood volume, cardiac function, and aerobic power. *Canadian Journal of Applied Physiology, 24*(1), 54-65.

Gleeson, M. (2000a). Mucosal immune responses and risk of respiratory illness in elite athletes. *Exercise Immunology Review, 6,* 5-42.

Gleeson, M. (2000b). Mucosal immunity and respiratory illness in elite athletes. *International Journal of Sports Medicine, 21*(Suppl. 1), S33-S43.

Gleeson, M., Ginn, E., & Francis, J.L. (2000). Salivary immunoglobulin monitoring in an elite kayaker. *Clinical Journal of Sports Medicine, 10,* 206-208.

Gleeson, M., McDonald, W.A., Cripps, A.W., Pyne, D.B., Clancy, R.L., & Fricker, P.A. (1995). The effect on immunity of long-term intensive training in elite swimmers. *Clinical Experimental Immunology, 102,* 210-216.

Gleeson, M., McDonald, W.A., Pyne, D.B., Cripps, A.W., Francis, J.L., Fricker, P.A., & Clancy, R.L. (1999). Salivary IgA levels and infection risk in elite swimmers. *Medicine and Science in Sports and Exercise,* 31, 67-73.

Harre, D. (1982). *Principles of sports training: Introduction to the theory and methods of training* (English version, 1st ed.). Berlin: Sportverlag.

Hawley, J.A., Myburgh, M., Noakes, T.D., & Dennis, S.C. (1995). Training techniques to improve fatigue resistance and enhance endurance performance. *Journal of Sports Sciences, 15,* 325-333.

Haymes, E.M., & Lamanca, J.J. (1989). Iron loss in runners during exercise: Implication and recommendations. *Sports Medicine, 7,* 277-285.

Hill, A.V. (1925). The physiological basis of athletic records. *Lancet, 2,* 481-486.

Hiscock, N., & Mackinnon, L.T. (1998). A comparison of plasma glutamine concentration in athletes from different sports. *Medicine and Science in Sports and Exercise, 50*(12), 1693-1696.

Hooper, S.L., & Mackinnon, L.T. (1995). Monitoring overtraining in athletes. *Sports Medicine, 20,* 321-327.

Hooper, S.L., Mackinnon, L.T., Howard, A., Gordon, R.D., & Bachmann, A.W. (1995). Markers for monitoring overtraining and recovery. *Medicine and Science in Sports and Exercise, 27,* 106-112.

Jeukendrup, A.E., Hesselink, M.K.C., Snyder, A.C., Kuipers, H., & Keizer, H.A. (1992). Physiological changes in male competitive cyclists after two weeks of intensified training. *International Journal of Sports Medicine, 13,* 534-541.

Jones, G.R., & Newhouse, I. (1997). Sport-related hematuria: A review. *Clinical Journal of Sport Medicine, 7,* 119-125.

Kanstrup, I., & Ekblom, B. (1984). Blood volume and hemoglobin concentration as determinants of maximal aerobic power. *Medicine and Science in Sports and Exercise, 16,* 256-262.

King, P.A., Goldstein, L., & Newsholme, E.A. (1983). Glutamine synthetase activity of muscle in acidosis. *Biochemical Journal, 216,* 523-525.

Kingsbury, K.J., Kay, L., & Hjelm, M. (1998). Contrasting plasma free amino acid patterns in elite athletes: Association with fatigue and infection. *British Journal of Sports Medicine, 32,* 25-33.

König, D., Grathwohl, D., Weinstock, C., Northoff, H., & Berg, A. (2000). Upper respiratory tract infection in athletes: Influence of lifestyle, type of sport, training effort, and immunostimulant intake. *Exercise Immunology Review, 6,* 102-120.

Koutedakis, Y., Budgett, R., & Faulmann, L. (1990). Rest in underperforming elite competitors. *British Journal of Sports Medicine, 24,* 248-252.

Kraemer, W.J., Fleck, S.J., Callister, R., Shealy, M., Dudley, G.A., Maresh, C.M., Marchitelli, L., Cruthirds, C., Murray, T., & Falkel, J.E. (1989). Training responses of plasma beta-endorphin, adrenocorticotrophin, and cortisol. *Medicine and Science in Sports and Exercise, 21*(2), 146-153.

Krüger, A. (1973, December). Periodization, or peaking at the right time. *Journal of Technical Track & Field Athletics—Track Technique,* Issue 54, 1720-1724.

Kuipers, H. (1998). Training and overtraining: An introduction. *Medicine and Science in Sports and Exercise, 30,* 1137-1139.

Kuipers, H., & Keizer, H.A. (1988). Overtraining in elite athletes: Review and directions for the future. *Sports Medicine, 6,* 79-92.

Lehmann, M., Dickhuth, H.H., Gendrisch, G., Lazar, W., Thum, M., Kaminski, R., Aramendi, J. F., Peterke, E., Wieland, W., & Keul, J. (1991). Training—Overtraining. A prospective, experimental study with experienced middle- and long-distance runners. *International Journal of Sports Medicine, 12*(5), 444-452.

Lehmann, M., Foster, C., & Keul, J. (1993). Overtraining and endurance athletes: A brief review. *Medicine and Science in Sports and Exercise, 25*(7), 854-862.

Lehmann, M., Gastmann, U., Petersen, K.G., Bachl, N., Seidel, A., Khalaf, A.N., Fischer, S., & Keul, J. (1992). Training-overtraining: Performance and hormone levels, after a defined increase in training volume vs. intensity in experienced middle- and long-distance runners. *British Journal of Sports Medicine, 26,* 233-242.

Lemon, P.W. (1991). Effect of exercise in protein requirements. *Journal of Sports Sciences, 9,* 53-70.

Levando, V.A., Suzdal'nitskii, R.S., Pershin, B.B., & Zykov, M.P. (1988). Study of secretory and antiviral immunity in sportsmen. *Sports Medicine Training and Rehabilitation, 1,* 49-52.

Lipschitz, D.A., Cook, J.D., & Finch, C.A. (1974). A clinical evaluation of serum ferritin as an index of iron stores. *New England Journal of Medicine, 290,* 1213-1216.

Lydiard, A., & Gilmore, G. (1962). *Run to the top.* Wellington, NZ: A.H. and A. Reed.

Mackinnon, L.T. (1996). Immunoglobulin, antibody and exercise. *Exercise Immunology Review, 2,* 1-35.

Mackinnon, L.T., Chick, T.W., van As, A., & Tomasi, T.B. (1989). Decreased secretory immunoglobulins following intensive endurance exercise. *Sports Medicine Training and Rehabilitation, 1,* 1-10.

Mackinnon, L.T., Ginn, E., & Seymour, G.J. (1993). Decreased salivary immunoglobulin: A secretion rate after intensive interval training in elite kayakers. *European Journal of Applied Physiology, 67,* 180-184.

MacLennan, P.A., Brown, R.A., & Rennie, M.J. (1987). A positive relationship between protein synthetic rate and intracellular glutamine concentration in perfused rat skeletal muscle. *FEBS Letters, 215*(1), 187-191.

Matveyev, L. (1981). *Fundamentals of sports training* (English translation of the revised Russian edition). Moscow: Progress.

McKenzie, D.C. (1999). Markers of excessive exercise. *Canadian Journal of Applied Physiology, 24*(1), 66-73.

Morton, R.H. (1991). The quantitative periodization of athletic training: A model study. *Sports Medicine Training and Rehabilitation, 3,* 19-28.

Muhlbacher, F., Kapadia, C.R., Colpoys, M.F., Smith, R.J., & Wilmore, D.W. (1984). Effects of glucocorticoids on glutamine metabolism in skeletal muscle. *American Journal of Physiology, 247* (Endocrinol.Metab.10), E75-E83.

Naessens, G., Chandler, T.J., Kibler, W.B., & Driessens, M. (2000). Clinical usefulness of nocturnal urinary noradrenaline excretion patterns in the follow-up of training processes in high-level soccer players. *Journal of Strength and Conditioning Research, 14*(2), 125-131.

Nehlsen-Cannarella, S.L., Neiman, D.C., Fagoaga, O.R., Kella, W.J., Henson, D.A., Shannon, M., & Davis, J.M. (2000). Salivary immunoglobulins in elite rowers. *European Journal of Applied Physiology, 81,* 222-228.

Neiman, D.C. (1997). Exercise immunology: Practical applications. *International Journal of Sports Medicine, 18,* S91-S100.

Neiman, D.C. (1998). Effects of athletic training on infection rates and immunity. In R.B. Kreider, A.C. Fry, & M. O'Toole (Eds.), *Overtraining in sport* (pp. 193-217). Champaign, IL: Human Kinetics.

Neiman, D.C. (2000). Exercise immunology: Future directions for research related to athletes, nutrition and the elderly. *International Journal of Sports Medicine, 21*(Suppl. 1), S61-S68.

Newsholme, E.A., & Leech, A.R. (1983). *Biochemistry for the medical sciences.* Chichester, UK: Wiley.

Newsholme, E.A., Parry-Billings, M., McAndrew, N., & Budgett, R. (1991). A biochemical mechanism to explain some characteristics of overtraining. In F. Brouns (Ed.), *Advances in nutrition and top sport* (Vol. 32, pp. 79-93). Basel, Switzerland: Karger.

Nicholas, C.W., Williams, J.C., Lakomy, H.K., Philips, G., & Nowitz, A. (1995). Influence of ingesting a carbohydrate-electrolyte solution on endurance capacity during intermittent, high-intensity shuttle running. *Journal of Sports Sciences, 13,* 283-290.

Noakes, T.D. (1991). *Lore of running.* (3rd ed.). Champaign, IL: Human Kinetics.

Parry-Billings, M., Budgett, R., Koutedakis, Y., Bloomstrand, E., Brooks, S., Williams, C., Calder, P.C., Pilling, S., Baigrie, R., & Newsholme, E.A. (1992). Plasma amino acid concentration in the overtraining syndrome: Possible effects on the immune system. *Medicine and Science in Sports and Exercise, 24,* 1353-1358.

Peters, E.M. (1997). Exercise, immunology and upper respiratory tract infections. *International Journal of Sports Medicine, 18,* S69-S77.

Pyne, D.B., & Gleeson, M. (1998). Effects of intensive exercise training on immunity in athletes. *International Journal of Sports Medicine, 19*(Suppl. 3), S183-S194.

Pyne, D.B., McDonald, W.A., Gleeson, M., Flanagan, A., Clancy, R.L., & Fricker, P.A. (2001). Mucosal immunity, respiratory illness and competitive performance in elite swimmers. *Medicine and Science in Sport and Exercise, 33,* 348-353.

Roberts, D., & Smith, D.J. (1992). Training at moderate altitude: Iron status of elite male swimmers. *Journal of Laboratory and Clinical Medicine, 120,* 387-391.

Rowbottom, D.G., Keast, D., & Goodman, C. (1995). The haematological, biochemical and immunological profile of athletes suffering from the overtraining syndrome. *European Journal of Applied Physiology, 70,* 502-509.

Rusko, H.K., Härkönen, M., & Pakarinen, A. (1994). Overtraining effects on hormonal and autonomic regulation in young cross-country skiers. *Medicine and Science in Sports and Exercise, 26*(5), S64.

Schnabel, A., Kindermann, W., Schmitt, W.M., Biro, G., & Stegmann, H. (1982). Hormonal and metabolic consequences of prolonged running at the individual anaerobic threshold. *International Journal of Sports Medicine, 3*(3), 163-168.

Seiler, S. (1997). *Endurance training theory—Norwegian style.* Retrieved June 20, 2001, from http://home.hia.no/~stephens/-xctheory.htm

Shephard, R.J., & Shek, P.N. (1995). Heavy exercise, nutrition and immune function: Is there a connection? *International Journal of Sports Medicine, 16,* 491-497.

Shephard, R.J., & Shek, P.N. (1998). Acute and chronic over-exertion: Do depressed immune responses provide useful markers? *International Journal of Sports Medicine, 19,* 159-171.

Smith, D.J., & Norris, S.R. (2000a). Building a sport science program. *Coaches Report, 6*(4), 19-21.

Smith, D.J., & Norris, S.R. (2000b). Changes in glutamine and glutamate concentrations for tracking training tolerance in elite athletes. *Medicine and Science in Sports and Exercise, 32,* 684-689.

Steinhaus, A.H. (1933). Chronic effects of exercise. *Physiological Reviews, 13,* 103-147.

Stray-Gundersen, J., Videman, T., & Snell, P.G. (1986). Changes in selected objective parameters during overtraining [abstract]. *Medicine and Science in Sports and Exercise, 18*(Suppl.), 54-55.

Tharp, G.D., & Barnes, M.W. (1990). Reduction of salivary immunoglobulin levels by swim training. *European Journal of Applied Physiology, 60,* 61-64.

Tomasi, T.B., Trudeau, F.B., Czerwinski, D., & Erredge, S. (1982). Immune parameters in athletes before and after strenuous exercise. *Journal of Clinical Immunology, 2,* 173-178.

Urhausen, A., Gabriel, H., & Kindermann, W. (1995). Blood hormones as markers of training stress and overtraining. *Sports Medicine, 20,* 251-276.

Urhausen, A., & Kindermann, W. (2000). Aktuelle Marker für die Diagnostik von Überlastungszuständen in der Trainingspraxis [Current markers for the diagnosis of overtraining syndrome in the practice of training]. *Deutsche Zeitscrift für Sportmedizin, 5,* 226-233.

Viru, A. (1995). *Adaptation in sports training.* Boca Raton, FL: CRC Press.

Walsh, N.P., Blannin, A.K., Robson, P.J., & Gleeson, M. (1998). Glutamine, exercise and immune function. Links and possible mechanisms. *Sports Medicine, 26*(3), 177-191.

Weight, L.M. (1993). "Sports anaemia"—Does it exist? *Sports Medicine, 16*(1), 1-4.

Woodson, R.D., Willis, R.E., & Lenfant, C. (1978). Effect of acute and established anemia on O_2 transport at rest, submaximal and maximal work. *Journal of Applied Physiology, 44,* 36-43.

Zatsiorsky, V.M. (1995). *Science and practice of strength training.* Champaign, IL: Human Kinetics.

Steinacker, J.M., & Lehmann, M. (2002). Clinical findings and mechanisms of stress and recovery in athletes. In M. Kellmann (Ed.), *Enhancing recovery: Preventing underperformance in athletes* (pp. 103-118). Champaign, IL: Human Kinetics.

6

Clinical Findings and Mechanisms of Stress and Recovery in Athletes

Jürgen M. Steinacker and Manfred Lehmann

Athletic training consists of repetitive phases of normal training, high-load training, overload training, overreaching, and recovery. During a training program, training load—defined by the intensity, duration, and frequency of exercise—varies and should gradually increase in response to the training-induced adaptation of various physical systems. This increase in training load is necessary to ensure further responses to a training program.

Coaches often organize training in alternating cycles of increasing training load and enhancing regeneration. Such training cycles, which are relatively safe, allow the training load to reach a high, sustainable level for a short time. During the process (which is called supercompensation, or reaching) the exhaustion and fatigue resulting from the high-load training phases elicits corresponding cellular stresses and consecutively raises performance in the recovery phases as an adaptation to the training overload.

Overreaching, defined as short-term overtraining that can be compensated by adequate recovery, is associated with typical cellular (e.g., molecular, biochemical, and regulatory) findings, which are discussed in this chapter. Recovery should be closely matched with the type, intensity, and duration of previous training phases. Prolonged recovery can lead to a loss of performance, which is also called detraining (Banister, Morton, & Clarke, 1997; Budgett, 1998; Lehmann et al., 1992; Lehmann et al., 1997; Steinacker, Lormes, Lehmann, & Altenburg, 1998). Perfor-

mance incompetence, or underperformance, can also result from prolonged recovery, as it can from insufficient recovery. In a successful training program, performance should increase in the long term (Banister et al., 1997; Budgett, 1998; Fry, Morton, & Keast, 1992; Lehmann et al., 1992; Lehmann et al., 1997; Steinacker et al., 1998).

If the process of overreaching is adjusted to allow the athlete to attain the highest sustainable training loads and maximum progress in performance, the risk of overload of various molecular, biochemical, and regulatory mechanisms is increased. This may lead to disturbance of well-being, illness, and underperformance.

Overtraining is long-lasting performance incompetence due to an imbalance of sport-specific and nonsport-specific stressors and recovery with typical cellular adaptations and responses, which are discussed later in this chapter. From a clinical standpoint, performance incompetence is the key symptom of overtraining, the explanation of which is one of the most demanding tasks in athletic medicine (Lehmann et al., 1997; Lehmann, Gastmann, et al., 1999; Lehmann, Foster, Gastmann, Keizer, & Steinacker, 1999; Uusitalo, 2001). Besides performance incompetence, many other clinical problems may arise as a result of overtraining, including sports injuries, infections, or mood disturbances such as fatigue or depression.

Understanding the mechanisms of overreaching, overtraining, and recovery will help to enhance the efficiency of training and will help to

103

avoid overtraining and long-term staleness in athletes. In this chapter we will address the possibilities of new therapeutic approaches and the biological effects of regeneration processes, recovery, and detraining.

Model of a Biphasic Response to Overreaching and Overtraining

Israel (1986) classified the stress response as sympathetic or parasympathetic. The sympathetic type was defined as a general activity of all stress systems (e.g., metabolic, humoral, neural, mental) with increased sympathetic activity and symptoms such as palpitations, increased heart rate, sleep disturbances, and agitation. The parasympathetic type of stress response was defined as low activity of all stress systems, manifesting physiologically as exhaustion or psychologically as "burnout." However, there is no clear evidence for such clearly distinguished types of reaction to training and overtraining (Kuipers & Keizer, 1988; Lehmann, Foster, & Keul, 1993).

We proposed a model of a biphasic response to overload involving predominantly peripheral mechanisms (in the early phases of overload) and more central mechanisms (in more pronounced phases of overload and overtraining; Lehmann et al., 1997; Lehmann, Foster, et al.,

1999; Lehmann, Gastmann, et al., 1999; Steinacker et al., 1998). The balance of stress (training-specific, psychological, and nonspecific) and recovery determines the outcome of a given training situation (see figure 6.1).

The peripheral mechanisms, listed here, are normal results of the training process:

- Training myopathy
- Mild adrenal insufficiency
- Metabolic deficits
- Hematological deficits
- Peripheral hormonal deficits
- Immunological findings

Central mechanisms are as follows:

- Decreases in motoneuron activity
- Depressed hypothalamic-pituitary-hormonal axes
- Depressed hypothalamic-sympathoneuronal axis (Lehmann, Gastmann, et al., 1999)

Most clinical problems are observed in training with a high metabolic load of more than 4,000 kilocalories per day. Training with lower metabolic demands may also result in performance incompetence and clinical symptoms; however, these problems result mainly from nonmetabolic causes rather than sport-specific stressors and incomplete recovery.

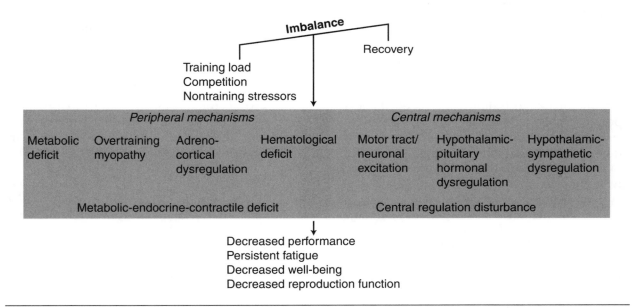

Figure 6.1 Balance between stress and recovery and the underlying pathophysiological mechanisms.

After Lehmann, Gastmann, et al., 1999.

The hypothalamus acts as a central integrator of all afferent signals to the brain and has an important role in the regulation of the central responses to stress and training. This integration involves information of neural, humoral, and autonomic nervous system afferents; direct metabolic effects; hormones and cytokines; and information from higher brain centers. We propose that studying the hypothalamic regulation will provide important clinical information in this processes (see figure 6.2). High information load on the hypothalamus during acute or chronic stress will activate excitatory neurons in the hypothalamic network (Baskin, Breininger, & Schwartz, 1999; Schwartz, Seeley, Campfield, Burn, & Baskin, 1996). This hypothalamic activation may then be related to effects on all efferents—autonomic nervous system, hormonal system, and motoneurons. The effects are likely to be more stimulating under conditions of acute stress and more inhibiting under conditions of chronic stress, overreaching, and overtraining (Lehmann et al., 1997; Lehmann, Gastmann, et al., 1999).

Metabolic-acting cytokines such as leptin or hormones such as insulin may provide a tissue signal of energy deprivation to the hypothalamus (Naveilhan et al., 1999; Wang, Liu, Hawkins, Barzilai, & Rossetti, 1998). The energy homeostasis of the adipose and muscle tissue is therefore linked to the hypothalamus, and consecutively, to sympathetic activity, hypothalamo-sympathoneuronal and hypothalamo-hypothalamic-pituitary axes, and the metabolism-dependent links of cell differentiation and cell growth involving adipo-hepatic links (Boden, Chen, Mozzoli, & Ryan, 1996; Considine & Caro, 1999; Heini et al., 1998; Steinacker, Lormes, Lui, et al., 2000). Local inflammatory cytokines such as tumor necrosis factor (TNF) and interleukin-1 (IL-1) have systemic effects and may be responsible for some symptoms of overtraining (Smith, 2000); interleukin-6 (IL-6) may act as a muscular cytokine (Nieman & Pedersen, 1999; Ostrowski, Rohde, Asp, Schjerling, & Pedersen, 1999; Ostrowski, Rohde, Zacho, Asp, & Pedersen, 1998).

Clinical Findings

The rate of various physical complaints rises with increased training load, as do objective clinical problems such as injuries or infections related to the training process. The following are typical clinical symptoms and findings (Kuipers & Keizer, 1988; Lehmann, Foster, et al., 1993; Lehmann, Gastmann, et al., 1999; Uusitalo, 2001):

- Underperformance
  - Maximum performance decreased or unchanged

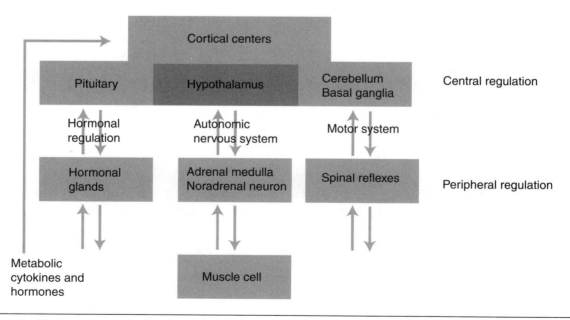

Figure 6.2 The important role of the hypothalamus in the regulation of the central response to training and overload. New peripheral links are proposed from the muscle cell to the other regulatory levels consisting of metabolic-acting cytokines.

- Rate of perceived exertion during submaximal load test increased
- Time to exhaustion during a constant load test decreased
- Mood and psychological parameters
  - Fatigue
  - Disturbances of mood and behavior
  - Psychosomatic or vegetative complaints (drowsiness, loss of appetite, palpitations, sweating)
  - Disturbance of sleep
- Muscle findings
  - Muscle weakness
  - Soreness, stiffness
- Cardiovascular findings
  - Increase or decrease of heart rate during exercise
  - Decreased heart rate variability
- Other findings
  - Increased rate of infections
  - Weight loss
  - Anorexia
  - Ammenorhea, decreased sexual function

These symptoms and findings can be monitored by the coach or a team doctor by interview, monitored by the athlete in a training log, or evaluated in a standardized questionnaire (see the following sections and Kellmann, this volume, chapter 3). The monitoring of clinical symptoms with one of these methods is essential for a successful training program. The documentation of the training by the athlete should contain information about volume and intensity of training, the aims and the achieved goals (times, speed, repetitions, etc.), and the time lag between training sessions. Training monotony is an independent risk factor for overtraining (Foster, 1998).

Infections and other medical illnesses are uncertain indicators of high training loads. In a five-week training camp of the German National Junior Rowing Team (1996), the male rowers showed a clear peak in visits to the doctor in the period with the highest training load (see table 6.1). These findings match those of previous studies that reported an increase of symptoms with increased training load (Nieman et al., 2000; Steinacker et al., 1999). However, in the phase with increased visits to the doctor, clearly no overload or overreaching situation was attained. In this study, the percentage of visits due to bacterial or viral infections varied between 12% and 47%, which is relatively high for a normal, healthy population. Although this infection rate can be related to the training load, other nontraining-dependent factors have to be considered, such as exposure to virulent agents (which can be high in the close-quarter conditions of a training camp), hygienic/sanitary conditions, and weather conditions.

Clinically Relevant Parameters of Stress and Regeneration

An athlete's complaints or clinical symptoms may give important information about his current status and level of stress and recovery. However, these complaints and symptoms are indirect signs and not specific (Lehmann, Foster, et al., 1999). Therefore, many parameters have been examined for their validity and relevance to the diagnosis of the recovery-stress status of an athlete (Lehmann, Foster, et al. 1999; Kuipers & Keizer, 1988; Steinacker, Lormes, Kellmann, et al., 2000; Uusitalo, 2001). In this chapter, selected clinically valid parameters are discussed.

Table 6.1   Total Number of Visits of the Male Rowers to the Doctor in the Training Period Before the Junior World Championships 1996 (n = 30)

Training phase	1 Preparation	2 Strength training	3 Intensive training	4 Tapering	5 Tapering
Total	8	28	13	19	12
Infection	1	11	4	9	5
Muscle/orthopedic	3	3	5	4	5
Other	4	11	4	7	1

Performance

Since improvement of physical performance is the specific goal of training, performance is the most important parameter for monitoring training adaptation. Changes in performance capacity can be analyzed during "all-out" exercise tests (over various distances or during ergometer tests). Maximum performance (Pmax) during a standardized test is therefore the gold standard for evaluating exercise capacity and monitoring training (Lehmann, Foster, et al., 1999; Lehmann et al., 1997). However, Pmax in a full-distance test is often subject to the athlete's present state of motivation and thus may not be sensitive enough for monitoring a complete training and competition season. Therefore, maximum underdistance tests may be useful (Steinacker, Lormes, Kellmann, et al., 2000); submaximum tests are generally not useful since they often give wrong predictions (Uusitalo, 2001).

We examined the rowing speed for the 2,000-meter total race distance as the performance parameter in the period before and during the Junior World Rowing Championships in 1995. Boat speed was slowest during the high-volume/high-intensity training phase, and fastest after the tapering period and at the World Championships (Steinacker et al., 1999; Steinacker, Lormes, Kellmann, et al., 2000). The importance of Pmax was also addressed in other studies. A decrease in performance was observed in recreational athletes after 7 to 10 successive days of unaccustomed prolonged training (Dressendorfer & Wade, 1991; Dressendorfer, Wade, Claybaugh, Cucinell, & Timmis, 1991). In swimmers, performance decreased after 10 days of intensified swimming training (Costill et al., 1991), and in cyclists, after 14 days of intensive training (Jeukendrup, Hesselink, Snyder, Kuipers, & Keizer, 1992). Decreased performance was followed by supercompensation after one to two weeks of recovery (Costill et al., 1991; Jeukendrup et al., 1992). Increases in training volume are generally considered to be more critical than increases in training intensity at moderate total training load (Lehmann et al., 1997; Steinacker et al., 1998).

In conclusion, performance is the gold standard parameter for the training and overtraining reaction and can be practically determined as maximum peak power, speed, or time for a race distance or underdistance, or time to exhaustion for a given speed or power. Submaximal tests are not recommended. Recovery can be indirectly assessed by monitoring the regain in performance after the recovery process.

Training Myopathy

Mammalian skeletal muscle tissue is highly heterogeneous. In fact, muscle fibers are composed of a series of contractile proteins with different molecular and biochemical characteristics that enable the muscles to fulfill a variety of functional demands. Fibers can be classified according to their contracting speed in slow and fast muscles. Furthermore, subgroups of fibers can be identified according to histochemical analysis, and it has been shown that myosin heavy chain (MyHC) isoforms represent this characteristic. However, more than one single isoform may exist in a single fiber (Pette & Staron, 1997; Termin, Staron, & Pette, 1989; Wada, Hämälainen, & Pette, 1995). Since MyHC content determines the metabolic and contractile properties of muscle fibers, understanding the changes of MyHC isoforms in the skeletal muscles of athletes may provide meaningful information about the functional state of the muscles. There is a close relation between functional variables and muscle morphology and biochemistry. Fast-type fibers (type II) are less efficient than slow-type fibers (type I), and they are more vulnerable to stress and energy deprivation (Pette & Staron, 1997).

The dominant phenotype of a muscle fiber is defined by predisposition, function, and neuronal innervation. However, fiber types are not unchangeable, but dynamic. Transition of muscle fiber type caused by changes in MyHC isoforms may take place depending on muscular adaptation. Many factors, including energy metabolism, blood flow, and exercise load, influence the MyHC isoforms and may thereby cause a transition of muscle fiber types due to changes in the content of MyHC II and MyHC I (Jaschinski, Schuler, Peuker, & Pette, 1998; Pette & Staron, 1997; Termin et al., 1989).

Type I fibers have a relatively higher efficiency of contraction than type II fibers (Bottinelli, Betto, Schiffiano, & Reggiani, 1994; Pette & Staron, 1997). Electrostimulation, training, and mechanical overload will lead to decreased cellular energy content and accordingly to increased expression of MyHC I and decreased expression of MyHC II fibers; in other words, there is a loss of type II fibers (Apoptosis of fibers; Podhorska-Okolow et al., 1998). Detraining, muscle disuse, and immobilization may lead to atrophic changes of muscle, but they may also lead to muscle fiber transition from type I to type II and respective changes in muscle fiber composition, for example, MyHC isoforms. Therefore, the expression of muscle fiber types depends on neuromuscular activity and cellular energy content (for a review, see Pette & Staron, 1997).

When metabolism is stressed and muscle and liver glycogen are deprived, as during acute exercise, the hormonal reaction involves hypercorticism and hypoinsulinism and, in the long term, deprivation of the hypothalamic-pituitary-adrenocortical (HPA) axis as discussed later. Furthermore, in the long term, peripheral thyroidal hormone levels, growth hormone (GH) levels, and levels of insulinlike growth factor-I all decrease. All of these hormonal effects together will cause a shift in expression of MyHC and other proteins in the direction of slow isoforms and will lead to the expression of slow-type fibers (Atalay, Seene, Hanninen, & Sen, 1996). Overtraining myopathy results from these metabolic and hormonal changes and may be diagnosed in muscle biopsies by a shift to slow-type myosins and decreased numbers and area of fast-type fibers. The athlete will experience these morphological changes as loss of sprinting and strength capabilities.

Heat-shock proteins are increased in muscle possibly as molecular chaperones. A single bout of exercise leads to the induction of heat-shock protein 70 (HSP70) transcription but not of effective protein production. Protein production rate is high after a week of training and peaks after approximately two weeks (Liu et al., 1999). High-intensity training leads to an induction of HSP70, while low-intensity endurance training does not. It can be concluded that HSP70 response to training is dependent on exercise intensity rather than exercise volume (Liu et al., 2000). Further studies are needed in order to determine whether the accumulation of heat-shock proteins is protective, indicates a training response, or is related to trainability or stress stability.

Biochemical values are often used to monitor muscular training load. Increases in serum creatine kinase (CK) activity at the beginning of a training cycle primarily reflect muscular damage, whereas normalization of CK activity during training reflects the muscular adaptation during that training cycle (see figure 6.3). Myoglobin levels will also reflect muscular damage, although the change in myoglobin levels seems to be faster than that of CK. Serum uric acid concentration can be used as an indicator of a lactic anaerobic load due to accumulation of adenosine monophosphate, which increases with weight training and sprint training in rowing. Since both parameters are less specific for detecting an overreaching or overtraining situation, they are instead used for analysis of the actual training load (Steinacker, 1993).

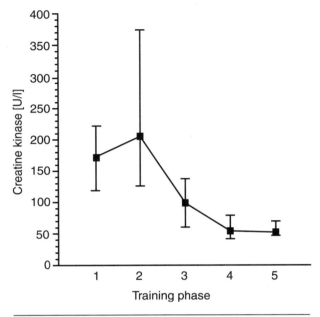

Figure 6.3 Creatine kinase during the training camp of the German Junior National Team 1996, at the beginning (1), and after training phases of approximately one week (2-5). Phases 2 and 3 are high-volume training phases, phase 4 is a tapering phase, and phase 5 is the training before the heats of the World Championships. [Median values and the interquartile range (25-75%)]

Adapted from Steinacker et al., 1999.

Hormonal Indices of Overreaching and Overtraining

Physical training and athletic performance are linked to, among others things, adaptations of tissue metabolism, somatic growth, body composition, and organ function. During prolonged heavy training periods muscle and liver glycogen stores are deprived. Correspondingly, the hormonal reaction involves hypercorticism and hypoinsulinism during acute exercise and the deprivation of the HPA axis and hypoinsulinism over the long term (Gastmann et al., 1998; Lehmann, Gastmann, et al., 1999). A similarity with the catabolic effects of calorie restriction is striking (Argente et al., 1997; Jenkins et al., 1993; Laughlin & Yen, 1996). The hypothalamic downregulation in overreaching and overtraining was first described by Lehmann and Barron, who observed that insulin-dependent hypoglycemia or corticotropin-releasing hormone (CRH) went along with a lower ACTH and/or cortisol response in the state of overtraining (Barron, Noakes, Levy, Smith, & Millar, 1985; Lehmann, Knizia, et al., 1993).

The HPA axis is biphasic regulated in the sense that (1) acute stress and high metabolic load during an overreaching training will lead to activation of the CRH-ACTH response and to a moderate adrenal desensitization, which means less cortisol response in relation to ACTH levels, and (2) chronic stress and overtraining will lead to central and peripheral downregulation (Lehmann et al., 1997). Therefore, basal cortisol levels may be used to analyze the effects of training (Steinacker, Lormes, Kellmann, et al., 2000). At an early stage during the 1996 training camp, when training load was highest, basal cortisol levels increased by 18% and decreased slightly afterwards (see figure 6.4). Increases in basal cortisol levels are indicative of a metabolic problem (e.g., glycogen deficiency) or of increased training-dependent stress (Lehmann, Knizia, et al., 1997). A common metabolic cause can be seen in glycogen depletion with increased counterregulatory activity of hormones such as cortisol, growth hormone, and catecholamines. Elevated basal cortisol levels are often seen as a normal stress response to high-intensity training, whereas decreased basal cortisol levels and decreased pituitary-adrenocortical responsiveness are a late sign of overreaching or overtraining (Lehmann, Knizia, et al., 1993). As discussed earlier, basal cortisol levels reflect an endpoint of the hypothalamic-pituitary-adrenocortical axis. Testing the axis with functional tests will give much more information, but they are time consuming, costly, and stressful for athletes (Kuipers & Keizer, 1988; Lehmann, Foster, et al., 1999).

The somatotropic growth hormone (GH)–insulinlike growth factor-I (IGF-I) axis is also involved in this hormonal regulation. The pulsatile pattern of GH is stimulated, and levels of GH rise by acute prolonged exercise (Fry & Kraemer, 1997; Kanaley et al., 1997). IGF-I levels increase, consecutively, after one to two weeks of training with moderate intensity and positive caloric balance (Engfred et al., 1994; Roelen et al., 1997; Roemmich & Sinning, 1997; Snyder, Clemmons, & Underwood, 1989) and decrease more profoundly when training is exhausting and catabolic mechanisms are predominant (Koistinen, Koistinen, Selenius, Ylikorkala, & Seppala, 1996). During prolonged exhausting training, the pulsatility of GH and IGF-I levels decrease simultaneously (Eliakim, Brasel, Mohan, Wong, & Cooper, 1998; Schmidt et al., 1995). Some researchers have found that depression of the GH–IGF-I axis is a common finding during overreaching. The effects are related to downregulation of the HPA axis (Barron et al., 1985; Steinacker et al., 1998). Furthermore, downregulation of the thyroid and gonadotropic axes will be observed (Lehmann et al., 1997).

Leptin as an adipocyte-derived hormone is involved in the hypothalamic regulation of appetite, thermogenesis, and metabolism (Friedman et al., 1997; Heiman et al., 1997). Leptin depresses the excitatory transmitter neuropeptide Y (NPY) expression in hypothalamic neurons (Carro et al., 1998). NPY neurons are activated by fasting and express leptin receptors to a high degree (Baskin et al., 1999; Schwartz et al., 1996). Increased NPY levels increase hypothalamic neuronal activity and therefore depress the HPA axis as described previously. Therefore, leptin is an example of a tissue hormone that directly impacts the hypothalamic regulation and provides information about the metabolic state to other tissues such as beta cells or liver cells. Whether leptin has the potential to be a marker for overreaching or overtraining has to be clarified in prospective studies.

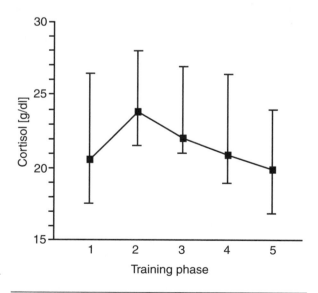

Figure 6.4 Resting morning cortisol concentrations at the beginning of a 1996 training camp (1) and after the training phases (2-5); 5 is before the World Championships. [Median values and the interquartile range (25-75%)] For further explanation, see figure 6.3.

Adapted from Steinacker et al., 1999.

Increased intrinsic sympathetic activity may be found in the early phase of heavy training (according to the previously mentioned classical model). This increase in sympathetic activity can be considered an adaptive regulatory process. However, if hypothalamic depression is more profound, intrinsic sympathetic activity decreases as indicated by decreased nocturnal catecholamine excretion and peripheral beta-receptor downregulation with compensatory increased plasma noradrenaline but ineffective catecholamine response (Lehmann, Foster, Dickhuth, & Gastmann, 1998; Wittert, Livesey, Espiner, & Donald, 1996). The excretion of free catecholamines during overnight rest can be seen as the basal renal (urinary) catecholamine excretion reflecting the intrinsic activity or tone of the sympathetic nervous system, as activating mechanisms are clearly reduced during night rest. Because noradrenaline concentrations in plasma and in cerebrospinal fluid are quite similar, circulating and excreted noradrenaline may also reflect the neuronal noradrenaline release in the brain. In overreaching and overtraining, resting and submaximal plasma noradrenaline concentrations might increase and beta-adrenoreceptor density might decrease (Jost, Weiss, & Weicker, 1990; Lehmann, Schmid, & Keul, 1984; see also figure 6.5). Downregulation of the intrinsic sympathetic nervous system activity is a late finding in

overtrained athletes and may be related to symptoms of fatigue (Lehmann et al., 1998). There is also indication of desensitization of the motoric end plate (for an overview, see Lehmann, Gastmann, et al., 1999). These findings are related to the subjective feeling of some overtrained athletes that their muscles are not responding normally and that they are experiencing peripheral weakness.

Immunological Findings

The immune system is closely related to the previously described central mechanisms in that it is influenced by sympathetic activity and hormones such as cortisol. In general, the status of the immune system is not very different between athletes and nonathletes, and the immune system is not much affected by regular athletic training. Natural killer cell activity tends to be enhanced, while neutrophil function is suppressed in response to training in athletes and nonathletes (Pedersen & Hoffman-Goetz, 2000) .

A commonly held belief is that regular physical activity may be beneficial in decreasing the risk of upper respiratory tract infections. Only a few studies have been undertaken in this field, and none are very substantial. However, there is indication that the positive effects of regular physical activity on immune function are mainly related to moderate intensities, whereas high training loads will increase the risk of infections. A J-shaped curve is proposed between the rate of upper respiratory tract infections and training load (see figure 6.6; Nieman et al., 2000; Pedersen & Hoffman-Goetz, 2000).

Reseachers have proposed that prolonged (exhaustive) endurance exercise leads to transient, but clinically significant, alterations in immune function, which are reflected by the upper range of the J-curve in figure 6.6. This altered immune function (persisting for 3-72 hours) may allow viruses and bacteria to enter the respiratory tract and to increase the risk of clinical and subclinical infections (Nieman et al., 2000). This depression of the immune function can be demonstrated, for example, for the overall cell-mediated hypersensitivity response, which is delayed in athletes after competing in a strenuous half-ironman triathlon race compared to resting triathletes and nonathletic controls (see figure 6.7; Bruunsgaard, Galbo, et al., 1997). This effect is related to the acute exercise response that includes hypercorticism, hypoinsulinism, and

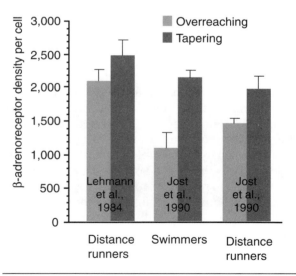

Figure 6.5 Downregulation of beta-adrenoreceptor density (quantitatively measured on granulocytes) after prolonged exhaustive training and overtraining and after recovery in distance runners and swimmers.

Data modified from Jost et al., 1990; Lehmann et al., 1984.

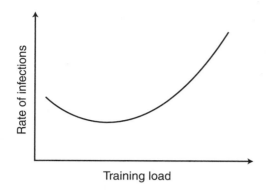

Figure 6.6 Proposed J-curve between rate of upper respiratory tract infections and training load. With moderate training load, infections may decrease; however, with high-volume and exhaustive training loads, rates of infection exceed those of nonathletic, sedentary persons.

After Nieman and Pedersen, 1999.

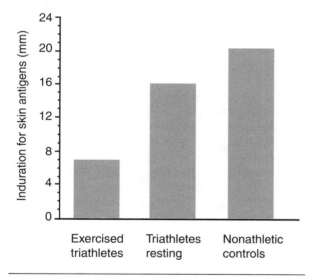

Figure 6.7 Skin-test response to recall antigens in 22 male triathletes 48 hours after competing compared with 11 nonexercising athletes and 22 controls. Reduced delayed-type hypersensitivity response in the exercised athletes compared to the other groups.

Adapted from Bruunsgaard, Galbo, et al., 1997.

sympathoadrenergic activation (Lehmann et al., 1992, 1997; Nieman et al., 2000). Close links clearly exist among the neuroendocrinological changes due to overload described earlier, the hypothalamic network, sympathetic activity, and the immune function (see figure 6.2, p. 105; Pedersen & Hoffman-Goetz, 2000; Pedersen, Rohde, & Zacho, 1996). During endurance exercise, proinflammatory cytokine production is downregulated and

anti-inflammatory cytokines such as interleukin-1 receptor-antagonist IL-1ra are upregulated as well as interleukin-6 (IL-6; Drenth et al., 1995; Nieman et al., 2000; Rohde, MacLean, Richter, Kiens, & Pedersen, 1997). Strenuous intensive exercise induces increases in the proinflammatory cytokines TNF alpha and IL-1 beta, as well as in IL-6. This is counterbalanced by cytokine inhibitors (IL-1ra, sTNF-r1, and sTNF-r2) and the anti-inflammatory cytokine IL-10 (Ostrowski et al., 1999).

What are the causes of these dramatic changes, and are they relevant to the clinical picture of overreaching and overtraining? There is indication that the hypothalamus contains receptors for several cytokines so that cytokines may impact the hypothalamic neuronal network (Nieman et al., 2000). Local inflammatory cytokines such as TNF-α have clear effects if they enter the circulation and may be responsible for some of the symptoms of overtraining (Smith, 2000). The systemic spillover of TNF-α marks the failure of local compensation mechanisms. Local inflammation reactions may be induced by muscle cell apoptosis or necrosis, by activated macrophages, and by inflammatory cytokines (Bruunsgaard, Hartkopp, et al., 1997; Podhorska-Okolow et al., 1998). Cytokines that act on peripheral and central organs, such IL-6 or IL-1, may have additional messenger functions (Nieman & Pedersen, 1999; Ostrowski et al., 1998, 1999; Pedersen & Hoffman-Goetz, 2000).

Carbohydrate supplementation during prolonged exercise will diminish the counter-regulatory activity of glucostatic hormones such as cortisol, growth hormone, and catecholamines (Lehmann et al., 1992, 1997). After exhaustive exercise with carbohydrate supplementation, cytokine levels are lower indicating lower metabolic stress, which is demonstrated in figure 6.8, a and b (Nehlsen-Cannarella et al., 1997; Nieman et al., 2000). Researchers have yet to investigate whether this decrease in cytokines is indicating a lower stress for the immune system and will result in lower rates of upper respiratory tract infections (Nieman et al., 2000).

How is the immune function measured in an athletic setting? In a study of swimmers salivary immune globuline A (IgA) levels correlated with the rate of infections, indicating that salivary IgA may be a potential marker of infection risk (Gleeson et al., 1995). However, until now, no really reliable markers are available related to the infection rate (Nieman et al., 2000).

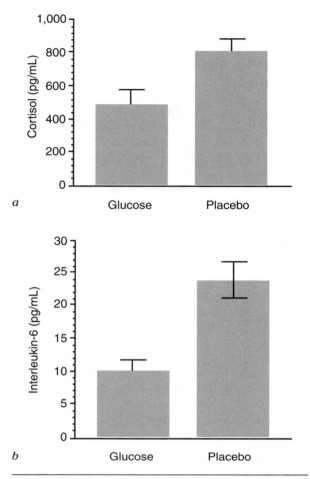

a — Glucose / Placebo (upper panel)

b — Glucose / Placebo (lower panel)

Figure 6.8 Plasma cortisol levels *(a)* and interleukin-6 expression *(b)* postexercise after 2.5 hours of cycling either with carbohydrate supplementation or with placebo.

Adapted from Nieman et al., 2000.

Mood State and Psychological Monitoring of Training Load

Monitoring athletes' mood states has also been introduced to rowing training. The Recovery-Stress Questionnaire for Athletes (RESTQ-Sport; Kellmann & Kallus, 2001) can be used to quantitatively measure the actual level of current stress imposed on athletes. A dose-response relationship was demonstrated among training load, performance ability, and physical components of stress and recovery in rowers (Kellmann, Altenburg, Lormes, & Steinacker, 2001; Kellmann

& Günther, 2000; Kellmann, Kallus, Günther, Lormes, & Steinacker, 1997).

A different approach is to monitor symptoms associated with overtraining and staleness (Hooper, Mackinnon, Howard, Gordon, & Bachmann, 1995; Morgan, Brown, Raglin, O'Connor, & Ellickson, 1987). Monitoring the current levels of both stress and recovery has the possible advantage of detecting problems before symptoms of overtraining and staleness (e.g., drowsiness, apathy, fatigue, irritability) appear. However, stress and recovery are often different in their time course. Figure 6.9, a and b, demonstrates data from a 1996 rowing training camp. The scores for *Physical Complaints* increased early and decreased afterwards with adaptation. The scores for *Fatigue* rose from low levels during the first two weeks to peak during the third week; they were at their lowest approaching the World Championships. In contrast to the scores for *Fatigue* and *Physical Complaints,* the scores for *General Stress* were low and quite stable during the training camp, with a small increase at the beginning and a decrease before the preliminary heats.

The changes in the recovery scales were also not uniform. No relevant changes are shown early except in the *Physical Recovery* score, which somewhat matches the stress score *Physical Complaints.* The scores of *General Well-Being* and *Social Recovery* show the lowest values at the fourth measurement and a small increase at time 5; however, basal values are not attained again. In general, recovery can be considered to be inadequate in this training camp. The interpretation of the indices of stress and recovery before the finals indicated low levels of stress but incomplete recovery. This is in accordance with the cortisol data shown in figure 6.4 (p. 109).

The relationship between psychological scales and physiological or biochemical parameters is not necessarily linear. For example, a U-shaped relationship is said to exist between specific fatigue ratings and sympathetic tone (e.g., basal noradrenaline excretion). That means that fatigue ratings are high during periods of (1) low sympathetic drive due to exhaustion of the sympathoneuroadrenergic system and (2) high sympathetic drive due to overstimulation of the sympathoneuroadrenergic system (with already decreased peripheral receptors).

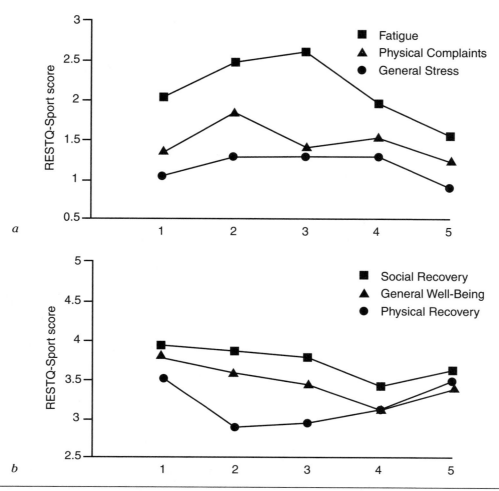

Figure 6.9   Results of the Recovery-Stress Questionnaire for Athletes (RESTQ-Sport) at the beginning of a training camp 1996 (1) and after the training phases (2-4); 5 is before the World Championships. Stress scales: *Fatigue, Physical Complaints, General Stress (a)*. Recovery scales: *Social Recovery, General Well-Being, Physical Recovery (b)*. Mean values, *n* = 20.

Adapted from Steinacker et al., 1999.

Summarized Approach to an Integrative Analysis of Training

The diagnosis of training adaptation and the clinical state of an athlete is a complex task. However, the underlying mechanisms are more and more understood, so that specific diagnostic tools can be used sufficiently for monitoring training. It is also evident that only a few parameters are reliable and specific enough. Therefore, there is a need for studies that evaluate further the prospective power of different variables for the diagnosis of overtraining.

Performance is the key parameter for analysis of the adaptive state of an athlete to a training program. Underperformance or performance incompetence is the key symptom of overreaching or overtraining and can be specifically tested using sport-specific performance tests (Lehmann, Foster, et al., 1993; Lehmann, Gastmann, et al., 1999; Steinacker, Lormes, Kellmann, et al., 2000).

Muscle function tests are not often included in the diagnostic process. Contraction mode is decreased in the overtrained state and is restored in recovery, as is neuromuscular excitability (Lehmann, Foster, et al., 1999). The parameters of MyHC and HSP70 are currently under investigation and need further evaluation (Liu et al., 1999, 2000; Lehmann, Gastmann, et al., 1999; Pette & Staron, 1997).

Nocturnal (basal) noradrenaline excretion is specific for the basal sympathetic tone and activation of the autonomic nervous system. Other more practically obtained variables, such as morning resting heart rate or heart rate variability, are often used as estimates of sympathetic activity, but these methods are of very limited value (Jost et al., 1990; Lehmann et al., 1992; Wittert et al., 1996).

The highest number of physical complaints corresponds with the highest training load in the different training studies, for example, of the effect of strength training. These complaints are not related to signs of overtraining. CK activity and myoglobin levels are elevated as a sign of muscle damage. In the data presented in figure 6.9, a and b, CK levels, as well as physical complaints, had already decreased when the *Fatigue* score increased. Therefore, CK is not a good predictor of overtraining and stress but may be used along with uric acid as an indicator of the acute load and damage (Lehmann, Gastmann, et al., 1999; Steinacker et al., 1998; Steinacker, Lormes, Kellmann, et al., 2000).

Metabolic strain is reflected in cortisol and insulin levels (Lehmann, Gastmann, et al., 1999). As discussed earlier, basal cortisol and insulin levels decrease when glycogen stores start to become depleted. However, acute stress of either physical or psychological origin will first elevate basal cortisol levels. With ongoing stress, cortisol will decrease as a sign of exhaustion from a decrease of sensitivity of the adrenals (Barron et al., 1985; Lehmann, Knizia, et al., 1993; Steinacker, Lormes, Kellmann, et al., 2000). Therefore, cortisol levels are difficult to interpret, and both absolute values and the time course should be considered. Practically, a decrease in cortisol levels and increase in fatigue-related symptoms indicate a high risk of exhaustion/overtraining, but is also found in normal overreaching cycles. In recovery, basal cortisol levels should normalize along with fatigue ratings (Lehmann, Foster, et al., 1999). Amenorrhea is an indirect sign of overtraining, and depressed pituitary-releasing hormones are a direct sign of overtraining (Laughlin & Yen, 1996). Metabolic state is also related to changes in body weight, which is a simple parameter that can be monitored easily in training.

Other typical neuroendocrinological findings and stress tests described in this chapter may also be used for the diagnosis of overtraining, although many are expensive and time consuming (Nieman & Pedersen, 1999; Pedersen & Hoffman-Goetz, 2000). Other parameters such as some cytokines (TNF-α or IL-6) and leptin may have potential value but need further evaluation.

Fatigue is one of the key findings in stress and overtraining situations, and recovery from these states is indicated by lower levels of fatigue. In general, mood state is correlated to physical performance ability, hormonal parameters, and metabolic data. However, this relation is not always linear, and different scales of questionnaires such as the RESTQ-Sport have different time courses (see also figures 6.3 on p. 108, 6.4 on p. 109, and 6.9, a and b, on p. 113; Kellmann & Kallus, 2001; Morgan et al., 1987).

In an integrative analysis of stress and recovery, this means that prolonged exhaustion, overreaching, or other stressors can be compensated for either by a reduction of these stressors or by an increase in different recovery measures (Lehmann, Gastmann, et al., 1999; Steinacker et al., 1999; Steinacker, Lormes, Kellmann, et al., 2000).

In summary, the clinical diagnosis of an athlete's current state of stress and recovery is possible by checking the clinically relevant parameters. This information may reveal disturbed organ or regulatory systems, however, making the diagnosis more difficult and complicated. Such information may also indicate important hints for therapeutic approaches.

Acknowledgments

We acknowledge the important support from Werner Lormes and Yuefei Liu from our study group and from Dieter Altenburg, head coach of the German National Junior Rowing Team. This work was substantially supported by various grants from the Bundesinstitut für Sportwissenschaft, Cologne, Germany.

References

Argente, J., Caball, N., Barrios, V., Munoz, M.T., Pozo, J., Chowen, J.A., Morande, G., & Hernandez, M. (1997). Multiple endocrine abnormalities of the growth hormone and insulin-like growth factor axis in patients with anorexia nervosa: Effect of short- and long-term weight recuperation. *Journal of Clinical Endocrinology and Metabolism, 82*(7), 2084-2092.

Atalay, M., Seene, T., Hanninen, O., & Sen, C.K. (1996). Skeletal muscle and heart antioxidant defences in response to sprint training. *Acta Physiologica Scandinavia, 158*(2), 129-134.

Banister, E.W., Morton, R.H., & Clarke, J.R. (1997). Clinical dose-response effects of exercise. In J.M. Steinacker & S.A. Ward (Eds.), *The physiology and pathophysiology of exercise tolerance* (pp. 297-309). London/New York: Plenum.

Barron, J.L., Noakes, T.D., Levy, W., Smith, C., & Millar, R.P. (1985). Hypothalamic dysfunction in overtrained athletes. *Journal of Clinical Endocrinology and Metabolism, 60*(4), 803-806.

Baskin, D.G., Breininger, J.F., & Schwartz, M.W. (1999). Leptin receptor mRNA identifies a subpopulation of neuropeptide Y neurons activated by fasting in rat hypothalamus. *Diabetes, 48,* 828-833.

Boden, G., Chen, X., Mozzoli, M., & Ryan, I. (1996). Effect of fasting on serum leptin in normal human subjects. *Journal of Clinical Endocrinology and Metabolism, 81,* 3419-3423.

Bottinelli, R., Betto, R., Schiffiano, S., & Reggiani, C. (1994). Unloaded shortening velocity and myosin heavy chain and alkali light chain composition in rat skeletal muscle. *Journal of Physiology, 478,* 341-349.

Bruunsgaard, H., Galbo, H., Halkjaer-Kristensen, J., Johansen, T.L., MacLean, D.A., & Pedersen, B.K. (1997). Exercise-induced increase in serum interleukin-6 in humans is related to muscle damage. *Journal of Physiology, 499*(Pt. 3), 833-841.

Bruunsgaard, H., Hartkopp, A., Mohr, T., Konradsen, H., Heron, I., Mordhorst, C.H., & Pedersen, B.K. (1997). *In vivo* cell-mediated immunity and vaccination response following prolonged, intensive exercise. *Medicine and Science in Sports and Exercise, 29,* 1176-1181.

Budgett, R. (1998). Fatigue and underperformance in athletes: The overtraining syndrome. *British Journal of Sports Medicine, 32*(2), 107-110.

Carro, E., Seoane, L.M., Senaris, R., Considine, R.V., Casanueva, F.F., & Dieguez, C. (1998). Interaction between leptin and neuropeptide Y on in vivo growth hormone secretion. *Neuroendocrinology, 68*(3), 187-191.

Considine, R.V., & Caro, J.F. (1999). Pleiotropic cellular effects of leptin. *Current Opinion in Endocrinology and Diabetes, 6,* 163-169.

Costill, D.L., Thomas, R., Robergs, R.A., Pascoe, D., Lambert, C., Barr, S., & Fink, W.J. (1991). Adaptations to swimming training: Influence of training volume. *Medicine and Science in Sports and Exercise, 23*(3), 371-377.

Drenth, J.P., Van Uum, S.H., Van Deuren, M., Pesman, G.J., Van der ven Jongekrijg, J., & Van der Meer, J.W. (1995). Endurance run increases circulating IL-6 and IL-1ra but downregulates ex vivo TNF-alpha and IL-1 beta production. *Journal of Applied Physiology, 79*(5), 1497-1503.

Dressendorfer, R.H., & Wade, C.E. (1991). Effects of a 15-d race on plasma steroid levels and leg muscle fitness in runners. *Medicine and Science in Sports and Exercise, 23,* 954-956.

Dressendorfer, R.H., Wade, C.E., Claybaugh, J., Cucinell, S.A., & Timmis, G.C. (1991). Effects of 7 successive days of unaccustomed prolonged exercise on aerobic performance and tissue damage in fitness joggers. *International Journal of Sports Medicine, 12,* 55-61.

Eliakim, A., Brasel, J.A., Mohan, S., Wong, W.L.T., & Cooper, D.M. (1998). Increased physical activity and the growth hormone-IGF-I axis in adolescent males. *American Journal of Physiology, 275*(1, Pt. 2), R308-R314.

Engfred, K., Kjaer, M., Secher, N.H., Friedman, D.B., Hanel, B., Nielsen, O.J., Bach, F.W., Galbo, H., & Levine, B.D. (1994). Hypoxia and training-induced adaptation of hormonal responses to exercise in humans. *European Journal of Applied Physiology, 68*(4), 303-309.

Foster, C. (1998). Monitoring training in athletes with reference to overtraining syndrome. *Medicine and Science in Sports and Exercise, 30* (7), 1164-1168.

Friedman, J.E., Ferrara, C.M., Aulak, K.S., Hatzoglou, M., McCune, S.A., Park, S., & Sherman, W.M. (1997). Exercise training down-regulates ob gene expression in the genetically obese SHHF/Mcc-fa(cp) rat. *Hormonal and Metabolic Research, 29*(5), 214-219.

Fry, A.C., & Kraemer, W.J. (1997). Resistance exercise overtraining and overreaching. Neuroendocrine responses. *Sports Medicine, 23*(2), 106-129.

Fry, R.W., Morton, A.R., Keast, D. (1992). Periodisation and the prevention of overtraining. *Canadian Journal of Sports Science, 17*(3), 241-248.

Gastmann, U., Dimeo, F., Huonker, M., Bocker, J., Steinacker, J.M., Petersen, K.G., Wieland, H., Keul, J., & Lehmann, M. (1998). Ultra-triathlon-related blood-chemical and endocrinological responses in nine athletes. *Journal of Sports Medicine Physical Fitness, 38*(1), 18-23.

Gleeson, M., McDonald, W.A., Cripps, A.W., Pyne, D.B., Clancy, R.L., Fricker, P.A. (1995) The effect on immunity on long-term intensive training in swimmers. *Clinical and Experimental Immunology, 102,* 210-216.

Heiman, M.L., Ahima, R.S., Craft, L.S., Schoner, B., Stephens, T.W., & Flier, J.S. (1997). Leptin inhibition of the hypothalamic-pituitary-adrenal axis in response to stress. *Endocrinology, 138*(9), 3859-3863.

Heini, A.F., Lara-Castro, C., Kirk, K.A., Considine, R.V., Caro, J.F., & Weinsier, R.L. (1998). Association of leptin and hunger-satiety ratings in obese women. *International Journal of Obesity Related Metabolism Disorders, 22*(11), 1084-1087.

Hooper, S.L., Mackinnon, L.T., Howard, A., Gordon, R.D., & Bachmann, A.W. (1995). Markers for monitoring overtraining and recovery. *Medicine and Science in Sports and Exercise, 27*(1), 106-112.

Israel, S. (1986) Zum Problem des Übertrainings aus internistischer und leistungsphysiologischer Sicht [Medical and physiological aspects of overtraining in Sport]. *Medizin und Sport, 16,* 1-12.

Jaschinski, F., Schuler, M., Peuker, H., & Pette, D. (1998). Changes in myosin heavy chain mRNA and protein isoforms of rat muscle during forced contractile activity. *American Journal of Physiology, 274,* C365-C370.

Jenkins, P.J., Ibanez-Santos, X., Holly, J., Cotterill, A., Perry, L., Wolman, R., Harries, M., & Grossman, A. (1993). IGFBP-1: A metabolic signal associated with exercise-induced amenorrhoea. *Neuroendocrinology, 57*(4), 600-604.

Jeukendrup, A.E., Hesselink, M.K., Snyder, A.C., Kuipers, H., & Keizer, H.A. (1992). Physiological changes in male competitive cyclists after two weeks of intensified training. *International Journal of Sports Medicine, 13,* 534-541.

Jost, J., Weiss, M., & Weicker, H. (1990). Sympatho-adrenergic regulation and the adrenoreceptor system. *Journal of Applied Physiology, 68*(3), 897-904.

Kanaley, J.A., Weltman, J.Y., Veldhuis, J.D., Rogol, A.D., Hartman, M.L., & Weltman, A. (1997). Human growth hormone response to repeated bouts of aerobic exercise. *Journal of Applied Physiology, 83*(5), 1756-1761.

Kellmann, M., Altenburg, D., Lormes, W., & Steinacker, J.M. (2001). Assessing stress and recovery during preparation for the World Championships in rowing. *The Sport Psychologist, 15,* 151-167.

Kellmann, M., & Günther, K. (2000). Changes in stress and recovery in elite rowers during preparation for the Olympic Games. *Medicine and Science in Sports and Exercise, 32,* 676-683.

Kellmann, M., & Kallus, K.W. (2001). *The Recovery-Stress Questionnaire for Athletes; User manual.* Champaign, IL: Human Kinetics.

Kellmann, M., Kallus, K.W., Günther, K., Lormes, W., & Steinacker, J.M. (1997). Psychologische Betreuung der Junioren-Nationalmannschaft des Deutschen Ruderverbandes [Psychological consultation in the German National Rowing Team]. *Psychologie und Sport, 4,* 123-134.

Koistinen, H., Koistinen, R., Selenius, L., Ylikorkala, Q., & Seppala, M. (1996). Effect of marathon run on serum IGF-I and IGF-binding protein 1 and 3 levels. *Journal of Applied Physiology, 80*(3), 760-764.

Kuipers, H., & Keizer, H.A. (1988). Overtraining in elite athletes. Review and directions for the future. *Sports Medicine, 6*(2), 79-92.

Laughlin, G.A., & Yen, S.S. (1996). Nutritional and endocrine-metabolic aberrations in amenorrheic athletes. *Journal of Clinical Endocrinology and Metabolism, 81*(12), 4301-4309.

Lehmann, M., Baumgartl, P., Wiesenack, C., Seidel, A., Baumann, H., Fischer, S., Spori, U., Gendrisch, G., Kaminski, R., & Keul, J. (1992). Training-overtraining: Influence of a defined increase in training volume vs training intensity on performance, catecholamines and some metabolic parameters in experienced middle- and long-distance runners. *European Journal of Applied Physiology, 64*(2), 169-177.

Lehmann, M., Foster, C., Dickhuth, H.H., & Gastmann, U. (1998). Autonomic imbalance hypothesis and overtraining syndrome. *Medicine and Science in Sports and Exercise, 30*(7), 1140-1145.

Lehmann, M., Foster, C., Gastmann, U., Keizer, H.A., & Steinacker, J.M. (1999). Definition, types, symptoms, findings, underlying mechanisms, and frequency of overtraining and overtraining syndrome. In M. Lehmann, C. Foster, U. Gastmann, H.A. Keizer, & J.M. Steinacker (Eds.), *Overload, performance incompetence, and regeneration in sport* (pp. 1-6). New York: Kluwer Academic/Plenum.

Lehmann, M., Foster, C., & Keul, J. (1993). Overtraining in endurance athletes: A brief review. *Medicine and Science in Sports and Exercise, 25,* 854-861.

Lehmann, M., Gastmann, U., Baur, S., Liu, Y., Lormes, W., Opitz-Gress, A., Reissnecker, S., Simsch, C., & Steinacker, J.M. (1999). Selected parameters and mechanisms of peripheral and central fatigue and regeneration in overtrained athletes. In M. Lehmann, C. Foster, U. Gastmann, H.A. Keizer, & J.M. Steinacker (Eds.), *Overload, performance incompetence, and regeneration in sport* (pp. 7-26). New York: Kluwer Academic/Plenum.

Lehmann, M., Knizia, K., Gastmann, U., Petersen, K.G., Khalaf, A.N., Bauer, S., Kerp, L., & Keul, J. (1993). Influence of 6-week, 6 days per week, training on pituitary function in recreational athletes. *British Journal of Sports Medicine, 27*(3), 186-192.

Lehmann, M.J., Lormes, W., Opitz-Gress, A., Steinacker, J.M., Netzer, N., Foster, C., & Gastmann, U. (1997). Training and overtraining: An overview and experimental results in endurance sports. *Journal of Sports Medicine and Physical Fitness, 37*(1), 7-17.

Lehmann, M., Schmid, P., & Keul, J. (1984). Age- and exercise-related sympathetic activity in untrained volunteers, trained athletes and patients with impaired left-ventricular contractility. *European Heart Journal, 5 Suppl E:1-7,* 1-7.

Liu, Y., Lormes, W., Baur, C., Altenburg, D., Lehmann, M., & Steinacker, J.M. (2000). Human skeletal muscle HSP70 response to physical training depends on exercise intensity. *International Journal of Sports Medicine, 21,* 351-355.

Liu, Y., Mayr, S., Opitz-Gress, A., Zeller, C., Lormes, W., Baur, S., Lehmann, M., & Steinacker, J.M. (1999). Human skeletal muscle HSP70 response to training in highly trained rowers. *Journal of Applied Physiology, 86* (1), 101-104.

Morgan, W.P., Brown, D.R., Raglin, J.S., O'Connor, P.J., & Ellickson, K.A. (1987). Psychological monitoring of overtraining and staleness. *British Journal of Sports Medicine, 21*(3), 107-114.

Naveilhan, P., Hassani, H., Canals, J.M., Ekstrand, A.J., Larefalk, A., Chhajlani, V., Arenas, E., Gedda, K., Svensson, L., Thoren, P., & Ernfors, P. (1999). Normal feeding behavior, body weight and leptin response require the neuropeptide Y Y2 receptor. *Nature Medicine, 5*(10), 1188-1193.

Nehlsen-Cannarella, S.L., Fagoaga, O.R., Nieman, D.C., Henson, D.A., Butterworth, D.E., Schmitt, R.L., Bailey, E.M., Warren, B.J., Utter, A., & Davis, J.M. (1997). Carbohydrate and the cytokine response to 2.5 h of running. *Journal of Applied Physiology, 82*(5), 1662-1667.

Nieman, D.C., Nehlsen-Cannarella, S.L., Fagoaga, O.R., Henson, D.A., Utter, A., Davis, J.M., Williams, F., & Butterworth, D.E. (2000). Influence of mode and carbohydrate on the cytokine response to heavy exercise. *Medicine and Science in Sports and Exercise, 30,* 671-678.

Nieman, D.C., & Pedersen, B.K. (1999). Exercise and immune function. Recent developments. *Sports Medicine, 27*(2), 73-80.

Ostrowski, K., Rohde, T., Asp, S., Schjerling, P., & Pedersen, B.K. (1999). Pro- and anti-inflammatory cytokine balance in strenuous exercise in humans. *Journal of Physiology, 515*(Pt. 1), 287-291.

Ostrowski, K., Rohde, T., Zacho, M., Asp, S., & Pedersen, B.K. (1998). Evidence that interleukin-6 is produced in human skeletal muscle during prolonged running. *Journal of Physiology, 508*(Pt. 3), 949-953.

Pedersen, B.K., & Hoffman-Goetz, L. (2000) Exercise and the immune system: Regulation, integration and adaptation. *Physiological Reviews, 80*(3), 1055-1081.

Pedersen, P.K., Rohde, T., & Zacho, M. (1996). Immunity in athletes. *Journal of Sports Medicine and Physical Fitness, 36,* 236-245.

Pette, D., & Staron, R.S. (1997). Mammalian skeletal muscle fiber type transitions. *International Review in Cytology, 170,* 143-223.

Podhorska-Okolow, M., Sandri, M., Zampieri, S., Brun, B., Rossini, K., & Carraro, U. (1998). Apoptosis of myofibres and satellite cells: Exercise-induced damage in skeletal muscle of the mouse. *Neuropathology and Applied Neurobiology, 24*(6), 518-531.

Roelen, C.A., de Vries, W.R., Koppeschaar, H.P., Vervoorn, C., Thijssen, J.H., & Blankenstein, M.A. (1997). Plasma insulin-like growth factor-I and high affinity growth hormone-binding protein levels increase after two weeks of strenuous physical train-

ing. *International Journal of Sports Medicine, 18*(4), 238-241.

Roemmich, J.N., & Sinning, W.E. (1997). Weight loss and wrestling training: Effects on growth-related hormones. *Journal of Applied Physiology, 82*(6), 1760-1764.

Rohde, T., MacLean, D.A., Richter, E.A., Kiens, B., & Pedersen, B.K. (1997). Prolonged submaximal eccentric exercise is associated with increased levels of plasma IL-6. *American Journal of Physiology, 273*(1), E85-E91.

Schmidt, W., Dore, S., Hilgendorf, A., Strauch, S., Gareau, R., & Brisson, G.R. (1995). Effects of exercise during normoxia and hypoxia on the growth hormone-insulin-like growth factor I axis. *European Journal of Applied Physiology, 71*(5), 424-430.

Schwartz, M.W., Seeley, R.J., Campfield, L.A., Burn, P., & Baskin, D.G. (1996). Identification of targets of leptin action in rat hypothalamus. *Journal of Clinical Investigation, 98*(5), 1101-1106.

Smith, L.L. (2000). Cytokine hypothesis of overtraining: A physiological adaptation to excessive stress? *Medicine and Science in Sports and Exercise, 32*(2), 317-331.

Snyder, D.K., Clemmons, D.R., & Underwood, L.E. (1989). Dietary carbohydrate content determines responsiveness to growth hormone in energy-restricted humans. *Journal of Clinical Endocrinology and Metabolism, 69,* 745-752.

Steinacker, J.M. (1993). Physiological aspects of training in rowing. *International Journal of Sports Medicine, 14* (Suppl 1), S3-10.

Steinacker, J.M., Kellmann, M., Böhm, B.O., Liu, Y., Opitz-Gress, A., Kallus, K.W., Lehmann, M., Altenburg, D., & Lormes, W. (1999). Clinical findings of stress and regeneration in rowers before world championships. In M. Lehmann, C. Foster, U. Gastmann, H.A. Keizer, & J.M. Steinacker (Eds.), *Overload, performance incompetence, and regeneration in sport* (pp. 71-80). New York: Kluwer Academic/Plenum.

Steinacker, J.M., Lormes, W., Kellmann, M., Liu, Y., Reissnecker, S., Opitz-Gress, A., Baller, B., Günther, K., Petersen, K.G., Kallus, K.W., Lehmann, M., & Altenburg, D. (2000). Training of Junior Rowers before World Championships. Effects on performance, mood state and selected hormonal and metabolic responses. *Journal of Sports Medicine and Physical Fitness, 40,* 327-335.

Steinacker, J.M., Lormes, W., Lehmann, M., & Altenburg, D. (1998). Training of rowers before world championships. *Medicine and Science in Sports and Exercise, 30*(7), 1158-1163.

Steinacker, J.M., Lormes, W., Liu, Y., Baur, S., Menold, E., Altenburg, D., Petersen, K.G., & Lehmann, M. (2000). Leptin and somatotropic hormones during intensive resistance training and endurance training in rowers (abstract). *International Journal of Sports Medicine, 20,* S52-S53.

Termin, A., Staron, R.S., & Pette, D. (1989). Myosin heavy chain isoforms in histochemical defined fiber types of rat muscle. *Histochemistry, 92,* 453-457.

Uusitalo, A.L.T. (2001). Overtraining. Making a difficult diagnosis and implementing targeted treatment. *Physician and Sportsmedicine, 29*(5), 35-50.

Wada, M., Hämäläinen, N., & Pette, D. (1995). Isomyosin patterns of single type IIB, IID and IIA fibers from rabbit skeletal muscle. *Journal Muscle Research Cell Motil, 16,* 237-242.

Wang, J., Liu, R., Hawkins, M., Barzilai, N., & Rossetti, L. (1998). A nutrient-sensing pathway regulates leptin gene expression in muscle and fat. *Nature, 393,* 684-688.

Wittert, G.A., Livesey, J.H., Espiner, E.A., & Donald, R.A. (1996). Adaptation of the hypothalamopituitary adrenal axis to chronic exercise stress in humans. *Medicine and Science in Sports and Exercise, 28*(8), 1015-1019.

Part III

Intervention of Underrecovery

Norris, S.R., & Smith, D.J. (2002). Planning, periodization, and sequencing of training and competition: The rationale for a competently planned, optimally executed training and competition program, supported by a multidisciplinary team. In M. Kellmann (Ed.), *Enhancing recovery: Preventing underperformance in athletes* (pp. 121-141). Champaign, IL: Human Kinetics.

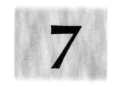

Planning, Periodization, and Sequencing of Training and Competition: The Rationale for a Competently Planned, Optimally Executed Training and Competition Program, Supported by a Multidisciplinary Team

Stephen R. Norris and David J. Smith

This chapter addresses the concepts of *planning, periodization,* and *sequencing* as they refer to training and competition, and as supported by a tiered and comprehensive ongoing monitoring program. Obviously, it is beyond the scope of a single chapter to examine every aspect of these topics extensively, particularly since other published works deal exclusively with planning and periodization. Therefore, in this chapter we will focus on the rationale surrounding the need for a systematic approach to the problem of effective training, the impact of effective recovery, and the preparation for high-performance execution regardless of the type of sport (power, technical, endurance, or various amalgams). Furthermore, we will advocate for support of a long-term developmental approach to potential athlete nurturing. Finally, we will present some case studies from the Human Performance Laboratory at the National Sport Centre Calgary that reflect typical sports with which we have been involved.

We will illustrate the need for an underlying philosophy that encompasses and drives the training and competition program. Indeed, this philosophy will be seen to influence virtually all areas of programming and support of the specific sport or event in question. We will also suggest that, rather than being some fixed and inflexible entity, the "optimal" program in the pursuit of excellence should encompass both general and specific elements; have short-, medium-, and long-term objectives; involve consistent and constant monitoring; incorporate the basic principles of training; be flexible and malleable; and use competitive experiences as well as appropriate rest and regeneration phases.

A fundamental component of all successful programs is individualization, that is, an attention to the requirements for, and reaction to, various stimuli by the individual, even in a team sport setting. Virtually all authors and groups identified worldwide as being authorities in the area of training-program design emphasize individualization (see appendix 7.A, p. 141).

A wealth of information, both documented and anecdotal, reveals, at least superficially, a massive range in the structure or type of training programs that have been successful in terms of elite competitive performance. This probably reflects the "elasticity" of response to various stimuli and human diversity (as largely dictated by the underlying genetic matrix and supported by the environment in which an athlete or team is immersed).

Another issue to consider in the process of eliciting "elite sport performance" is the fact that elite endeavors typically require a disproportionately large allocation of resources compared with average, good, or even high performance. This view does not align itself well with the notion of "sport for all," a notion that will likely lead to inappropriate resource allocation and an eventual dilution of the support structure required for truly elite performance. Although this may seem to be a hard-line standpoint, the stark reality is that there are only three places on the medalists' podium and a finite number of places in any international event final.

The progression to elite performance is a long-term affair that involves a "complicated pedagogic process in which pedagogic, biological, psychological and logical-epistemological laws manifest themselves at many levels" (Berger, Harre, & Ritter, 1982). Researchers have documented well that control and coercion of the training process "requires planning and design" (Nádori & Granek, 1989), that is, the training process depends on the current and future objectives and involves some element of future performance prediction.

Despite the rather sophisticated phraseology used in the previous paragraphs, we want to emphasize that planning, periodization, and sequencing with regard to training and competition is a straightforward concept. Essentially, these three concepts are intertwined within the "project management problem" of athlete development. A statement by Dawson (1996) highlights this point: "Periodization is no more than a technical term for adopting a sensible and well planned approach to training, which maximizes training gains and performance improvement" (p. 76). Of course, the considerable number of factors that must be taken into account when adopting such an approach is what leads to difficulties; confusion; and suboptimal design, implementation, and subsequent critique of the plan.

Planning and Periodization: Historical Perspective and Current Thought

The historical perspective concerning the planning and periodization of physical activity with regard to future performance is extensive. Although a great deal of attention is paid to "modern" (post-1960) authors, the premise for the planning and implementation of training programs can be found documented as far back as the ancient societies of China, Egypt, India, Greece, and Rome. Texts or writings from these societies often refer to the use of systematic training pro-

grams to improve strength, endurance, and general athletic ability. There are references to both males and females that transcend all socioeconomic strata of the societies. In addition, ancient training programs were not restricted to training athletes for military endeavors as one might expect initially. Indeed, motivation ranged from purely social standing and peer pressure, to basic health and functional preservation, and on to include sporting prowess and the obvious demands of military and combat-oriented groups.

Training methodologies over the last 2,000 years have led us to a complex and confusing position concerning planning and periodization. Among the issues that confuse current thinking are the historical development and ascension of the main points of training methodology, the adoption of various terminologies or jargon, political ideologies, influential individual biases, and even commercial pressures. However, recent authors have written extensively in this area and provide interested readers with great insight into the historical origins and overall development of training methodology. Excellent examples of these publications include those by Bompa (1999) and Siff and Verkhoshansky (1999).

Planning and Training

Siff and Verkhoshansky (1999) wrote a succinct and well-researched perspective that presents a balanced critique of the historical development of modern training thought, particularly with regard to the divergence of classical Western and Eastern philosophies and doctrines. Essentially, the divergence of East and West is often simplified by cursory inspection into a muscular strength (East) versus cardiovascular (West) bias, although the underlying mechanisms relative to the political hemispheres were far more complex and consequential (Siff & Verkhoshansky, 1999). Indeed, through the third quarter of the 20th century this divergence led to substantially different research directions, training knowledge (quantitative and qualitative), and training philosophies between the two main sociopolitical groups.

Siff and Verkhoshansky (1999) further suggested that the West's preoccupation with the "performance-enhancing" substance use of former Eastern Bloc athletic programs actually led to a reluctance by Western countries to effectively examine the underlying sport training philosophy and knowledge base that had been developed by the East. This is particularly ironic since Western European, Scandinavian, and North American researchers were undertaking a substantial amount of research into exogenous pharmaceutical use for training and competition, and athletes in these areas have also used such substances, particularly over the last 25 years (Burkett & Falduto, 1984; MacDougall, 1983; Wilson, 1988; Yesalis, Kennedy, Kopstein, & Bahrke, 1993). Perhaps of even greater consequence is the fact that the knowledge base and availability of information concerning the training methodology of the Eastern Bloc and allied nations in the West, particularly with regard to planning and periodization, has been slow to build, leading to the belief that planning, periodization, and sequencing of training is some recent theory that is untested and perhaps unnecessary for elite sport performance.

Typically, the core references that are cited in English publications are translations of the work of authors such as Matveyev, Nádori, Granek, Verkhoshansky, and Harre. Arguably, the earliest references to periodization in the modern era of training (for the sake of discussion, 1960 onward) belong to Matveyev (i.e., 1966, 1977, 1981) and Nádori (1962). Indeed, Matveyev has often been referred to by some as the "father of periodization." Clearly this author's influence on the current structure and content of much of the recent literature concerning this topic has been profound. The "classic" works by Harre (1971, 1982), Verkhoshansky (1985), and Nádori and Granek (1989), together with more recent additions by Wilke and Madsen (1986), Bompa (1999), and Siff and Verkhoshanky (1999), have all been shaped to some degree by Matveyev's thinking.

However, this is not to lessen the originality of the "modern" authors. In fact, it is interesting to see how several have clearly moved the field substantially forward in terms of basic understanding, application and implementation, creativity, and original thought. Aside from those previously mentioned, notable additions to this exclusive list are Viru (1995), Zatsiorsky (1995), Balyi (1995), and Platonov (1996). Balyi (e.g., Balyi, 1997, 1998; Balyi & Hamilton, 1999a, 1999b), in particular, has had an increasing level of influence in recent years by combining a comprehensive understanding of the available literature in several languages with a unique ability to bring together the relevant components required for practical application in a clearly communicated manner. Balyi (1993) described four major historical models of the theory of training that may be distinguished from an examination of the literature—namely, the early "classical" models through various adaptations

focusing on exercise physiology and finally into truly integrated and sequenced versions involving sport science, sports medicine, and sport techniques.

Periodization

One of the most common definitions given to periodization by prominent authors in the field is the predetermined sequence of training sessions and competitions (Nádori & Granek, 1989). The fundamental purpose of this sequence is to recognize the partial and complete goals or objectives for a given athlete and to implement interventions that will positively affect these goals within assigned time frames. Most readers familiar with periodization literature will recognize the typical division of time periods as follows:

Nádori (1962)	Matveyev (1966)
Foundation or preseason period	Preparation period
Maintenance period	Competition period
Transition period	Transition period

These divisions of the available time span, typically molded around the notion of the annual, or yearly, training plan (which itself may be part of some multiyear program), have been further clarified, expanded, and refined by modern authorities (Balyi, 1995; Bompa, 1999).

Essentially, periodization is a systematic and methodical planning tool that serves as a directional template for the specific athlete, athletes, and/or team in question. Diagrammatic templates are often used as tools in the planning process. The most widely published of these templates may be found in Bompa (1999). Bompa's template uses a linear format that lends itself well to expansion over several training plans or years, as well as being easily adapted to suit the requirements of any athletic or training and competition situation (see figure 7.1).

The basic concept of periodization is sometimes misunderstood, particularly by some North American coaches and authors. The concept is not a rigid one with only one form of approach; rather, it is a framework within and around which a coach and sport science/sports medicine team can formulate a specific program for a specific situation. The periodized plan is therefore only limited by the underlying tenets of scientific knowledge in the relevant areas and the resources available, and not by and of itself (Smith & Norris, 1999). Of course, the art of coaching involves the

Yearly training plan					
Phases of training	Prepatory		Competitive		Transition
Subphases	General preparation	Specific preparation	Pre-competitive	Competitive	Transition
Macrocycles					
Microcycles					

Figure 7.1 Typical periodization and planning template.

Adapted, by permission, from T.O. Bompa, 1999, Annual training plan. In *Periodization theory and methodology of training*, 4th ed., edited by T.O. Bompa (Champaign, IL: Human Kinetics), p. 16.

interweaving of scientific knowledge with a plan based on the specific circumstances and environment within which the coach operates.

Pyne (1996) listed the common features of periodized training programs as follows:

1. The training program is designed based on the long-term performance goal for the season.
2. Training loads are increased progressively and cyclically.
3. The training phases follow a logical sequence.
4. The training process is supported by a structured program of scientific monitoring in the areas of physiology, biomechanics, psychology, and physiotherapy.
5. Recovery or regenerative techniques are used intensively throughout the training program.
6. Emphasis on skill development and refinement is maintained throughout the training program.
7. The improvement and maintenance of general athletic abilities is an underlying component of the training program.
8. Each phase of the training program builds on the preceding phase.

Points similar to Pyne's list may be found permeating the thoughts and writings of most periodization experts. It is well supported by the principles of athletic training described by Harre (1982) and the synopsis by Siff and Verkhoshansky (1999) of contributions made in this area by Vorobyev (1978), Schneidman (1979), Matveyev (1981), and Yessis and Trubo (1987). In contrast to these extensive listings, typical exercise physiology texts refer to only four basic principles: (1) overload, (2) specificity, (3) individual differences, and (4) reversibility (McArdle, Katch, & Katch, 1991). Overall, it may be inferred from much of the material previously mentioned that the success of any training program is closely linked to the underlying philosophy that shapes the sport program in the first place and that there are "at least eight interrelated principles" in scientific sport preparation that should be incorporated into a periodized plan (Siff & Verkhoshansky, 1999). These are as follows:

1. *The Principle of Awareness.* Essentially this refers to the ideological and philosophical aspects of the situation as well as the need for the athlete to become an educated participant in the training process.

2. *The Principle of All-Around Development.* This point embodies the need for an underlying general athletic ability that is supported by a strong psychological profile.

3. *The Principle of Consecutiveness (or Consistency).* This "classic" overloading principle addresses the progressive increasing of the intensity and volume of physical work, as well as the degree of difficulty of motor skills.

4. *The Principle of Repetition.* This component is founded on "Pavlov's 3-stage theory for development of conditioned reflexes" (Siff & Verkhoshanksy, 1999) and is similar to the stages applied in teaching sports skills:

a. Development of knowledge

b. Development of motor ability

c. Development of automatic motor response

5. *The Principle of Visualization.* The ability of the athlete to "visualize" the correct technical movements of the activity in question is extremely important in the training process. This process is aided by personal and expert demonstrations and tools such as film and video analyses.

6. *The Principle of Specialization.* This principle emphasizes the need to be exposed to and practice under similar conditions to those operating during competition. This recognizes the fact that competition is extremely important in the training process. In addition, special exercises or drills to aid in the development and honing of motor skills, tactics, and other specific components required to compete efficiently and effectively in the sport should be included in a well-designed program.

7. *The Principle of Individualization.* As mentioned previously, the concept of athletes as distinct individuals is a central scientific tenet. Athletes will react and adapt differently and over individual time frames even when presented with "identical" training regimes. Hence, trainers must formulate individualized training programs with sound monitoring systems to evaluate individual responses to the training load.

8. *The Principle of Structured Training.* This central principle suggests that the training process should be arranged as a "system of cycles, centred upon periodic cycles" (Harre, 1982), as described by Matveyev (1970, 1977, 1981). As stated earlier, training design will tend to follow preparatory, competitive, and transition stages of varying duration and it is this principle that has generated the term *periodization.*

Harre's original terminology differs somewhat from those listed here; however, readers will recognize the similarities between those listed here and the factors Harre described.

Difference in Terminology

The difference in terminology used to describe the actual structural components of a cyclical plan leads to some confusion when discussing periodization. Matveyev (1981) listed the major elements as the *microstructure* (microcycle), the *mesostructure* (mesocycle), and the *macrostruc-*

ture (macrocycles). According to this terminology, *microstructure* refers to the structure of separate training sessions and of short groupings of several sessions (microcycles); *mesostructure* involves the grouping of a distinct number of microcycles leading to the realization of a predetermined and specific training or performance goal(s); and *macrostructure* is concerned with larger time periods (groupings of mesocycles) such as semiannual, annual, and those of many years. This terminology is widely understood and used throughout the European literature, whereas other geographical areas (e.g., Australia and the United States) occasionally use slightly different definitions. For example, Pyne (1996) stated that the "meso cycle" represents the entire swimming season (16-24 weeks) for club to national level performers, but that international-level swimmers with longer seasons would require two "meso cycles." Pyne (1996) also defined a "macro cycle" as a major phase of training "within a season or meso cycle," with typical durations of between 3 and 10 weeks (typically 3-4 weeks in Australia). Pyne's "micro cycle" remains the term used for the weekly training plan. We will use the European terminology in this chapter for the sake of consistency.

Various authors have classified Matveyev's three terms (macro-, meso-, and microcycle) into distinct subcategories (Balyi, 1995; Bompa, 1999; Harre, 1982; Matveyev, 1981). Examples include developmental, shock, regeneration, and peaking/unloading microcycles or macrocycles (Bompa, 1999), or introductory, basic, control, supplemental, preparatory, and competitive mesocycles (Harre, 1982). Such terms may also precede macrocycles depending on the plan. Although these phrases are fairly self-explanatory, these authors (and others) usually describe them in some detail. See appendix 7.A (p. 141) for a list of authors who have contributed important research in this area.

Despite the variations described earlier, periodization is a planning tool that a coach, athlete, sport science/sports medicine team may use to organize training and competition. The terminology used is somewhat immaterial as long as the group in question acts consistently. The program and time frame must be divided into manageable units with distinct objectives for each unit, as well as an overall goal, depending on the situation (developmental stage, unique athlete or team needs). The length of time (weeks, months, or even years) available to achieve the relevant and identified objectives for the situation, together with the competition calendar, sets the overall structure and tone for the periodized plan. Obviously, the single-year plan for a senior-level athlete competing in a specific "power event" would look considerably different from the plan for a developing athlete currently engaged in multiple activities.

It's interesting that in a 1999 paper Verkhoshansky vehemently attacked the underlying premises to the postulations of Matveyev (1981) on the grounds that Matveyev's stance has little scientific support. Although many of Verkhoshanky's (1999) comments may be well founded, we believe that the concept of periodization has grown beyond the actual specific recommendations of Matveyev. When an integrated scientific approach is used for planning periodization, the concept reflects more the philosophy of the need for planning and addressing the core components in order to maximize or optimize future performance than adherence to a central methodology. In fact, Balyi[1] (1995, p. 40) summarized the overview well when remarking that "failure to plan is planning to fail."

Although the groundwork of Matveyev's original periodization concepts had been in existence for over a decade, the athletic "Russian machine" recognized by the end of the 1970s the need for a more scientifically integrated format involving specialists in several fields, rather than leaving all the responsibility to a single coach (Schneidman, 1979; Haljand, personal communication[2]). Several countries or specific national sport federations have tried to adopt and implement this fundamental concept in recent times (e.g., Australia, see Gore, 2000). A heavy commitment of resources and central government aid together with a supportive philosophical/cultural presence is necessary to do this effectively, however, which is not always forthcoming in both established and emerging nations. Nevertheless, it is exactly this approach and the notion of an educated and receptive coaching staff working with a team of specialists and support staff to guide and monitor the training and competition plan that we wish to emphasize.

Figures 7.2 and 7.3 illustrate the athlete-focused/coach-centered/team-supported approach whereby specialists meet regularly to discuss the specific and general state of the ongoing program and provide the coach with detailed information at both the individual athlete and group levels in order to help the coach make more informed (better) coaching decisions. Figure 7.2 displays both positive and negative aspects of having an array of experts available to the coach. The coach may find himself either the recipient of valuable information or bombarded with extraneous information from this intellectual group. It is therefore advisable to have a qualified individual (overall sport scientist) with a good working relationship with the coach act as a filter of information in order to provide the coach with an ongoing synopsis of the circumstances surrounding a training group, team, or individual.

A multidisciplinary team approach is a core aspect of the modern philosophy of a planned, periodized, and sequenced approach to training and competition. At the heart of this emphasis is a research- and knowledge-based core that constantly strives to improve the information provided to coaches concerning any facet of the athletic training and competition. This emphasis also serves to dispel further the notion that periodization in modern terminology refers to a single, fixed form of training methodology.

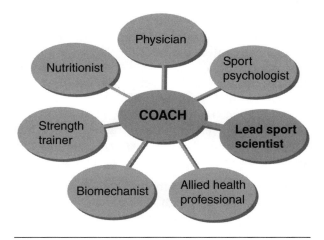

Figure 7.2 Coach-centered model to support an athlete-focused system.

Adapted from Smith, 1999.

---

1. Istvan Balyi is a respected authority on planning, periodization, and long-term development. This statement, although relatively common in coaching circles, was first heard by Norris in a coaching presentation by Balyi.

2. Rein Haljand is professor of biomechanics at the Tallinn University of Educational Sciences, Tallinn, Estonia. This personal communication took place during the European Swimming Championships in Helsinki, Finland, in June 2000.

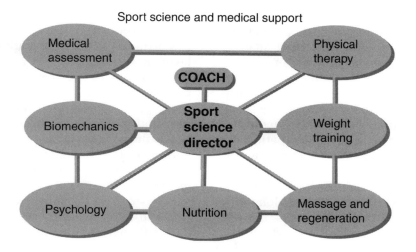

Sport science and medical support

Figure 7.3 Multidisciplinary team approach.

Adapted from Smith, 1999.

Components of Training

The previous section and the Smith and Norris chapter (this volume, chapter 5) introduced various principles of training. Beyond these points are factors that could be considered to be the fundamental components of training. For example, MacDougal and Wenger (1991) stated that genetics, training, and health status all underscore athleticism. In addition, several years ago Balyi created a list of determining components for both current and future training and competition, which has since been amended (Balyi, 1997; Smith, 1999; Smith & Norris, 1999) and is presented as a checklist for coaches and sport scientists to consider (see figure 7.4). This list, referred to as the eight S's, compartmentalizes the aspects required for effective training, recovery, regeneration, and subsequent competition performance. These S's—skill, speed, strength, stamina, suppleness, psychology ('sych), stature, and sustenance (which incorporates all aspects of nutrition, recovery, and regeneration—hence, "sustenance" in the broadest sense)—may be applied to any physical endeavor regardless of the nature of the activity. That is, the components may be applied to short-duration, high-intensity individual sports or, at the other end of the spectrum, to long-lasting, submaximal team games.

The components of skill, speed, strength, and stamina are relatively simple to comprehend. Suppleness, however, is somewhat more broadly defined than just as straightforward static flexibility, as it involves the aspect of dynamic actions (both specific and nonspecific) that may or

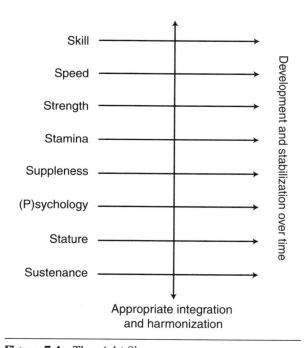

Figure 7.4 The eight S's.

After Balyi, 1997; Smith and Norris, 1999.

may not have been rehearsed prior to event participation.

The psychological component is extremely important and yet is often left to the individual athlete to deal with. This is in spite of the obvious recognition of the impact of this component on training and competition by a succession of authors (e.g., Balyi, 1995; Harre, 1982; MacDougal & Wenger, 1991; Matveyev, 1981; Smith, 1997; Wilke & Madsen, 1986).

Smith (1997), an exercise physiologist, stated during an oral presentation to the IOC Congress that, with regard to the competitive performance, "the psychological state of an athlete on a given day will define the outcome of a performance, all other things being equal." It should be clearly understood that unless the athlete has the "will" (Matveyev, 1981) to undertake the planned training or to deal with the demands of competing at a high level, the other components of training will have little effect. Matveyev (1981) stated that the "moulding" of the will should be integrated into the overall long-term training program along with any of the other more tangible aspects, despite the fact that entities such as "purposefulness, initiative, resolution, courage, self-control, persistence and staunchness" are somewhat intangible.

The component of stature is often misconstrued as the measurement of adipose tissue, particularly the catchall, popular percent body fat (%fat) figure. Although this may have some merit in certain instances, aspects such as total body mass, lean tissue mass, and fat-to-muscle ratio are probably of greater interest to those involved in high-performance sport training, training design, and training and competition monitoring. In addition, the use of segmental lengths and proportions may also provide useful tools in the evaluation of stature, particularly during training phases that coincide with periods of rapid growth and development. However, because the aspect of anthropometry is fraught with the potential for less-than-adequate measurement techniques, some level of quality assurance of the measurements sought must be established via sound methodology and the determination of appropriate levels of technical error (see Gore, 2000).

Finally, the sustenance term is focused on the need for sound nutritional practices and recovery/regeneration strategies that aggressively counter the prior training or competition stress or at least aid the restorative processes that the specific loading has induced. This component also must be built into the periodized plan, not just from an educational point of view, but also from the standpoint of the sequence of training and competition proposed. In addition, special scenarios such as especially demanding training phases, camps, travel, environmental demands (i.e., altitude or hypoxic exposures, heat and humidity situations, cold and dry scenarios), recovery from illness, and readiness for competition also warrant careful planning with regard to sustenance (before,

during, and after such episodes). Keep in mind too that a comprehensive and adequate diet that is well timed in its administration (at the hour/day level) is the building block for a stable health platform and a sound recovery program, as well as for growth and maturation.

Integral to a systematic approach to the planning and periodization of training and competition is the need to document carefully the quality and quantity of training and competition undertaken. Quantification is one of the most important elements in the area of training methodology, and yet it is one of the most neglected and poorly understood areas. This is probably due to the fact that although it is relatively easy to track the volume of training performed, it is frustratingly difficult to examine the element of intensity of training and particularly the summation of these elements ([volume × intensity] × "impact on the athlete" quotient), which represents the actual impact, or effect, on the individual. That is, volume of training is easily tracked by monitoring suitable units such as hours of training, miles or kilometers covered, number of repetitions performed, amount of weight lifted, number of ski runs or gates taken, number of ground contacts made, balls hit, and so on. However, because the issue of intensity is extremely complex, to date no single physiological variable has been identified that can unequivocally act as *the* marker of intensity.

Smith and Norris (this volume, chapter 5) introduced some of the pertinent aspects regarding potential indicators or markers of intensity, however. The diagram in figure 7.5 illustrates in a succinct and clear manner the idea that the potential performance gain from a given training or intervention load acts in summation with the level of fatigue or homeostatic disruption associated with that load to establish a pathway for the level of preparedness (or readiness) of the athlete to perform at any moment in time. This two-factor model, proposed by Zatsiorsky (1995), is similar to the one proposed by Banister (1991); both emphasize the complexity of the interaction between fitness and fatigue. Fry, Morton, and Keast (1992) and Morton (1992) are examples of other researchers working in this area of training analysis and quantification. The question that remains to be answered, however, concerns the exposure of definitive and easily measurable variables concerned with training impact.

Figure 7.5 illustrates that in the period immediately after completing the training load, the level

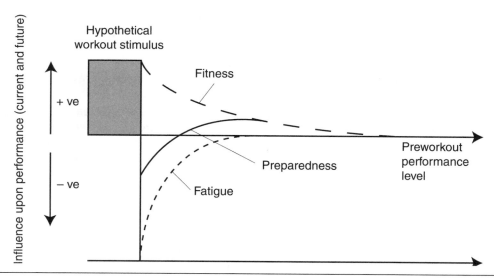

Figure 7.5   Two-factor model contributing to preparedness for competition.

Adapted, by permission, from V.M. Zatsiorsky, 1995, Basic concepts of training theory. In *Science and practice of strength training*, edited by V.M. Zatsiorsky (Champaign,IL: Human Kinetics), 16.

of fatigue tends to outweigh the ability to actually attain the performance potential gained. This is clearly shown by the line of preparedness. As time progresses, however, the level of fatigue diminishes such that the level of preparedness rises. This occurs despite a loss in the potential gain from having done the particular training load in the first place. In fact, the available literature tends to suggest that, when comparing the fitness component with the fatigue component, the rate of decay is three-to-one in favor of the fitness component. That is, the fitness component will take three times as long to decay back to the previous level than the fatigue component. This construct alone demonstrates the need for systematic and appropriate recovery practices. Viru (1995) stated that the main functions of the recovery period are as follows:

- "A normalization of functions" (essentially the transition from some exercising level back to the preexercise state)

- "Replenishment of energy resources together with temporary supercompensation for them"

- "Normalization of homeostatic equilibriums"

- "Reconstructive function, particularly in regard to cellular structures and enzymes systems"

Further, it should be understood that Viru's components follow different time spans; that is, the first and third components are likely to be achieved within a relatively short period of time (minutes to some hours). The other two components, however, tend to require much longer periods of time to return to what would be characterized as their preexercise conditions. Viru (1995) also suggested that the time element basically follows a two-stage path, *a stage of rapid recovery* and *a stage of delayed restitution of bodily resources and working capacity,* although both stages are not necessarily exclusive of each other.

In practical terms, all of the preceding information points clearly to the need to incorporate recovery periods (rest, recovery, and regeneration) into the training process and the periodized plan that are sequenced to reflect the bias of the previous training period. Basically, the message is that such recovery periods are an integral part of the format of training design and that unless designers of training regimes understand this aspect, the final performance outcome is likely to be compromised.

The usual breakdown of physical recovery involves either *active* or *passive* forms, or a combination of the two, together with the recognition of the need for psychological recovery. *Active recovery* typically follows a pattern of low intensity and low volume in relation to the current capacity and training load of the individual athlete. Such recovery may be used in the period immediately following sustained high-intensity training or competition, particularly when the anaerobic glycolytic energy pathway has been substantially involved.

In addition, this level of activity may also be incorporated into a longer period of time (perhaps several days) to aid recovery from an extended period of intense training, competition, or other nontraining stressors (e.g., travel).

In practical terms, for well-trained individuals with sound aerobic backgrounds, active recovery from performances producing peak postexercise blood lactate levels of approximately 14 to 18 mmol · L^{-1} typically have to last 20 to 40 minutes to even begin to approach preexercise levels. An example intensity for this active recovery would be exercise resulting in a heart rate of around 135 to 140 b · min^{-1} for an athlete with a maximal heart rate of 195 to 200 b · min^{-1} and a resting heart rate of 40 to 60 b · min^{-1}.

Passive (or *static*) *recovery,* on the other hand, refers to periods that do not involve any form of activity. These may be of short duration (e.g., a few minutes) through to several days (e.g., 1-10 days) after the completion of extended periods of arduous training and competition, or as part of the preparation for peak performance. This form of recovery is preferred when the priority is to restore adenosine triphosphate (ATP) and the high-energy phosphagens after short-duration, high-intensity efforts (typically less than 15 seconds in duration). It may also be used when the priority is to restore macronutrients and essential substances such as water, carbohydrate, protein, and fat. Additionally, passive recovery measures may also be used to allow for neuromuscular recovery and a restoration of neural movement pattern execution after intense exercise or loading. Massage and other physical manipulative techniques can be helpful in aiding recovery from training and competition.

Several authors have emphasized clearly the need for a systematic and planned inclusion of rest and recovery periods within each training phase or cycle (Kraemer & Nindl, 1998; Rowbottom, Keast, & Morton, 1998; Lehmann et al., 1998). Kraemer and Nindl (1998) asserted that "mistakes in training" (leading to the potential for some realization of underperformance) are typically the result of inappropriate levels of intensity and/or volume of training. The publication *Overtraining in Sport* (Kreider, Fry, & O'Toole, 1998) provides an extensive examination of a multitude of relevant components and published literature covering both endurance and power/strength activities and is recommended for those interested in the etiology, concepts, and potential identifiers of overtraining that leads to underperformance.

Model of Global Performance

The complex interrelationship of variables involved in training and competition has been discussed in previous sections as well as by Smith and Norris (this volume, chapter 5), who also displayed a full version of the schematic shown in figure 7.6. This schematic attempts to communicate the point that although several cooperating and competing variables are involved, they have a high degree of association among them.

This schematic model illustrates that performance is not simply isolated to physiological, biomechanical, or psychological elements, but involves a complex matrix of all stressors acting on the individual (or team), including components that would be viewed as nontraining stressors. That is, the stress placed on an athlete at any

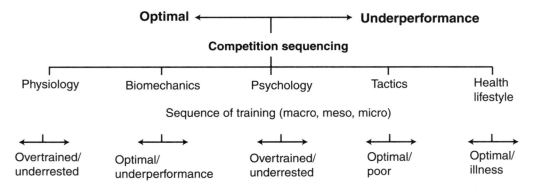

Figure 7.6 Abridged global performance model.

Adapted from D.J. Smith and S.R. Norris, 2000, Physiology. In R. Jackson (Ed.), *Sport medicine manual 2000, International Olympic Committee Medical Commission* (Lausanne, Switzerland: International Olympic Committee).

one moment or over a particular period is made up of many factors, all of which have an implication for the recovery of that athlete and her readiness for further training loads or competitive performance. Stress is a cumulative process.

Long-Term Planning and Perspective

When dealing with planning, periodization, and sequencing issues, as indeed with training and competition in general, there is a tendency to focus on relatively short-term time frames. However, it is important to understand the longer-term ramifications since the overall training strategy should reflect the natural course of maturation factors as well as the final goal or objective. Viru (1995) presented an overview of the stages of long-term development—in other words, the career of an athlete from the developmental stage through to senior-level performance. This is presented in figure 7.7 alongside the similar but more user-friendly version by Balyi and Hamilton (1999a, 1999b).

Since both Viru's and Balyi and Hamilton's versions occupy time frames of around 10 to 15 years, further expansion is not necessary. Both versions assume that to reach some level of consistent mastery of performance requires a substantial period of deliberate practice. A distinct characteristic of such models is the extensive general athletic preparation and multiactivity base that is suggested. This is in contrast with the tendency toward early (young age) specialization and intense competition that is seen widely in North America. An extensive body of literature demonstrates that supreme athletic performance typically occurs between approximately ages 21 and 35, with only a few notable exceptions such as in female Olympic gymnasts (Fomin, Filin, & Tschiene, 1975; Platonov, 1994).

Long-term plans, rather than a series of truncated shorter ones, allow the training and competition exposures of the athlete to be seamlessly merged as the athlete develops. Also, with a sound understanding of biological and physical maturation processes, the coach and team of experts may be able to design a more individualized and pertinent program, which again recognizes the differences between the individual and the norm. Another key tenet of the periodization stance is that long-term developmental progress should not be subordinated to short-term competitive events (Zatsiorsky, 1995). Since very different maturation processes are at work, particularly from birth through the late teens, researchers have suggested that training programs for developing athletes should reflect these events rather than be tempered versions of adult or senior-level programs.

The work of Scammon (1930) is often cited to illustrate the previous points since it is noticeable that elements of nervous system development are established early in life, as compared to the development of muscle mass, which must wait well beyond the onset of the hormonal disturbances associated with puberty. Such scientific literature has prompted some authors to design relatively detailed long-term training regimes that address these different developmental time frames (Balyi & Hamilton, 1999a; Wilke & Madsen, 1986).

Balyi instigated a terminology and long-term athlete participation structure revolving around the following "seamless" chronological and developmental categories; FUNdamental, Training to

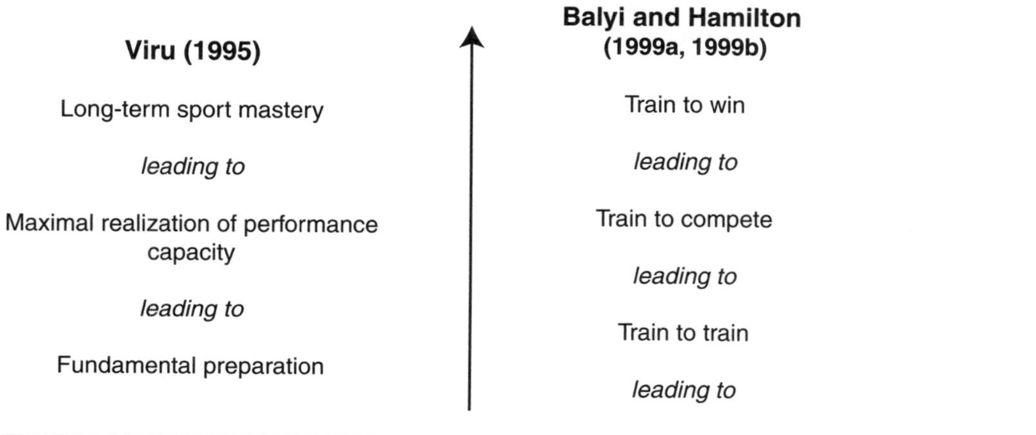

Viru (1995)

Long-term sport mastery

leading to

Maximal realization of performance capacity

leading to

Fundamental preparation

Balyi and Hamilton (1999a, 1999b)

Train to win

leading to

Train to compete

leading to

Train to train

leading to

Figure 7.7 Long-term planning stages of development.

Train, Training to Compete, and Training to Win (1999). Such terminology and structure is well supported by the literature in the areas of human growth and development, training development, and the empirical information of states that have embarked on guided child/youth athletic programs. A hallmark of such systems is the deliberate inclusion of a comprehensive and evolutionary ongoing monitoring system examining a broad spectrum of current and potential performance characteristics and psychological traits.

Monitoring System

While the aspects of individualization and long-term development have already been discussed, another factor weaves a path between these two in a manner that is both integrated and objectively separate. This is the commitment to an ongoing monitoring program. Although competition is the "highest form of training," it is also the "highest form of testing and monitoring" (Smith, 1999). However, relying solely on competitive performance for monitoring purposes and program evaluation is an inadequate and naive approach.

Because of the number of variables involved and the time span of development of the components (both positive and negative) involved in athletic performance, coupled with the individual response to training, coaches and sport scientists should use a battery of monitoring protocols to assess the status of the athlete. Among useful protocols are a hierarchy of monitoring procedures that range from the whole competitive performance, to isolated but sport-specific "field tests," to invasive and intrusive physiological protocols. The fundamental base test will, of course, revolve around a thorough health screening, since maintenance of a stable health platform is imperative when embarking on or engaged in a strenuous training and competition program.

A comprehensive monitoring program will follow an "entry/exit" format for each variable over a given time period; each variable is appropriately matched to a phase of training, competition, or transition. The exit tests should be performed after a recovery and regeneration period in order to allow maximal positive changes to occur as well as to facilitate the eradication of any residual fatigue due to the previous training intervention. It is also suggested that rather than relying on clinical, normative, or typical data for comparative or evaluative purposes, each athlete have a database built around him so that over time the

coach, athlete, and sport science/sports medicine team will be able to describe accurately specific states of preparedness for that athlete. This database would cover a multitude of aspects that fall under the eight S's described earlier, including such elements as physiology, biomechanics, psychology, anthropometry, nutrition, and basic health characteristics. Furthermore, such a profile should also address the following specific athlete situations (see figures 7.8, 7.9, and 7.10):

- When the athlete is well rested and healthy prior to serious training (i.e., following a transition period)
- When the athlete is fatigued yet basically healthy following a strenuous training phase
- When the athlete is well rested, healthy, well trained, and able to complete a good performance
- When the athlete produces an unexpected "underperformance"
- When the athlete is experiencing the onset of infection or transient illness
- When the athlete is experiencing acute and chronic responses to specific training and competition elements (i.e., altitude or hypoxic exposures, international travel, closely repeated competitive events)

The profile should also include the athlete's upper and lower limits of particular variables (especially bloodborne parameters) to establish an individual's range of response for "reference" use with the scenarios listed above.

To aid in the process of identifying the level of preparedness or residual fatigue in an athlete, we suggest a tiered approach that is coupled with the developmental age and performance capability of the athlete. By this we mean a system that has at its base a fundamental level of frequently examined simple measures (e.g., resting heart rate, body weight, lean mass measurements, psychological questionnaires) together with standard field tests (i.e., a sport-specific test set) and careful tracking of the training and competition load (i.e., quantification of volume and intensity—to whatever degree is possible).

This first tier of criterion measures is characterized by its minimally intrusive and sport-specific nature. These measures should be able to provide the coach and sport science team with the necessary early warning signs of a buildup in residual fatigue components before

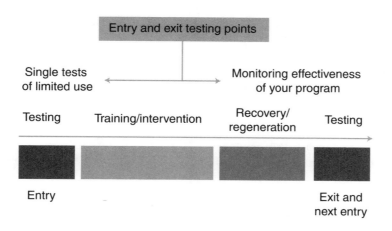

Figure 7.8 Ongoing monitoring: entry and exit testing.

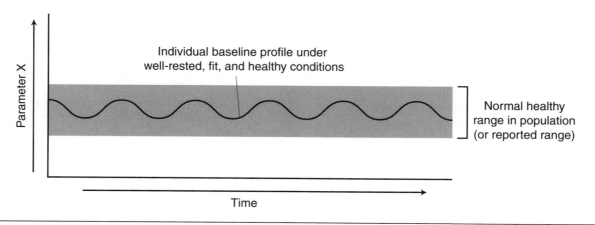

Figure 7.9 Ongoing monitoring: establishing athlete profiles.

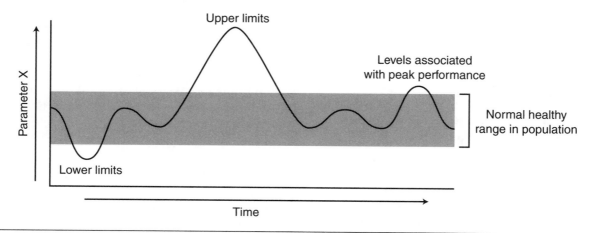

Figure 7.10 Ongoing monitoring: effect of various stages of training/competition load.

the need for drastic supplementary recovery practices. In addition, during periods of planned high stress during particular training and competition phases (e.g., increases in training volume, intensity, combinations of these, travel, repeated competition) this level of monitoring also provides the first stage of training response information. Depending on observations by the coach and the results of the first-tier measures, the athlete may then access subsequent levels of monitoring or investigation, particularly those involving health.

In situations of more substantial funding and/ or higher training and competition demands, a program of more sophisticated and invasive procedures may be warranted. These tiers will encompass aspects such as blood lactate monitoring, as well as the frequent examination of an athlete's blood profile involving parameters ranging from those indicating immune function and health status to the family of variables examining the continuum between anabolic and catabolic conditions persisting in the athlete. Again, Kreider and colleagues (1998) offered an excellent synopsis of recent discussions concerning overtraining etiology, identifying characteristics and potential markers for activities falling at both ends of, and along, the endurance/power continuum.

Errors of Training Sequencing

The fundamental element here is the recognition of the "interplay between work and recovery" (Harre, 1982). As presented earlier, the workload undertaken and recovery process associated with that workload can be considered to be an integrated manifestation. Harre (1982) described the following "errors of training" together with associated factors that lead to reduced performance and the signs that may be apparent under such circumstances:

- Recovery is neglected.
- Training demands are increased too rapidly for the athlete to adequately adapt.
- After a break in regular training due to illness or injury, the workload is inappropriately high.

- The overall volume of training (both at maximal and submaximal levels) is too high.
- The overall volume of intense[3] work is too great when primarily engaged in endurance training.
- Excessive attention and time are spent practicing highly complex technical aspects with little opportunity for less-intense aspects.
- Excessive numbers of high-level competitions are coupled with little supportive training.
- Direction of training is extremely biased (i.e., very high-volume or very high-intensity work).
- The athlete lacks confidence in the coach, who sets goals inappropriately high (leading to repeated performance failure on the part of the athlete).

Although these errors are largely self-explanatory, it is appropriate to dwell on some of them to emphasize the philosophical basis that permeates this chapter. For example, the inadequate use of recovery and regeneration periods as integral tools in the training process is a major oversight and demonstrates a number of possible problems with a particular training situation. These problems may include poor understanding by both the coach and the athlete of the need for suitable recovery strategies, coupled with a lack of, or inadequate, monitoring of pertinent variables capable of identifying excessive fatigue. The strategy involved for identifying excessive fatigue will, of course, be related to the nature of the predominant form of training undertaken in the particular training phase in question (i.e., an endurance, strength/resistance training, or power/speed bias).

Additionally, the suggested testing/monitoring battery must retain as a priority a suitable level of practicality in terms of the commitment of resources, such as time utilization, financial cost, equipment required, and the information produced. Obvious parameters for potential inclusion in such a battery of variables (depending on the form of training) are orthostatic heart rate responses; neuromuscular excitation factors; overall bloodborne iron status; hormonal and other blood indicators of the balance between possible anabolic/catabolic conditions; markers of immune

---

3. *Intense* is defined as the power output ranging from immediately above a sustainable workload and conducted for an extended period of time until fatigue through to short-duration/high-power output repetitions. The definition should include the individualized aspect of both a relative and an absolute dimension to the continuum.

function and inflammatory responses; examination of the individual's power output/time relationship, efficiency, and economy capability; as well as a multifactorial analysis of psychological factors.

It should also be noted that since the competitive performance itself is both the highest form of training and the highest form of monitoring (due to the integration of all facets involved in the task), this too is a primary monitoring tool. The problem with relying on competitive performance (or *in-season* performance) as a major marker is one of timing; that is, the definitive indicator of an error in the training, planning, and periodization construct is underperformance, worsened only if it is seemingly unexpected and occurs at a time in the process that leaves no time for rectification.

Another error is the imposition of an inappropriately high training volume for an athlete with an unsubstantial history or "critical mass" of training prior to this new loading level, which leads to too great a demand on the athlete's resources and a subsequent failure of adaptation unless the stimulus is removed or reduced. A further example of incorrect training design is the incorporation of too much intense work when actively pursuing a high-volume, endurance focus. In this case, the problem is that intensity loading does not increase in a linear fashion (as might be assumed from a simple heart rate profile during a simple incremental test to maximal heart rate), but rather in a nonlinear path whereby the cost to, or impact on, the athlete rises in some excessive way. At less than maximal intensities, this nonlinear stress loading may lead to an accumulation of intense training (a high volume of intense work) that cannot be recovered from due to the sheer volume of endurance work concurrently being undertaken. Again, appropriate monitoring techniques would aid in avoiding such occurrences. Previous sections of this chapter have illustrated the key elements that coaches, athletes, and sport scientists should incorporate into their programs.

A basic tenet that should be emphasized is that the vast majority of biological adaptation takes place during the recovery/regeneration phases. This supports the notion that recovery and regeneration are not only integral to the overall process leading to elite performance, but they are also pivotal elements in the attainment of peak performance. Indeed, continual training or training without regard for the processes of adaptation demonstrates a distinct naivete at best, or a serious lack of understanding at worst, about the main components leading to improved performance. Recovery and regeneration practices, including the allocation of sufficient time to these ends, should be viewed by the coach as an integral part of the training and competition process, particularly when supported by a knowledgeable sport science and sports medicine team.

Case Studies From the National Sport Centre Calgary

This section provides typical real-life scenarios of training and monitoring aimed at maximizing the training response while minimizing the associated level of fatigue, thereby facilitating conditions for an optimal performance outcome in the future. We will use examples from the sport disciplines of swimming, speedskating, and cross-country skiing.

Case Study 1

This first example is based on a senior member of Canada's National Swimming Team during the spring/summer of 1999. Figure 7.11 gives the overall information concerning the volume of sport-specific training (meters swum), as well as the sequence of competitions. This specific section is of a 19-week macrocycle that culminated in two major competitions at weeks 16 and 19 (the Pan-American Games in Winnipeg, Canada, and the Pan-Pacific Swimming Championships in Sydney, Australia, respectively). The 19 weeks were broken into two mesocycles, with the first running from weeks 1 to 8 and the second from weeks 10 to 19, with week 9 being a planned recovery week. The major volume of training was accomplished between four and five weeks out from each competition, as had been previously practiced and assessed. This meant that the peak volumes occurred in weeks 3 and 4 for the competition in week 8, and in weeks 11 and 12 for the competition in week 16. The competitions prior to week 16 were the Mel Zajac Meet in Vancouver, Canada, the Mare Nostrum (two meets in close proximity) in southern Europe, and the Janet Evans Meet in Los Angeles (United States).

The taper for the in-season competitions was approximately 5 to 7 days, whereas for the major competitions it was approximately 10 to 12 days. The main problem faced by this swimmer was the need to revitalize the aerobic system with some work after the main competition in week 16 in

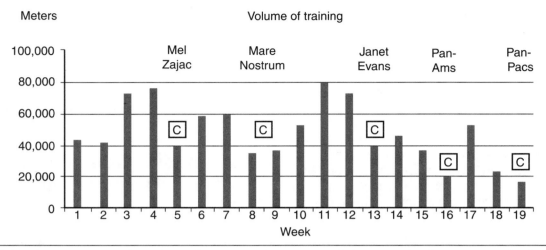

Figure 7.11 Swimming example: volume of sport-specific training and the sequence of competitions leading to two major events.

preparation for the final competition of the season in week 19. In addition, this final competition was further complicated by the fact that it involved a significant amount of travel and time zone crossing (Canada to Australia), as well as the shortness of time between major efforts (13 days).

The actual results of the key performances as a percentage of personal best time were 97.4%, 97.8%, 100.3%, and 99.5%, respectively, across the competitions (Mare Nostrum, Janet Evans, Pan-Ams, and Pan-Pacs). This 19-week cycle illustrates the necessity to select the in-season competitions carefully and to challenge the aerobic system significantly with training volume four to five weeks out from the selected competitions. It should also be noted that this swimmer was supported by the coach and sport scientist–led team approach described throughout this chapter.

Case Study 2

This second example is of the periodization plan for the Canadian Sprint Speed Skating Team for the 1999-2000 season. The plan was built around the international competition schedule with mesocycles of recovery/preparation incorporated into the periods between competition phases (keep in mind that this format is clearly for established athletes as opposed to those in developmental phases of their careers). At the microcycle level, five physiological parameters considered to be essential components to speed skating success were prioritized for each microcycle week. Once this basic plan was established, the coach set the daily detail of training for

each microcycle, together with a preplanned alternative for each session in order to react to specific aspects, such as extended training fatigue. The plan required a peaking system for the World Cup competitions, as well as a major priority emphasizing the final two competitions of the major season, the World Sprint Championships in Seoul (Korea), followed by the World Single Distance Competition in Nagano (Japan).

Although sprint speed skating over 500 and 1,000 meters is predominantly an anaerobic activity (typically 35-77 seconds), these physiological components are supported by aerobic training of both capacity and power. Figure 7.12 illustrates the priority of training components in each microcycle of training. The important elements are safeguarding of opportunities to truly train at highly intense effort levels with sound technical execution and incorporating planned periods of recovery and regeneration, while at the same time retaining a degree of flexibility within the preplanned model that allows for unforeseen eventualities without adversely affecting the predetermined objectives of the overall program.

Case Study 3

This final example concerns frequent (in this case, daily) ongoing monitoring and the role this has in the avoidance of training errors and the creation of flexible training plans. The sport group in question is a developing group of male cross-country skiers (aged 18-22 years) undergoing a sport-specific training camp at moderate altitude (approximately 1,600-1,900 meters) with a high-volume training

Sprint speed skating																					
Month	October			November					December				January					February			
Week date	11	18	25	1	8	15	22	29	6	13	20	27	3	10	17	24	31	7	14	21	28
Traveling																						
Location							World Cup Berlin	World Cup Warsaw	World Cup Pine					Canadian champs	World Cup Butte	World Cup Calgary				World Sprints Seoul	Single Dist. Nagano
Training phase																						
Macrocycle	Preparation					Competition																
Mesocycle	1						2		3					4				5			6	
Microcycle	1	2	3	4	5	6	1	2	3	1	2	3	4	1	2	3	1	2	3	1	21
Priority 1, 2, 3																						
Aerobic capacity	1	1	M	M		R	R	R	R	1	1			R	R	R	1		R	R	R
Aerobic power			2		2							1						1			
Lactate power		2	3	2		3					2		3			2			3		
Lactate capacity			1	1	3	1	2	2	2	3	3	1	2	2	2			3	1	2	2
Max speed				3	1	2	1	1	1		2	2	1	1	1				2	1	1

R = Recovery
M = Maintenance

Figure 7.12 Speed skating example: process of prioritizing training components and implementing the training program to meet predetermined objectives.

emphasis. Although the camp had a duration of 19 days, only 4 days are shown here for the purposes of this illustration.

Figure 7.13 shows the Rusko Heart Rate Test profile (Rusko, Härkönen, & Pakarinen, 1994) of a 19-year-old skier. This particular test involves an examination of heart rate response to the transition from lying to standing positions and is typically carried out early in the day by this particular training group. The day 3 profile for this individual would normally be associated with a positive adaptation response to the environmental and training stressors in this situation. The team coach then had to examine the morning profile on day 4 and assess the situation prior to embarking on the day's planned training load. In this instance, the profile can be seen to be clearly elevated in the standing phase of the test; the coach assessed this as "some form of negative influence" and changed the planned workout for this individual to one that would allow for

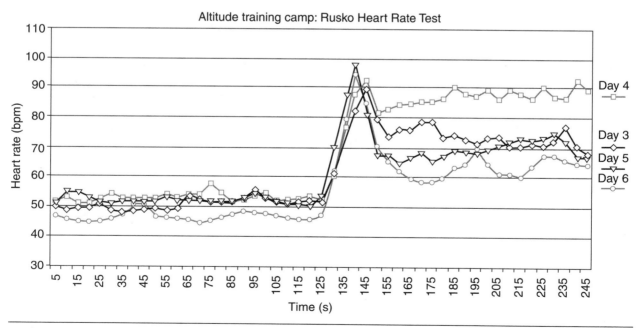

Figure 7.13 Cross-country skiing example: use of frequent ongoing monitoring to avoid training errors.

greater adaptation to the environmental conditions and the loading thus far in the camp. The heart rate profiles for day 5 and day 6 supported the coach's decision since they revealed a restoration of, and indeed improvement in, the adaptation and level of preparedness of the athlete.

Case Study Summaries

Although these three examples are specific and relatively straightforward, they all serve to illustrate the importance of sound planning incorporating a degree of flexibility supported strongly by a practical and adequately implemented monitoring program. In addition, even though these examples reflect sport activities undertaken in specific situations, it should be clear that the underlying tenets can be extended to other sport activities.

Summary and Guideline Framework for Planning

The objective of this chapter has been to provide some perspective on the concept of periodization of training together with the view that the training process should be supported by a multifaceted ongoing monitoring regime that provides relevant and timely information that the coach can use to evaluate and, where appropriate, adjust the training and competition program. Furthermore, the realization that recovery and regeneration is an integral component of the overall training process should be apparent; indeed, it may be argued that the correct timing, structure, and use of recovery strategies is the most potent weapon in a coach's arsenal of training methodologies.

A possible framework to tackle the problem of suitable planning has been the topic of much discussion among several conductors[4] of the course titled Task 12 Program Design (Planning and Periodization) of the Coaching Association of Canada's (CAC's) National Coaching Certification Program. In terms of a step-by-step approach, C. Cardinal (personal communication) suggested the

stages described here and we have expanded them to provide greater detail and direction:

Analysis
- Demands of the sport
- Phase of athletic career (FUNdamental, Train to Train, Train to Compete, Train to Win, and beyond—Balyi terminology)
- Athlete's current performance level and all relevant components

Forecast
- Establish the objectives of the training cycles or periods (micro-, meso-, macro-, annual, or multiyear cycles) based on the prior analysis. That is, short-, mid-, and long-term objectives have to be set in order to determine a scientifically based agenda of priorities, particularly in situations in which the short-term competitive calendar may interfere or mask the longer-term goals.

Prescription
- Develop the programs and activities required to achieve the objectives of the FORECAST.

Implementation
- The correct execution of the prescription is probably the most difficult aspect of the overall process, particularly when dealing with a large number of athletes. This will involve careful ongoing monitoring of all areas of the program, such as appropriate intensity levels (physical and cognitive), as well as group and individual recovery and regeneration periods.

Evaluation and Assessment
- As stated in Implementation, a need exists for ongoing monitoring (evaluation) of each phase of training (micro-, meso-, macro-, yearly, and multiyear cycles). This evaluation should examine all aspects of programming and performance, not just the athlete's.

Adjustment(s)
- If the evaluation and assessment concludes that adjustment is warranted, this should be

---

4. Particular recognition should be acknowledged to Istvan Balyi, Charles Cardinal, Alain Marion, and Michael Poortmans for their influential and significant contribution to this discussion concerning Task 12, Level 4/5 NCCP (2000, 2001).

carried out in an appropriate fashion and within a suitable time frame.

Finally, it is important to note that a successful sport science/sports medicine team of experts to support the coach requires sound and experienced leadership. All those concerned have to understand clearly the role of being a "service provider" to a coach and the sport in question. Service provision is not always an easy role to adopt or even understand for those traditionally engaged in research or university-based positions, and yet it is vital if the team is to have real impact and longevity. Gaining the trust of the coach and athlete and helping them see periodization as worthwhile are as important as the process of periodization itself.

References

Balyi, I. (1993, February). Beyond Barcelona: A contemporary critique of the theory of periodisation. *Queensland Pistol News,* 15-17.

Balyi, I. (1995). Planning, periodisation, integration and implementation of annual training programs. Presentation to and in proceedings of the *Australian Strength and Conditioning Association National Conference* (pp. 40-66). Gold Coast, Australia.

Balyi, I. (1997, June-September). *NCCP level 4/task 12 planning, periodization & integration lecture and workshop series.* Hong Kong, China, and Canada.

Balyi, I. (1998, December). Long-term planning of athlete development. Part 2: The training to compete phase. *FHS (Faster, Higher, Stronger), 2,* 8-11.

Balyi, I., & Hamilton, A. (1999a, April). Long-term planning of athlete development. Part 3: The training to win phase. *FHS (Faster, Higher, Stronger), 3,* 7-9.

Balyi, I., & Hamilton, A. (1999b, September). Alpine Integrated Model (AIM; ACA High Performance Advisory Committee). Based extensively on I. Balyi and A. Hamilton's unpublished paper and presentation: *ACA long-term athlete development project.* Ottawa, ON: Alpine Canada.

Banister, E.W. (1991). Modeling elite athletic performance. In J.D. MacDougal, H.A. Wenger, & H.J. Green (Eds.), *Physiological testing of the high-performance athlete* (2nd ed., pp. 403-424). Champaign, IL: Human Kinetics.

Berger, J., Harre, D., & Ritter, I. (1982). Principles of athletic training. In D. Harre (Ed.), *Principles of sports training: Introduction to the theory and methods of training* (English version, 1st ed., pp. 73-94). Berlin: Sportverlag.

Bompa, T.O. (1999). *Periodization: Theory and methodology of training.* Champaign, IL: Human Kinetics.

Burkett, L.N., & Falduto, M.T. (1984). Steroid use by athletes in a metropolitan area. *Physician and Sportsmedicine, 12,* 69-70.

Dawson, B. (1996). Periodisation of speed and endurance training. In P. Reaburn & D. Jenkins (Eds.), *Training for speed and endurance* (pp. 76-96). St. Leonards, Australia: Allen & Unwin.

Fomin, N.A., Filin, V.P., & Tschiene, P. (1975). Altersspezifische Grundlagen der körperlichen Erziehung [Age-specific foundation of physical education] (Translation of a book published by Fizkultura i sport, Moscow, 1972). Schorndorf, Germany: Hofmann.

Fry, R.W., Morton, A.R., & Keast, D. (1992). Periodisation of training stress: A review. *Canadian Journal of Sport Sciences, 17,* 234-240.

Gore, C.J. (2000). Quality assurance in exercise physiology laboratories. In C.J. Gore (Ed.), *Physiological tests for elite athletes* (pp. 3-11). Champaign, IL: Human Kinetics.

Harre, D. (Ed.). (1971). *Trainingslehre* [Training teaching]. Berlin: Sportverlag.

Harre, D. (1982). *Principles of sports training: Introduction to the theory and methods of training* (English version, 1st ed.). Berlin: Sportverlag.

Kraemer, W.J., & Nindl, B.C. (1998). Factors involved with overtraining for strength and power. In R.B. Kreider, A.C. Fry, & M.L. O'Toole (Eds.), *Overtraining in sport* (pp. 69-86). Champaign, IL: Human Kinetics.

Kreider, R.B., Fry, A.C., & O'Toole, M.L. (Eds.). (1998). *Overtraining in sport.* Champaign, IL: Human Kinetics.

Lehmann, M., Foster, C., Netzer, N., Lormes, W., Steinacker, J.M., Liu, Y., Opitz-Gress, A., & Gastmann, U. (1998). Physiological responses to short- and long-term overtraining in endurance athletes. In R.B. Kreider, A.C. Fry, & M.L. O'Toole (Eds.), *Overtraining in sport* (pp. 19-46). Champaign, IL: Human Kinetics.

MacDougal, J.D., & Wenger, H.A. (1991). The purpose of physiological testing. In J.D. MacDougal, H.A. Wenger, & H.J. Green (Eds.), *Physiological testing of the high-performance athlete* (2nd ed., pp. 1-5). Champaign, IL: Human Kinetics.

MacDougall, D. (1983). Anabolic steroids. *Physician and Sportsmedicine, 11,* 95-99.

Matveyev, L.P. (1966). Cited in L. Nádori, & I. Granek, I. (1989), *Theoretical and methodological basis of training planning with special considerations within a microcycle* (pp. 11). Lincoln, NE: National Strength and Conditioning Association.

Matveyev, L.P. (1970). Probleme der Untersuchung der Trainingsstruktur [Problems of investigation in the training structure]. *Teoriya I praktika fizical kulture, 33,* 51.

Matveyev, L.P. (1977). *Fundamentals of sports training* (Russian). Moscow: Fizkultura i Sport.

Matveyev, L.P. (1981). *Fundamentals of sports training* (English translation of the revised Russian version). Moscow: Progress.

McArdle, W.D., Katch, F.I., & Katch, V.L. (1991). *Exercise physiology: Exercise, nutrition, and human performance* (pp. 423-427). Philadelphia: Lea & Febiger.

Morton, A.R. (1992). The quantitative periodization of athletic training: A model study. *Sports Medicine, 3,* 19-28.

Nádori, L. (1962). Cited in L. Nádori, & I. Granek, I. (1989), *Theoretical and methodological basis of training planning with special considerations within a microcycle* (pp. 11). Lincoln, NE: National Strength and Conditioning Association.

Nádori, L., & Granek, I. (1989). *Theoretical and methodological basis of training planning with special considerations within a microcycle.* Lincoln, NE: National Strength and Conditioning Association.

Platonov, V.L. (1994). I principi della preparazione a lungo termine [Principles of long-term preparation]. *SDS, Rivista di Cultura Sportiva (Roma), 13,* 2-10.

Platonov, V.L. (1996). Formation of athletes preparation within a year. *Athletic Asia, 21,* 37-74.

Pyne, D. (1996). The periodisation of swimming training at the Australian Institute of Sport. *Sports Coach, 18,* 34-38.

Rowbottom, D.G., Keast, D., & Morton, A.R. (1998). Monitoring and preventing of overreaching and overtraining in endurance athletes. In R.B. Kreider, A.C. Fry, & L. O'Toole (Eds.), *Overtraining in sport* (pp. 47-66). Champaign, IL: Human Kinetics.

Rusko, H.K., Härkönen, M., & Pakarinen, A. (1994). Overtraining effects on hormonal and autonomic regulation in young cross-country skiers. *Medicine and Science in Sports and Exercise, 26,* S64.

Scammon, R.E. (1930). The measurement of the body in childhood. In J.A. Harris, C.M. Jackson, D.G. Paterson, & R.E. Scammon (Eds.), *The measurement of man* (p. 193). Minneapolis: University of Minneapolis Press.

Schneidman, M. (1979). Cited in Siff, M.C., & Verkhoshansky, Y.V. (1999). *Supertraining* (4th ed., p. 22). Denver: Supertraining International.

Siff, M.C., & Verkhoshansky, Y.V. (1999). *Supertraining* (4th ed.). Denver: Supertraining International.

Smith, D.J. (1997, October). Preparation of teams for international competition. Invited presentation, Fourth IOC World Congress on Sport Sciences, Monte Carlo, Monaco.

Smith, D.J. (1999, October). Building a sport science program. Invited presentation, Investors Group National Coaching Conference, Toronto, Canada.

Smith, D.J., & Norris, S.R. (1999, October). Issues of sequencing. Invited presentation, Investors Group National Coaching Conference, Toronto, Canada.

Verkhoshansky, Y.V. (1985). *Programming and organisation of training.* Moscow: Fizkultura i Sport.

Verkhoshansky, Y.V. (1999). The end of "periodisation" of training in top-class sport. *New Studies in Athletics, 47,* 14-18.

Viru, A. (1995). *Adaptation in sports training.* Boca Raton, FL: CRC Press.

Vorobyev, A. (1978). *A textbook on weightlifting.* Budapest: International Weightlifting Federation.

Wilke, K., & Madsen, O. (1986). *Coaching the young swimmer.* London: Pelham.

Wilson, J.D. (1988). Androgen abuse by athletes. *Endocrine Reviews, 9,* 181-199.

Yesalis, C.E., Kennedy, N.J., Kopstein, A.N., & Bahrke, M.S. (1993). Anabolic-androgenic steroid use in the United States. *Journal of the American Medical Association 270,* 1217.

Yessis, M., & Trubo, R. (1987). *Secrets of soviet sports fitness and training.* New York: Arbor House.

Zatsiorsky, V.M. (1995). *Science and practice of strength training.* Champaign, IL: Human Kinetics.

Author Recognition List

The following alphabetical list of names is provided as a guide for those wishing to read further on the topics presented in this chapter. The list is by no means definitive; however, it does provide a starting point for those interested and in some way acknowledges those who have influenced the authors of this chapter.

Balyi, I.	Seiler, S.
Banister, E.W.	Siff, M.C.
Bompa, T.O.	Verkhoshansky, Y.V.
Harre, D.	Verontsov, A.
Lehmann, M.	Viru, A.
Matveyev, L.	Weiss, M.
Medvedev, A.N.	Zatsiorsky, V.M.
Platonov, V.	

Botterill, C., & Wilson, C. (2002). Overtraining: Emotional and interdisciplinary dimensions. In M. Kellmann (Ed.), *Enhancing recovery: Preventing underperformance in athletes* (pp. 143-159). Champaign, IL: Human Kinetics.

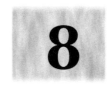

Overtraining: Emotional and Interdisciplinary Dimensions

Cal Botterill and Clare Wilson

Coaches and military leaders around the world have striven for decades to optimize training and preparation for competition or battle. Probably the most important initial lesson dedicated athletes or soldiers need to learn is that they can work harder than they thought possible. Dan Millman (1985) uses over half of his epic novel *The Way of the Peaceful Warrior* to depict the main character—a dedicated student-athlete named Dan—learning how hard he can work at his sport. Having finally learned this lesson, Dan's next critical insight is balance—the need to balance work with adequate rest, nutrition, and recovery. From there Dan goes on to learn critical social, mental, and emotional lessons that help him realize much more of his potential. Critical lessons, such as accepting people for what they are, letting certain things go, and recognizing that every moment is special, enable Dan to focus better, train hard, and recover effectively.

Millman does a great job of communicating that people are not just physical beings. Our ability to focus, work, perform, and recover is related to mental and emotional factors as well as physical factors. Performance and recovery are clearly interdisciplinary phenomena, with fairly complex relationships in every individual.

This chapter describes some of the Canadian history on recovery and then outlines a model that illustrates the interactive and multidisciplinary dimensions of total fitness. A brief description of training demands today is followed

by nine descriptive illustrative case studies on overtraining and recovery.

Case studies have played a critical role in the history of medicine and medical research. Since the phenomena involved in overtraining and recovery are clearly multifactorial, qualitative descriptive case studies and research can assist us in understanding the complex relationships involved.

Related topics such as training addiction, modern competitive demands, early warning signs of overtraining, monitoring and assessment, energizing techniques, emotional management, character development, self-awareness, interdisciplinary implications, and Canadian Sport System initiatives are discussed.

Canadian History

Eric Banister (1991) was one of the first sport scientists in Canada to explore individual differences in recovery rates of hard training in middle-distance athletes. Both blood tests and the Rating of Perceived Exertion (Borg, 1998) confirmed individual differences in time needed for recovery. Ironically, with experience, the Borg Scale (Psychological Perception Measure) became a more reliable early predictor of impending overtraining than other physiological testing.

Sport Canada commissioned an interdisciplinary study on overtraining in the 1980s, and Belcastro, McKenzie, and Smith (1989) identified some general guidelines and simple monitoring suggestions

143

for Canadian coaches, athletes, and applied sport scientists. Interest in "overtraining prevention" and recovery has increased in Canada over the last decade as specific monitoring strategies have become known and dramatic cases of overtraining have been observed. Perhaps Canadian athletes have always been slightly more prone to the phenomenon of overtraining than their international competitors. Being a small country of recent "pioneers" with a "New-World" ethic and strong desire to compete presents cultural and identity factors that may fuel proneness to overtraining. Certainly individuals differ in the extent to which these cultural and identity factors might be significant. At the same time, the intensity, passion, and work ethic that is credited for Canada's success in the 1972 Hockey Summit versus the Soviet Union, the five consecutive World Junior Hockey Championships, and the six consecutive Women's World Hockey Championships are constantly paraded as critical elements in our identity and approach to sport. In the cases observed by the authors at the National Sport Centre Calgary, "work ethic and intensity guilt" often appeared to be important factors in the path to overtraining. Guilt about not working hard enough and being intense all the time seemed to be a complicating factor in recovery and rehabilitation.

An important connection on this topic occurred at the 1996 conference of the Association for the Advancement of Applied Sport Psychology in Williamsburg, Virginia (United States). Cal Botterill (1996a) presented a keynote address entitled "Emotion as a Factor in Health and High Performance," and Michael Kellmann presented on his developing research and findings on the Recovery-Stress Questionnaire for Athletes (RESTQ-Sport; Kellmann & Kallus, 2001) and its potential to predict performance and possibly to prevent overtraining (Kellmann, Kallus, & Kurz, 1996). Participants at the conference began to explore the important connections among the topics. Kellmann expressed an interest in the possibilities for research and interventions at the National Sport Centre Calgary. Shortly after, David Smith (an applied exercise physiologist at the National Sport Centre Calgary) came across a fascinating article by Kenttä and Hassmén (1998) of Sweden on the topic of preventing overtraining in elite athletes (see also Kenttä & Hassmén, this volume, chapter 4). The interdisciplinary sport science support team at Calgary was impressed with the conceptualizing of Kenttä and Hassmén (1998) and with the RESTQ-Sport that had been developed by Kellmann and Kallus (2001).

Kellmann was invited to the National Sport Centre Calgary in 1999 to administer the RESTQ-Sport to interested coaches and athletes and to educate sport science professionals, coaches, and athletes on monitoring and recovery techniques. Highlights of the interventions and experiences in the Canadian system follow along with case studies of particular interest. In 1999 members of the Canadian Interdisciplinary Sport Science Support Team from Calgary participated in an International Symposium in Banff (Canada), coordinated by Kellmann, on overtraining in sport (Botterill & Wilson, 1999; Smith, 1999). The "Team Approach to Interdisciplinary Sport Science Support" was presented at the National Coaching Seminar later the same year (Smith, Norris, Maki, & Botterill, 1999).

Total Fitness Model

The work of Kellmann (cf. Kellmann et al., 1996; Kellmann & Günther, 2000; Kellmann & Kallus, 1999) as well as Kenttä and Hassmén (1998) helped sensitize the professionals at the National Sport Centre Calgary to the importance of an interdisciplinary approach to preventing overtraining. As well, a dramatic case brought to sport psychology consultant Botterill's attention early in his tenure at the National Sport Centre Calgary by physiologist Smith in 1997 also pointed to important interdisciplinary links.

Case Study 1

Vicki, a volleyball player at the National Sport Centre Calgary, had shown an "overtraining profile" repeatedly over several blood test batteries despite what was considered a very reasonable training load. An interview with Vicki revealed a lot of emotional and mental turmoil that was obviously affecting her focus and ability to recover. Three weeks of counseling and support produced a healthier mental and emotional "perspective," a significant turnaround in the blood test profile, and a dramatic shift in her ability to handle and recover from even heavier workloads!

Cases like this and the work of Kellmann (cf. Kellmann et al., 1996; Kellmann & Günther, 2000; Kellmann & Kallus, 1999) and Kenttä and Hassmén (1998) point to the importance of an interdisciplinary model of total fitness. Total fitness involves at least three major components—physical, mental, and emotional—which are dynamically related (see figure 8.1).

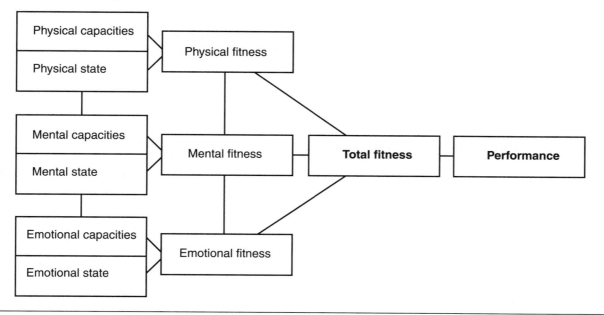

Figure 8.1   Total fitness model.

As well as being related, each domain of fitness (physical, mental, and emotional) involves both a set of capacities and a state. Athletes work hard to develop their physical capacities, but we know if their state is not good due to lack of rest, nutrition, hydration, or recovery, their capacities will be "masked" or lost. Similarly, elite performers develop impressive mental skills or capacities to facilitate training, performance, and recovery. If the athlete is feeling mentally "overloaded" or exhausted due to "overanalysis" or mental fatigue, these important capacities (focusing, goal setting, visualizing, relaxing, relating, communicating, energizing) will be eroded or dramatically limited.

Probably the most powerful domain of total fitness is the emotional domain (Goleman, 1995). When individuals are emotionally healthy, they have tremendous capacities to process and harness emotions. They usually enjoy extensive "natural" energy, and the tasks in the physical and mental domains are handled with enjoyment, gratitude, and efficiency; recovery is also usually proactive and efficient. In addition to being powerful, the emotional system is also tremendously resilient, as long as it is managed properly. On the other hand, when "emotional exhaustion" occurs, the consequences are usually very dramatic. As mentioned earlier, top performers often learn that they can work harder than they thought both physically and mentally, but when they are emotionally drained, they are usually "toast"!

When the emotional domain is exhausted, the performer's capacities in all three domains can be affected, and feelings of burnout, guilt, indifference, anxiety, and depression can occur. The degree of exhaustion and the length of the period over which it developed will probably influence how quickly recovery can occur. The good news is that once physical and mental recovery is accomplished, the emotional system is often amazingly resilient. It may, however, require proactive "recovery management" just like the other systems. Emotional management will be addressed later in the chapter.

The important thing to respect is that the capacities and state in any one domain can greatly affect the capacities and state in any other domain. Complex relationships among these factors are more likely than not, and an individual's "nature" and experiential history are inevitably significant. Finally, these complex relationships are important not only in the ability to perform, but also in the ability to recover.

Training Demands Today

Most physical training programs today are designed to be of high enough quality training and sufficient volume to push the athlete right to the edge of overtraining when recovery is optimal. The reality is that most athletes are also facing more daily mental and emotional demands than ever before. The heavy training loads put more pressure on personal relationships than ever before, and "personal space" for recovery and reflection is often disappearing in a world of media demands, sponsor needs, cellular phones, e-mail, and information overload (McGovern, 1998).

Case Study 2

Julie illustrates how mental and emotional demands on top of intensive training can contribute to feelings of burnout (Weinberg & Gould, 1999). Julie was one of Canada's top international cyclists. Despite her success, she worked closely with a physiologist as well as her coach to increase the quality of her training in the off-season. As the season approached, Julie felt good about her training but experienced increased media, public, and sponsor demands. All of these demands started to affect her personal relationships, and powerful emotional feelings and uncertainty added to the drain.

Athletes are tough; Julie hung in there until the first major competition of the season. Performance was even quite good for so early in the season. A few days later, however, Julie reported virtually a total loss of motivation; she was unsure whether she might even be "done" and maybe whether she should retire. All this from a top athlete who seemed "hyped" about the next Olympics only a few weeks before.

Julie's sport psychology consultant encouraged her not to make major decisions if she was tired. She was encouraged to adjust her schedule, give up some of her competition opportunities, and trust that she would know better what she wanted to do when rested. Part of the advice was not only to get more rest, but also to do things she loved doing—on her own and with others. Finally, Julie was cautioned that if she was really exhausted, recovery might take a bit of time.

Julie loved painting—she painted at home and then out in the wilderness. A week of creative recovery effort stretched to almost two weeks with little sign of a desire to train. Relationship stress, however, began to dwindle, and Julie began to hang out and enjoy coffee with her favorite people and friends. Finally, as week 2 was stretching into the middle of week 3, signs of "the Julie people knew" began to resurface. The energy and drive began to return, and she started to get hungry to train and compete again.

Despite close to a three-week disruption in her training and competitive program, Julie went on to have the most successful season and following season in her storied career. Recovery is obviously extremely important, and if a multidisciplinary type of overtraining or exhaustion has developed, even creative recovery can take some time.

Not many coaches, athletes, and trainers are comfortable with this kind of recovery break, but demanding year-round training over several years can make breaks of this magnitude essential for health and high performance. Optimizing daily and weekly recovery is also very important, but our systems may really benefit from periodical macro-recovery breaks (Norris & Smith, this volume, chapter 7).

Training Addiction

Once athletes learn how hard they can work (and how this is related to development), it is not unusual for them to become addicted to training. As well as giving them a feeling of accomplishment, training can become "therapeutic" and a "conditioned response" to setback, guilt, or failure. At times this developing addiction can be productive, but at other times it can lead to serious overtraining.

Case Study 3

Kim sensitized us to the role that a "work ethic obsession" or "training addiction" can play in a young athlete. Kim was a National Junior Team speed skater who had shown great promise and came from a large, conscientious, hard-working family. In this case, the coach became concerned and referred Kim to the sport psychology consultant at the National Sport Centre Calgary. A lot of interactive teamwork takes place at the National Sport Centre Calgary, and a high trust level develops among athletes, coaches, and support staff. This facilitated the referral to the consultant (see Canadian Athlete Support System, p. 155).

Kim began meeting with the consultant and discussing her situation. By the time the sport psychology consultant had been sensitized to Kim's plight, she had lost considerable weight (despite nutritional counseling), and her performances had fallen far below expectations. After much discussion and conversation, Kim finally was able to see that she was in a state of overtraining. Because fatigue, fear, and frustration seemed unusually high, the consultant recommended stepping away from competition immediately to try to regain perspective and develop strategies to recover physically, mentally, and emotionally (see figure 8.1).

Through counseling, Kim came to realize that she is a highly motivated individual with lots of potential in her life beyond sport. She is extremely bright as well as motivated and plans a career in medicine as well as sport. Her drive, though, had become her own enemy. During the previous two or three years her response to disappointment was always to get on the bike and weights and work harder. She had progressively pushed herself into a seriously overtrained state. Worry and guilt only added to the overload and contributed to the exhaustion. Nutritional counseling alone was not enough to keep her healthy.

Kim was scheduled to compete in the World Junior Championships two weeks after connecting with the counselor. The first job was to convince Kim that her health and well-being were much more important than the World Junior Championships (her first lesson in medical health care started with herself). She finally agreed that a fairly dramatic change in her attitude, training, and recovery schedule might be important. She agreed to a rest and recovery strategy for most of the two weeks prior to the championships. Most important, the counselor wanted Kim to start enjoying performing for its own sake again.

Kim's participation in the World Championships produced some better, more encouraging moments, but the recovery was clearly not complete. Upon return, Kim was supported through a coaching change; a strong, perceptive coach kept Kim's training loads dramatically reduced and encouraged her to focus on recovery for the rest of the year. Close to two months after diagnosis, Kim finished the season with personal best performances. Her recovery was clearly physical, mental, and emotional.

Kim is an exceptional human being who now knows herself much better and has an exciting future in sport, medicine, and life. When one is in the bottom of an overtraining tunnel, however, it can be hard to see any of that potential or find strategies that can help.

Competition Today

According to Gould and Dieffenbach (this volume, chapter 2) a high percentage of U.S. athletes report "perceived overtraining" after the Olympics. Since top professional coaches are highly unlikely to prescribe excessive physical demands prior to such intense competition, athletes' feelings of overload are more likely the result of increased emotional and mental demands.

Competition in sport today has grown in stature and significance so much that some authors (i.e., Botterill, 1996b) are suggesting that emotional preparation and emotional management are often the keys to success. Feelings run high, and this can lead to enhanced performance, distraction, or exhaustion. When the increasing mental and emotional demands of competing are added to the physical demands of preparing and performing, it is not surprising that athletes often experience a form of overtraining during or just after a big competition (Gould & Dieffenbach, this volume, chapter 2). The increasing public and media interest, national expectations, the "fish bowl" feeling, and the many distractions just add to the focus and recovery challenges.

Case Study 4

Heidi provides evidence that major competition on top of a demanding program can lead to feelings of exhaustion and overtraining. Heidi had a history of handling high loads in several sports as well as excelling in school. Upon reaching college age, she enrolled in a top academic university and played on their varsity team as well as maintaining a role on the Canadian National Team.

The first year was demanding but extremely enjoyable with a feeling of success and accomplishment on all three fronts—national team, college team, and academics. Year 2 started in a similar way for Heidi, but new challenges soon arose. She was pressured to choose an academic major, two veteran leaders from the college team had graduated, and most significant, Heidi was being courted for a much more significant role on the national hockey team.

A major international tournament before Christmas turned out to be highly successful for Heidi but also extremely exhausting. She performed at a new level in the tournament, enjoying the role and the opportunity. The first signs of emotional exhaustion, however, were evident immediately following the tournament. Even the elation of winning and celebration gave way quickly to the need for rest. Despite her success, returning to college was not easy. Her energy was low, her attention seemed to wander, and guilt seemed to build when feelings weren't right. A four-day block of rest at Christmas proved not to be enough. Although her persistence resulted in academic and athletic obligations being met, her energy was low and a nagging injury developed (probably from fatigue).

Heidi's midterm break of eight or nine days proved to be the salvation. She turned down a National Team Camp opportunity and returned home for recovery. Rules were simple: Rest as much as possible and do things that are personally enjoyable. She averaged 11 hours of sleep per night for eight nights. Injury treatments and walks in her home community were the main activities. Home-cooked meals and visits with friends completed the restoration. Heidi began to show her old energy in the last couple of days before returning to college.

Coaches and trainers were patient in facilitating her return to action, and Heidi went on to have the best three months of her career—winning several major awards and a World Championship. Her enthusiasm academically and athletically had never been higher. Recovery at the right time and in the right way was obviously critical.

Early Warning Signs

Canadian coaches, athletes, and support personnel in general found the RESTQ-Sport (Kellmann & Kallus, 2001) monitoring/evaluation instrument very valuable, and several National Team programs have used it in conjunction with periodic blood and fitness tests. Nevertheless, a simpler, less time-consuming instrument was needed that could be used for weekly (maybe even daily) monitoring to try to pick up early warning signs regarding possible overtraining or underrecovery in individuals and teams.

The result was a simple seven-item self-monitoring and evaluation instrument, the Recovery-Cue (Kellmann, Botterill, & Wilson, 1999; see also Kellmann, this volume, chapter 3 and Kellmann, Patrick, Botterill, & Wilson, this volume, chapter 12). The Recovery-Cue reflects some of the progressive conceptualization of Kenttä and Hassmén (1998); the key questions of the RESTQ-Sport; and the educational/monitoring interests of Canadian athletes, coaches, and support staff. Three items on the Recovery-Cue reflect perceived exertion, perceived recovery, and recovery effort. These hint at progressively earlier warning signs regarding possible overtraining effects. The three key components of these are described as follows:

- *Perceived Exertion:* How difficult was it to perform normal workloads? (Backlog of fatigue starting to affect performance capacity)
- *Perceived Recovery:* How refreshed did you feel prior to your workouts? (First perceived

signs of physical, mental, or emotional fatigue)
- *Recovery Effort:* How successful were you with activities that optimize recovery for you? (First sign that recovery activities may not be adequate)

When the Recovery-Cue is administered weekly and collected by support staff for analysis, both individual and team fluctuations in scores can be identified and appropriate interventions planned. This Recovery-Cue also seems to have strong educational value. The regular reminders to optimize recovery can help educate performers on issues that have been taken pretty casually. Because athletes differ in what is most regenerating for them, especially emotionally, it takes a while to identify the best strategies.

Often, proactive recovery is every bit as important as rest. For example, going to a good movie is not physically much different from sitting in front of a TV watching soap operas. If the movie is good, however, the recovery and reenergizing effect can be much greater in emotional, mental, and physical systems. Similarly, after a lot of travel or mental stress, a light physical workout can have an energizing, regenerating effect. If combined with inspiring music and video highlights, the effect on all systems can be quite profound.

Case Study 5

Chris admitted that for him the first sign of possible overtraining was the tendency to become totally passive versus active in recovery. As he reported, "rest is important, but when you start feeling like a sloth or pig in a hammock, it is not often optimal recovery!" Chris has learned to adjust his training load slightly or to work more actively during recovery when he notices these signs of passivity. He is a great young developing speed skater and has learned some important lessons to enhance his future.

As with so many things, early warning signs are important. Educating athletes to respond and not overreact can make a big difference in preventing overtraining and optimizing performance. The next step is to educate more performers on ways to optimize recovery so they can handle their demanding jobs, stay healthy, and perform well. Kallus (this volume, chapter 16) explores the important implications of recovery for air traffic controllers and other professionals.

Energizing Techniques

Botterill and Patrick (1996) outlined a wide range of energizing techniques and activities that athletes can use to maximize recovery. If managed creatively, all four components of total behavior (doing, thinking, feeling, and physiology) identified by Glasser (1984) can contribute to recovery or reenergizing. Certainly things we think and do can have an energizing effect and influence our feelings and physiology. An inspiring movie, light exercise, and music are examples of activities that can influence our emotional and physiological states. In addition, we can actively manage our physiological well-being through massage, hydration, nutrition, and "power naps" (Glasser, 1984). Emotional management, discussed next, can play a big role in recovery and performance.

Emotional Management

Effective emotional management probably involves emotional preparation, emotional management, and emotional health (Botterill, 1996a, 1996b). All are important and affect our ability to perform, recover, and stay healthy. Emotions can have powerful, fairly spontaneous effects, which can be a challenge to prepare for and manage (Hanin, 2000). The inability to manage emotions can lead to major performance and health problems.

Emotional preparation involves anticipating the key feelings (emotions) one is likely to experience and rehearsing effective responses. The result is a form of "emotional inoculation" that produces a much more effective and efficient response under pressure. The efficiency results in a more manageable, less stressful performance demand, and recovery is less difficult.

Top performers should probably prepare for the seven basic human emotions identified by Vallerand (1984). Fear, anger, guilt/embarrassment, surprise, sadness, happiness, and interest are all likely and possible in performance environments. Identifying situational possibilities for each emotion and rehearsing effective responses can dramatically improve emotional preparation, performance, and recovery. In fact, life itself also involves a lot of emotional management!

All basic emotions have functional values. Fear triggers preparation, or readying. Anger mobi-lizes fighting for what you think is right. Guilt/embarrassment motivates us to act for significant others. Surprise keeps us from becoming complacent. Sadness is a type of grieving that facilitates recovery. Happiness is the joy of life. Interest prevents boredom and indifference. Despite the functional significance of emotions, emotional mismanagement costs society immensely. Fear out of control leads to anxiety. Anger out of control leads to violence. Guilt and sadness out of control lead to depression. These three social problems point to the tremendous financial and human cost of emotional mismanagement. Despite this reality, it is amazing how few young people are taught emotional management as part of their early education.

The first critical element in effective emotional processing is acceptance. When strong feelings are not accepted and shared, denial and repression can begin to affect one's health and ability to focus and recover. Personal honesty; integrity; and the confidence to accept, share, and process emotions can be a great start toward emotional health and dynamic recovery. Just accepting one's feelings can lead to a release and the beginning of a functional adaptation or response.

After accepting and sharing strong emotions, most of us need help with rational constructive interpretation and response possibilities. Friends, family, or colleagues that can help us see the big picture and bring perspective are a big help. Perspective is an important concept that involves how we feel about ourselves, our significant others, our activities, and life values (Brown, Cairus, & Botterill, 2001; Newburg, 1999). When we have a healthy perspective, emotional management is more likely to go well. Like everything, though, our sense of perspective is vulnerable and very much related to "inner peace" and emotional health.

The final phase of emotional management is channeling the energy created in an effective way. All emotions either produce energy or contribute to recovery. Harnessing this energy in constructive ways is critical for enhancing performance and avoiding fatigue. Everyone has experienced the power of emotions, but few really appreciate how exhausting emotions can be if not managed effectively. Repression and denial often add significantly to the buildup of fear, guilt, anger, and frustration. Fatigue, depression, and performance/recovery problems usually follow. Regular emotional processing with people one trusts can make a big difference in enhancing emotional health, performance, and recovery.

Most performers have not had much help with emotional management. A person who is "emotionally retarded" is limited in the ability to process emotions effectively and optimize health and high performance. When one develops or regains a strong, clear perspective, recovery is amazingly effective, and natural energy flows freely. Being and feeling genuine and at peace can make a big difference with recovery, processing, and performance. It has long been suspected that repressed, denied, or unprocessed emotions can be the source of subconscious and conscious stress and dissonance. The logical extension of this is a related effect on focus, performance, and, eventually, health. Hopefully, in the future there will be much more assistance in learning and mastering "emotional intelligence" (Goleman, 1995).

Team emotional dynamics can be powerful, contagious, and complex (Botterill & Brown, 2001). Groups trying to optimize training and recovery should work on creating "real" versus "pseudo" team dynamics (Werthner & Botterill, 2000). The emotional climate for work, performance, and recovery is dramatically superior when there is a high level of trust, respect, and support in the team (Robertson, 2000). Emotions can be very contagious, escalating, and distracting, and there is a much better chance that they will be harnessed and accepted if trust, respect, and team perspective are strong (Botterill & Patrick, in press). Our situational beliefs, focus, and capability are often affected by the beliefs of those around us (Riley, 1993). Team building, emotional preparation, and emotional management are well worth investing in, if we are trying to optimize team and individual health and performance. As others have discovered, though (Hanin, 2000; Kellmann, this volume, chapters 1 and 3), assessment and management of emotions is often a very individual and situational challenge. Teamwork and a real sense of team can help, but it is important to never overlook the personal response or challenge.

Character Development

The issue of whether sport involvement builds character in young athletes has been debated for many years and extensively in the literature (Beller & Stoll, 1994; Decker & Lasley, 1995; Dickey, 1979; Eitzen, 1989; Galasso, 1986; Miracle & Reese, 1994; Sage, 1998; Tutko & Bruns, 1979). One question that often arises is whether sport actually does develop athletes into responsible, self-aware, and independent adults. "Recent research (Beller &

Stoll, 1994; Decker & Lasley, 1995) actually suggests that organized sport for youth may actually be detrimental to moral development, a key component of character" (Sage, 1998, p. 17). Some argue that athletes at various levels can become more dependent and less responsible for their own lives and development. They are told when to eat, where and when to sleep, what their training should be, when and how to rest and recover, and when to get on the bus. George Sauer, the former All-Pro receiver for the New York Jets was quoted to have said

> College and professional level coaches still treat you like an adolescent. They know damn well that you were never given a chance to become responsible or self-disciplined. Even in the pros you are told when to go to bed, when to turn your lights off, when to wake up, when to eat and what to eat. You even have to live together like you were in a boys' camp. (Tutko & Bruns, 1979, p. 233)

Athletes often seem to become dependent on other people to prepare them, and ultimately they do not learn to make their own decisions. Even when they do make a decision, they are not confident and need to be reassured.

On the other hand, some argue that involvement in sport does build character. Sport involvement develops an independent, responsible, and self-aware individual, an individual who is now ready to tackle the rest of the world and life. Educating athletes and support staff on rest and recovery and promoting self-awareness and responsibility for recovery needs may actualize more independent individuals and athletes. The RESTQ-Sport and Recovery-Cue are tools that can be used to educate and sensitize athletes and support staff about individual rest and recovery needs. Educating both the athlete and the support staff about the importance of rest and recovery is crucial when working with an interdisciplinary team.

National Sport Centre Calgary System

The National Sport Centre Calgary has a team of support staff that works closely together. This team helps coaches become more aware and sensitive to fluctuations in an athlete through regular monitoring. In many cases the athletes are comfortable in this environment, working closely with coaches and sport psychology consultants as a team to help them become better performers. They share information with the coaches and support staff in order to create and follow the rest and recovery plan that is best for them. With regular monitoring, coaches become aware that each athlete is unique and therefore has different rest and recovery needs and strategies.

The term *overtrained* may be used loosely in the sport environment and without important relevant information due to a lack of knowledge, inconsistent terminology, and undefined symptoms or diagnoses (Hooper & Mackinnon, 1995). At times the term *overtrained* is used when *underrecovered* may be more suitable (see Kellmann, this volume, chapter 1). This can be difficult for an athlete who is uneducated and unfamiliar with the concepts of rest and recovery. For example, when an athlete starts to get tired, support staff or others who are uneducated in rest and recovery might suggest that the athletes is overtrained and should take time off. This is sometimes the case; however, it might also be that the athlete is in an overreaching phase of training, or that the athlete needs to be more active in the recovery efforts (see Kellmann, this volume, chapter 1; Smith & Norris, this volume, chapter 5).

Self-Awareness

In his 1983 research on Ideal Performance States, Loehr suggested that the first step in optimizing one's state for many athletes is self-awareness. Once athletes have learned about the importance of the total fitness model (see figure 8.1, p. 145), and that rest and recovery play an essential role, they can bring their training to a new level. They can increase their body awareness. They will also know when to increase or implement certain recovery techniques and have confidence in their decision. This next case is an example of this situation with a young athlete.

Case Study 6

Leanne, a young swimmer, was in the process of becoming aware of many different aspects about her training, the amount of stress she could endure, and her individual rest and recovery needs. Nearing the end of the season, but with some major competitions still to come, the consultant received an e-mail message from this panic-stricken athlete who was not enjoying training or anything to do with her sport. She was feeling overwhelmed with schoolwork, training, and other personal

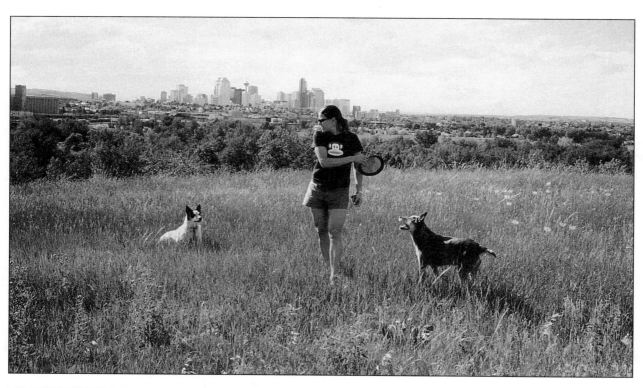

Emotional recovery strategy can take place with reenergizing activities, such as playing outside with pets.

development extracurricular activities. Due to her busy days, she was not finding enough time to get the appropriate amount of sleep or relaxation time. She still was getting up early for her morning training sessions.

After some interventions and conversations with the consultant regarding listening to her body and some education about total fitness, Leanne was willing to try some recovery strategies. However, she was concerned that her coach would not respect her decision and think she was "slacking." Fortunately, one day the coach pulled her aside at training and gave her permission to take some time off if she was tired and not enjoying herself. She spent the next week of training time lying in the sun, reenergizing, and sleeping. A week later, her attitude and performance were dramatically improved. With education and self-awareness she is now able to make those decisions with confidence and feel she is fulfilling her individual needs.

A self-aware athlete will not only know when to increase or implement the recovery techniques, but also know which recovery strategies will be most useful at that particular time in life and training. The strategies could range from passive recovery such as sleeping or refraining from train-

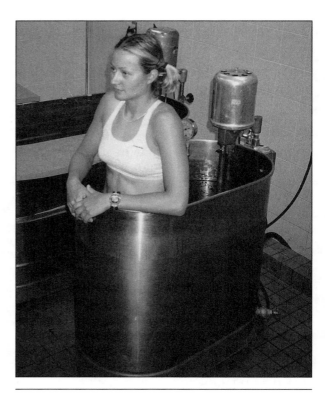

Proactive physiological recovery can be assisted with hot and cold baths.

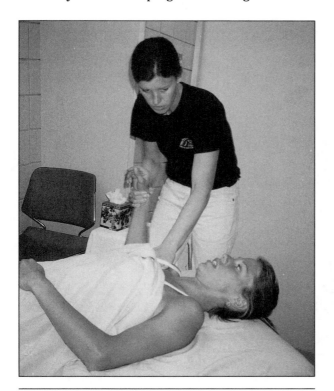

Actively managing the physiological well-being through massage is an excellent recovery strategy.

ing to various forms of active recovery. Active recovery could include strategies such as hot and cold baths, massages, spending more time warming up and cooling down, or doing more enjoyable energizing and regenerating activities (Rattray & Ludwig, 2000; Sedergreen, 2000).

When a monitoring tool is in place, the athlete, coaches, and support staff can be aware of when the "active" recovery pursuits start to drop off. A simple discussion with the athlete about her RESTQ-Sport profile can help in detecting overtraining and planning recovery.

Case Study 7

While discussing her profile, which showed poor physical recovery effort, with her consultant, Angela (a speed skater) explained how the tool was useful for her. She described how she was too tired to be proactive with her recovery and make the effort to do hot and cold baths, go for massages, or do any type of actively planned recovery. While completing the RESTQ-Sport, she realized and became aware that her recovery was not where it should be and that her recovery strategies were seriously lacking (see figure 8.2).

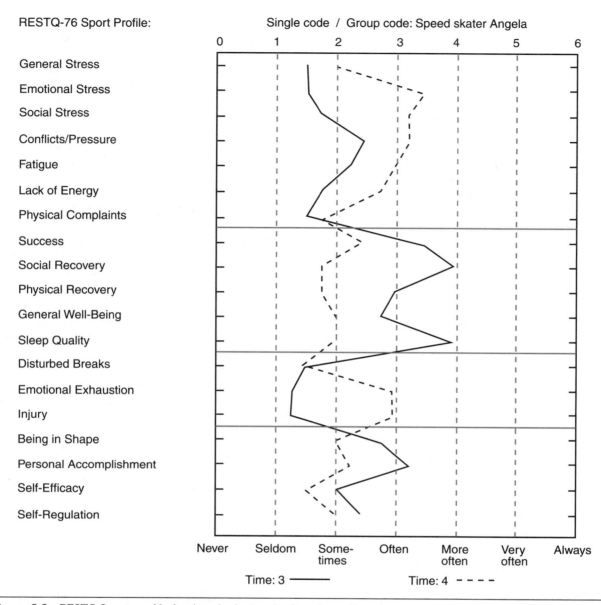

Figure 8.2 RESTQ-Sport profile for Angela during the first (time 3) and second (time 4) hard training phase.

Angela's profiles provide information about her recovery effort and general stress level. Testing time 3 was during a hard training phase (solid line); however, Angela was able to maintain her recovery efforts. Testing time 4 (broken line) was also during a hard training phase; however, she also had some other aspects of her life that were causing more general stress.

After completing the RESTQ-Sport and then seeing the profile, Angela knew that this was the time to take more time for active recovery. Following this, her training started feeling better and she was able to reenergize in order to recover for the next training session.

Self-aware athletes are more likely to take responsibility for their own development and growth as individuals and as athletes. As stated at the beginning of the chapter, athletes' most important lesson is to learn that they can work harder than they thought possible. With education and awareness of rest and recovery strategies, they will know when to push themselves and realize that it is appropriate to push as long as the necessary rest and recovery efforts are being made. Though athletes will continue to push themselves, they will also give themselves permission to take the necessary rest and recovery measures in order for optimal quality training and performance enhancement to occur. Such an attitude can help prevent staleness, overtraining, and fatigue buildup.

Athletes at all levels of competition will sometimes attend a competition or training camp without their coaches. If they are self-aware and educated in rest and recovery, and understand the importance of monitoring themselves regularly, they will be able to make some of their own decisions and take more responsibility for their own actions, training, and successes.

Of course this self-awareness and education may take time and effort. It takes days, months, and years for athletes to learn and perfect what works well in terms of physical, technical, and tactical preparation. They will also need to learn what type of recovery techniques to use, when to use them, and how to use them most effectively and efficiently. All of this information can promote a better training program, a more independent athlete, and ultimately the desired performances.

In addition to understanding the importance of rest and recovery, athletes should be educated in the many different forms of rest and recovery. These can include going to a movie, spending time in the mountains, sleeping, changing activities (e.g., a swimmer may choose to go for a hike or a bike ride), spending time with friends or family, taking hot and cold baths, getting massages (relaxation and sport related), writing, reading, and so on. Clearly athletes—indeed, all people—need to recover physically, mentally, and emotionally. At times even social and spiritual recovery needs to be facilitated if the athlete is spending considerable amounts of time away from friends and family and other support networks. The case of Trevor that follows illustrates the significance of the environment and emotional climate.

Case Study 8

Trevor was a longtime elite short-track speed skater who started training with a new group of athletes and a new coach and spending a lot of time learning new techniques. The new group of athletes and the coach had been working closely together for a number of years. Trevor found it very difficult to receive the attention he needed, and his perception was that the other athletes were annoyed with him. They did not appear to be very open to newcomers, and he found it difficult to connect with them. Trevor felt his needs were not being met by the coach or by the team, and he was beginning to lose confidence in his own training methods and preparation. He worried constantly about fairness, fitting in, and being himself, and he began to feel extremely worn out. His life felt like an emotional roller-coaster ride. Although the physical training had been difficult, Trevor and his consultant came to the conclusion that the mental and emotional struggle was causing these feelings of exhaustion, lack of desire and motivation, and wanting to quit.

Trevor spent some time away from the group and started to do things and be with people that bolstered his confidence. As time went on, he started to remember the fire and desire that had made him great before; ultimately, he remembered who he was. His energy returned, and the natural determination that he had enjoyed in previous years returned with it. He trained, competed, and recovered with a new sense of confidence and vigor.

Athletes differ in the amount and kind of physical, mental, and emotional recovery needed to restore themselves (see figure 8.1, p. 145). After a major competition, athlete A might need to spend a couple of days away from training to hang out with friends before being ready to get back into the thick of things. After the same major competition, on the other hand, athlete B might need a few more days to spend some alone time in the mountains or a large amount of time with family (spouse and kids) and friends. Coaches and support staff, therefore, must be aware of athletes' different requirements. By considering the athletes' whole lives, not just their lives as athletes, coaches are in a better position to understand each athlete's unique recovery needs. As such, they are better able to formulate strategies to meet those needs.

Interdisciplinary Approach and Issues

While coaches play a crucial role in the development of an athlete, other support staff might be assisting the athlete in the pursuit of excellence. The support staff might include sport psychology consultants, psychologists, exercise physiologists, athletic therapists, strength coaches, physiotherapists, doctors, nutritionists, and administrators. Each of these people plays an important role in the world of the athlete. Together they make up a team that can help the athlete from many different perspectives, a concept referred to as the interdisciplinary approach.

In this section we will discuss the interdisciplinary approach, the interdisciplinary support system in Canada, and the challenges and benefits of implementing this approach.

Interdisciplinary Versus Multidisciplinary approach

The terms *interdisciplinary* and *multidisciplinary* are often used interchangeably. In his article on interdisciplinary research in sport, Mills (1996) suggested that these two terms have very different meanings and should not be used interchangeably.

> Multidisciplinary research constitutes a group of people from different subdisciplines working on a common topic in parallel. Interdisciplinary research involves an integration of ideas from various subdisciplines to answer a question that could not be answered from a monodisciplinary approach. (Mills, 1996, p. 2)

Professionals from a variety of disciplines are increasingly working together on the same research/service projects, bringing their resources to improve the quality of a project. An example of interdisciplinary research is a project in which researchers from the medical profession work with exercise physiologists to determine how exercise programs can benefit women with breast cancer. Everyone is working together to uncover contributing factors and collective conclusions. The same research project from a multidisciplinary approach would find a physiologist, sport psychology consultant, and physician all making different conclusions and then coming together to collaborate. The article "Creating a Multidisciplinary Team to Promote the Mental and Physical Well-Being of College Dance Students" (Davis, Stombaugh, & Tenley, 1992) is an example of a multidisciplinary approach in practice. A variety of professionals, including psychologists, nutritionists, instructors, and exercise physiologists worked independently with the dancers.

Interdisciplinary collaborations that happen early on decrease the occurrence of half-truths (Mills, 1996). A recommendation may seem appropriate from one discipline but might only be a half-truth when information from other disciplines is considered. Interdisciplinary input is necessary to optimize advice and minimize inappropriate and dangerous half-truth suggestions. Professionals working together from such an approach are better able to view the athlete as a whole person as they consider insights and relationships from all disciplines and systems. The interdisciplinary approach can be of considerably greater value when intervening to help athletes reach their fullest potential by taking into consideration the total fitness model (see figure 8.1, p. 145).

Canadian Athlete Support System

The Canadian athlete support system has gradually developed a series of National Sport Centres across the country to better serve athletes' needs. Resources are still limited in comparison with countries like Australia, but a high percentage of Canada's elite athletes and coaches are starting to take advantage of interdisciplinary support services. Athletes have the opportunity to work with strength coaches, exercise physiologists, sport psychology consultants, nutritionists, and a variety of other professionals in pursuit of their fullest potential. At the National Sport Centre Calgary the interdisciplinary teams collaborate regularly on issues, situations, and effects that might be affecting an individual athlete or a team of athletes. Interdisciplinary meetings might include the coach, a sport psychology consultant, a strength coach, an exercise physiologist, a nutritionist, and sometimes administrators, all of whom are looking out for the best interests of the athlete. Regular phone, e-mail, and personal contact between support team members is also encouraged.

Knowledge from the various subdisciplines can be combined to more accurately and comprehensively understand an athlete's problems. For example, the sport psychology consultant may have a RESTQ-Sport profile that suggests that recovery is insufficient. The exercise physiologist may have data from a blood test suggesting that underrecovery may be taking place, and the coach may be noticing that performance is decreasing. A sharing and brainstorming session with all the information might be necessary in order to provide the athlete with the most important information to return him to a state of optimal training, performance, and recovery.

When implementing an interdisciplinary approach, some important issues must be taken into consideration. First, unless there is a regular dialogue between the athlete and all team members, this approach might lead to less independence on the part of the athlete as she perceives that many people are taking responsibility for her. Second, the issue of confidentiality must be considered when working closely with an athlete or team.

Interdisciplinary Challenges

If the support staff is not educated on how to reduce the dependency of the athlete, the athlete can ultimately have difficulty making his own decisions and may depend too much on other people to achieve high performance. This can happen easily in the area of rest and recovery. Athletes should be invited to have input in all assessments and decisions and be provided with inter-disciplinary rationale for all advice so they become self-aware and educated about rest and recovery. Howe (1980) suggested that in order to have an athlete reach the highest potential performance, it is crucial that the coach reduce the dependency of the athlete on the coach or other support staff. Educating the athlete and support staff about rest and recovery could reduce this dependency, as discussed in the previous section.

As interdisciplinary athlete support programs become more prevalent all over the world, issues such as role clarification, conflict, and confidentiality become more important. Collins, Moore, Mitchell, and Alpress (1999) brought this to the forefront and suggested some solutions and steps that can be taken in order to have an effective and efficient team working for the well-being of the athlete or performer.

Benefits of the Interdisciplinary Team Approach

The interdisciplinary team approach to rest and recovery can also enhance an athlete's performance. Working closely as a unit allows the entire team of support staff to be aware of the individual athlete's needs and also her emotional, mental, and physical states when she is performing at her best. This allows all support staff to be aware if something is not going well with the athlete. The support staff can collaborate and find out if all things are running smoothly mentally, physically, and emotionally (see figure 8.1, p. 145), and if not, where things can be changed, altered, or improved.

The RESTQ-Sport and Recovery-Cue monitoring tools are useful for integrating athletes' self-management with the interdisciplinary approach. When an athlete is showing signs of underrecovery, which can be clearly identified on a RESTQ-Sport profile or various other physiological testing, the interdisciplinary team can work together to figure out what needs to happen. Along with the athlete, the coach, the sport psychology consultant, the exercise physiologist, and other members of the interdisciplinary team collaborate on some of the

desired changes that will bring the athlete back to a position in which quality training, sufficient recovery, and enhanced performance can take place. Regular monitoring of rest and recovery strategies is essential for this to work most effectively and efficiently. The following case illustrates how important situational monitoring and interdisciplinary discussion can be.

Case Study 9

Canada's National Speed Skating Team returned from a demanding road trip in Europe the year before the Olympics. Dialogue with athletes and coaches revealed a host of concerns about training loads, recovery, nutrition, and hydration as well as team building and emotional fatigue.

The sport psychology consultant immediately invited the physiologist, strength coach, and nutritionist to a meeting that had been primarily scheduled for psychological issues. As the physiologist became more aware of the emotional and competitive demands of the trip, he began to adjust training guidelines and recommend recovery strategies. From there, the team had an interactive interdisciplinary discussion of possible individual and team strategies and adjustments. Tremendously relieved and much more confident, the athletes and coaches then participated in some highly effective team building and emotional preparation activities.

Interdisciplinary meetings with performers can be extremely valuable for staff and coaches as well as for the performers themselves. Confidence and insight regarding programming and recovery can be dramatically enhanced. Also, support staff can gain insights from performers, coaches, and professionals in other disciplines that can make their advice and adjustments much more appropriate and effective. Clearly, performance enhancement continues to be an art as well as a science. Multiple sources of input are often necessary to make good decisions.

Although athletes must take responsibility for themselves, the support staff must also support the total fitness model and the rest and recovery necessary for all systems, including the physical, mental, and emotional. Small reminders by the coaches or other support staff will help the athlete make a routine of evaluating the rest and recovery strategies that they are implementing or should be implementing. Regular sharing of insights and concerns by support staff personnel is critical for the interdisciplinary approach to work most effectively and efficiently.

Recovery-Cue in Canadian Sport

Over the past year the Recovery-Cue, discussed in chapters 3 and 12 of this volume, has been implemented with a variety of national teams in Calgary. The interest in the Recovery-Cue has grown over the past year, and it will be implemented with more teams with increased structure and follow-through. In the past year athletes and coaches were given a chance to try the Recovery-Cue to evaluate whether it would be a useful tool for them. Now, the coaches and athletes have become great supporters of the instrument. Each year more teams are using the Recovery-Cue as part of a regular monitoring system. Some of them are including the Recovery-Cue as part of their logbooks, whereas others will complete it as a separate entity that will be discussed with the consultant or trainer. Using this tool in conjunction with periodically administering the RESTQ-Sport facilitates regular monitoring and education that will assist athletes in becoming more self-aware and confident in their programs and individual rest and recovery needs.

In addition to daily or weekly monitoring with the Recovery-Cue, the coaches and support staff of the teams have found periodically administering the more comprehensive RESTQ-Sport to be a valuable supplement. National Sport Centre staff and coaches have explored different beneficial times to administer the RESTQ-Sport. Currently they suggest: during a hard training phase, just after a hard training phase, while traveling or at camps, following camps, and immediately before two or more competitions. Attaining results from a wide variety of phases allows the athlete and support staff to become more aware of the needs of the athlete. After regular use of the RESTQ-Sport, athletes develop a common profile of when they are feeling great and performing well. This allows them and their support staffs to see clearly when there are deviations (highs or lows) from this ideal profile. If a deviation occurs, clear communication with the athlete determines what is happening and then suggestions of how to return to an ideal state are discussed.

The RESTQ-Sport is now available for coaches and athletes as a manual (Kellmann & Kallus, 2001). This is especially helpful in situations in which a support staff is not within the budget. Coaches can work closely with athletes on a regular basis to learn how to read the RESTQ-Sport

profile and the Recovery-Cue. After some time working with these tools, and with good communication, the coach and athlete can become very aware of the athlete's needs. In some cases, with the Recovery-Cue specifically, the athlete can determine if some recovery issues need to be dealt with. Although the athlete may know what to do to alter this, good communication with the coach or support staff, if available, will provide the athlete with educated information.

The beauty of the Recovery-Cue is that it is a simple, noninvasive method of monitoring that acts as an early warning system. Athletes can learn to monitor themselves and know when to work closely with the coach or support staff to get some help. Ideally, a trainer or sport psychology consultant is also monitoring the data each week for individual or team implications. At times there may be coaching, psychological, medical, massage, nutrition, hydration, sport science, or team building implications. This instrument can help sensitize performers to how best to optimize health, recovery, and performance.

Summary

Overtraining prevention in top performers is a complicated task. It involves espousing a concept called total fitness and optimizing physical, mental, and emotional recovery as well as workload. Today's demands, in and out of sport, make it an important topic. Athletes and their supporters must respect individual differences and detect and respond to early warning signs.

Emotional management plays a major role in overtraining prevention and long-term performance enhancement. While interdisciplinary support teams can be a great help, performer awareness, education, and independence are critical objectives. Canadian experience in overtraining prevention has been very sensitizing, and responses to date have been encouraging. Nevertheless, many aspects of optimizing recovery and adjusting training loads and strategies still need to be researched, refined, and implemented.

Acknowledgments

The authors acknowledge the athletes, coaches, and support staff of the National Sport Centre Calgary, whose testimonies, observations, and monitoring made a critical contribution to the data and insights in this chapter.

References

Banister, E.W. (1991). Modelling elite athletic performance. In J.D. MacDougall, H. Wenger, & H.J. Green (Eds.), *Physiological testing of the high-performance athlete* (2nd ed., pp. 103-129). Champaign, IL: Human Kinetics.

Belcastro, A., McKenzie, D., & Smith, M. (1989). *Assessing and monitoring of overtraining in elite Canadian athletes.* Unpublished Study. Ottawa: Sport Canada.

Beller, J.M., & Stoll, S.K. (1994). Sport participation and its effect on moral reasoning of high school student athletes and general students. *Research Quarterly for Exercise and Sports* (Suppl. A), 94.

Borg, G. (1998). *Borg's Perceived Exertion and Pain Scales.* Champaign, IL: Human Kinetics.

Botterill, C. (1996a). *Emotion as a factor in health and high performance.* Keynote address at the Association for the Advancement of Applied Sport Psychology Conference, Williamsburg, VA.

Botterill, C. (1996b). Emotional preparation for the Olympic Games. *Coaches Report 2*(1), 26-30.

Botterill, C., & Brown, M. (2001). Emotion & perspective in sport. *International Journal of Sport Psychology, 32,* 352-374.

Botterill, C., & Patrick, T. (1996). *Human potential.* Winnipeg, ON: Lifeskills.

Botterill, C., & Patrick, T. (in press). Emotion in sport. In K. Henschen & R. Lidor (Eds.), *Psychology of team sport.* Morgantown, WV: Fitness Information Technology.

Botterill, C., & Wilson, C. (1999, September). *Overtraining prevention.* Symposium presentation at the Association for the Advancement of Applied Sport Psychology Conference, Banff, AB.

Brown, M., Cairus, K., & Botterill, C. (2001). The process of perspective: The art of living well in the world of elite sport. *Journal of Excellence, 1*(5), 5-38.

Collins, D., Moore, P., Mitchell, D., & Alpress, F. (1999). Role conflict and confidentiality in multidisciplinary athlete support programmes. *British Journal of Sports Medicine, 33,* 208-211.

Davis, K.M., Stombaugh, I.A., & Tenley, K. (1992). Creating a multidisciplinary team to promote the mental and physical well-being of college dance students. *Kinesiology and Medicine for Dance, 14*(1), 126-132.

Decker, D., & Lasley, K. (1995). Participation in youth sports, gender, and the moral point of view. *The Physical Educator, 53,* 14-21.

Dickey, G. (1979). Athletes and the self-discipline myth. In D.S. Eitzen (Ed.), *Sport in contemporary society* (pp. 237-245). New York: St. Martin Press.

Eitzen, D.S. (1989). The dark side of coaching and the building of character. In D.S. Eitzen (Ed.), *Sport in contemporary society* (2nd ed., pp. 133-138). New York: St. Martin Press.

Galasso, P.J. (1986). *The autonomous athlete: More gold, better citizen.* Unpublished manuscript. Canadian Track and Field Association Symposium, Toronto, ON.

Glasser, W. (1984). *Control theory.* New York: Harper and Row.

Goleman, D. (1995). *Emotional intelligence.* New York: Bantam Books.

Hanin, Y.L. (Ed.). (2000). *Emotions in sport.* Champaign, IL: Human Kinetics.

Hooper, S.L., & Mackinnon, L.T. (1995). Monitoring overtraining in athletes. *Sport Medicine, 20,* 321-327.

Howe, B. (1980). Reducing independence in the high level performer. *Recreation Research Review, December, 8*(2), 45-49.

Kellmann, M., Botterill, C., & Wilson, C. (1999). *Recovery-Cue.* Unpublished Recovery Assessment Instrument. Calgary, AB: National Sport Centre.

Kellmann, M., & Günther, K.-D. (2000). Changes in stress and recovery in elite rowers during preparation for the Olympic Games. *Medicine and Science in Sports and Exercise, 32,* 676-683.

Kellmann, M., & Kallus, K.W. (1999). Mood, recovery-stress state, and regeneration. In M. Lehmann, C. Foster, U. Gastmann, H. Keizer, & J.M. Steinacker (Eds.), *Overload, fatigue, performance incompetence, and regeneration in sport* (pp. 101-117). New York: Plenum.

Kellmann, M., & Kallus, K.W. (2001). *Recovery-Stress Questionnaire for Athletes: User manual.* Champaign, IL: Human Kinetics.

Kellmann, M., Kallus, K.W., & Kurz, H. (1996). Performance prediction by the Recovery-Stress Questionnaire. *Journal of Applied Sport Psychology, 8* (Suppl.), S22.

Kenttä, G., & Hassmén, P. (1998). Overtraining and recovery: A conceptual model. *Journal of Sport Medicine, 26*(1), 1-16.

Loehr, J.E. (1983). The ideal performance state. *Sports: Science Periodical on Research and Technology in Sport, Sport Psychology* BU-1. Jan 1983, 1-8.

McGovern, S. (1998). An evaluation of services provided to elite athletes at a multi-sport training facility: A model of excellence (Doctoral Dissertation, Boston University, 1998). *Dissertation Abstracts International,* No. 9901948.

Millman, D. (1985). *The way of the peaceful warrior.* New York: New World Library.

Mills, B.D. (1996). Interdisciplinary research: An old idea revisited. *Journal of Interdisciplinary Research in Physical Education, 1*(1), 1-6.

Miracle, A. Jr., & Reese, C.R. (1994). *Lessons of the locker room: The myth of school sports.* Amherst, NY: Prometheus Books.

Newburg, D. (1999). *Resonance: Keeping desire greater than fear.* Charlottesville: University of Virginia School of Medicine.

Rattray, F., & Ludwig, L. (2000). *Clinical massage therapy.* Toronto, ON: Talus Incorporated.

Riley, P. (1993). *The winner within.* New York: Putnum's Sons.

Robertson, S. (2000). Creating an Olympic success story. *Coaches Report, 6*(3), 9-13.

Sage, G. (1998). Does sport affect character development in athletes? *The Journal of Physical Education, Recreation and Dance, 69*(1), 15-18.

Sedergreen, C. (2000). Massage therapy: A review. *British Columbia Medical Journal, 42,* 342-344.

Smith, D. (1999, September). *Monitoring an athlete's tolerance for training.* Symposium presentation at the Association for the Advancement of Applied Sport Psychology Conference, Banff, AB.

Smith, D., Norris, S., Maki, B., & Botterill, C. (1999, October). *The team approach to interdisciplinary sport science support.* Presentation at Canadian National Coaching Seminar, Toronto, ON.

Tutko, T., & Bruns, W. (1979). Sports don't build character—they build characters. In D.S. Eitzen (Ed.), *Sport in contemporary society* (pp. 232-236). New York: St. Martin Press.

Vallerand, R. (1984). Emotion in sport: Definitional, historical, and social psychological perspectives. In W. Straub & J. Williams (Eds.), *Cognitive sport psychology* (pp. 65-78). Lansing, NY: Sport Science Associates.

Weinberg, R., & Gould, D. (1999). *Foundations of sport and exercise psychology.* Champaign, IL: Human Kinetics.

Werthner, P., & Botterill, C.(2000). On sport psychology. *Coaches Report, 6* (4), 28-29.

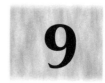

9

Mood and Self-Regulation Changes in Underrecovery: An Intervention Model

Henry Davis IV, Cal Botterill, and Karen MacNeill

Vince Lombardi (as cited in Maraniss, 1999, p. 217) is quoted as having said in 1959, "Fatigue makes cowards of us all." Did Lombardi know about underrecovery back then? The athlete in high-intensity training provides a wonderful example for the elucidation of psychological factors that can adversely affect performance when the athlete is underrecovered. Lombardi knew well that fatigue can trigger many emotions. During training camps high-performance athletes incur training loads that surpass general training levels; this high-intensity training compromises physiological recovery and can bring a deterioration of mood (Kellmann & Kallus, 1999). Such loads demand physical and psychological adaptive responses to restore homeostasis as described in chapter 1 of this volume. However, when the recovery of consumptive resources is inadequate, the athlete is said to be in a state of underrecovery (UR), and return to psychological homeostasis is impaired. When this happens, various negative psychological states become possible.

The model outlined in this chapter describes a triad of negative psychological responses in the UR[1] athlete: depressed-tone (negative affect) responses, anxiety-like mood responses, and a constellation of various fear responses each arising as a consequence of nonspecific arousal and low self-regulation factors. Each of the members of this triad is subclinical (i.e., not a diagnosable mood disorder) and has thought, affect, and be-

havioral components. This chapter identifies empirical research that serves as the scientific base for the responsible intervention in UR; case examples follow. We begin by elaborating on the concept of empirically supported treatment as it applies to intervention in UR.

Our position on cause and effect is that poor self-regulation and low mood may sometimes *result in* poor athletic performance and prolong inadequate recovery; at other times, these factors may directly *result from* inadequate recovery. Recovery occurs at physical, psychological, and social levels. We therefore propose continuous two-way interactions between psychological and physiological states.

The Need for an Empirically Derived Intervention Model

Empirical research on depressive mood, anxiety, and fear provides for the development of scientifically and professionally acceptable interventions that can hasten the return to balance and homeostasis in the UR athlete. A chapter on methods for intervention would imply that UR can be reliably diagnosed and that an empirically validated model has already spawned *theory-driven interventions* that have themselves been subjected to investigation. Unfortunately, this is not the case. The interventions that are herein proposed are intended to serve as examples of applications of the current

---

1. We will use *UR* for both *underrecovered* and *underrecovery* in this chapter.

model. There are no treatment manuals. The term *empirical construction,* resting at the foot of treatment planning in the absence of model and method validation, must be understood at the outset. Wilson (1996) cautions the psychologist that clinical judgment is never preferable to the rigorous application of science to treatment planning. Empirical construction refers to such use of empirical research to establish a scientific basis for intervention in a context, such as sport, in which there may be few if any tested interventions (Gaskovski, 1999).

Applied sport psychologists generally use empirical construction. On the basis of theory, they teach strategies for coping with fear, for dealing with precompetitive anxiety, for modifying negative thinking, and for altering communication patterns with coaches when no treatment manuals exist. For example, a high-functioning UR athlete in a training camp might (with no history of psychological disorder) start to socially withdraw, cry, or talk self-critically. Research on depression would not apply to this individual since he is not depressed, and research on the acute effects of crisis would not apply to this individual since he is not in the aftermath of a traumatic event. Neither does the literature on overtraining apply (Weinberg, 1990). There is little empirical evidence that methods intended to alter a UR-evoked mood state would be appropriate, necessary, or relevant, let alone efficacious. In sum, therefore, we do not yet have empirically supported psychological interventions for UR athletes.

Caveats for Ethical Intervention

Consecutive American Psychological Association (APA) task forces have confirmed the obvious by stating that psychology is a science and that the ethical practitioner uses interventions that possess a foundation in science. In 1996 one APA task force noted the following in its report:

> Whatever interventions that mysticism, authority, commercialism, politics, custom, convenience, or carelessness might dictate, clinical psychologists focus on what works. They bear a fundamental ethical responsibility to use where possible interventions that work and to subject any intervention they use to scientific scrutiny. (American Psychological Association, 1996, p. 7)

Recently, Hunsley, Dobson, Johnston, and Mikail (1999) added their weight to this position by

reiterating that the services provided by psychologists are ethically founded on a base of scientific evidence; with Chambless and Hollon (1998), they advocated a step further in requiring that interventions be based on manual-based clinical trials. These are obvious challenges for the applied sport psychologist working with UR athletes, and, as some will quickly point out, the working relationship between the athlete and the sport psychologist still remains one of the most powerful predictors of mastery (Bachelor & Horvath, 1999). Empiricism will probably never overtake the human element as one of the most powerful factors in the facilitation of change.

The Model

Sport psychological intervention with the UR athlete promotes emotional management and self-regulation. Our intervention model, as delineated in this chapter, builds on the following factors and their interactions: (1) fatigue as a trigger for self-regulation failure and (2) fatigue and neurochemical responses to stress and fatigue as related to three forms of mood disturbance—(1) low positive affect (depression, helplessness, and low self-efficacy), (2) anxiety, and (3) fear.

Definition of Negative Mood

Underrecovery can evoke acute and brief (negative) emotional changes as well as transient but more stable (negative) mood states. After Rosenberg (1998) and numerous others we see emotions and moods as brief adaptations to a situation lasting more than a few hours. The present UR model uses Watson and Clark's (Clark & Watson, 1991; Mineka, Watson, & Clark, 1998; Watson & Clark, 1984) framework for negative affect (NA) even though their model addresses affects that are typically more stable and more pervasive in scope than negative affects characteristic of UR; these include subjective nervousness, tension, and worry (anxiety) combining in NA with anger, scorn, revulsion, guilt, self-dissatisfaction, low positive affect, and sadness. Transient NA, or negative moods, are common in UR; one should note that they lack the stability that is necessary for a clinical diagnosis. In exception to the model of Lane and Terry (2000), we urge the use of the terms *low positive affect, negative affect,* and *negative mood* in order to denote ephemeral states as contrasted with clinical states, such as depression (e.g., Major Depressive Disorder). Watson and Clark (1984) write:

"NA will be significantly related to transient discomfort at all times and regardless of the situation, even in the absence of any overt distress" (p. 471).

Following the tripartite model of anxiety and depression (clinical states) (Clark & Watson, 1991; Mineka, Watson, & Clark, 1998), our construct of UR places the nonspecific distress of arousal (e.g., irritability and disturbed sleep) in a position where it plays a nonspecific etiological role in low self-regulation, low positive affect (depression, low self-efficacy, helplessness), anxiety, and fear. In UR, as in the tripartite model, anxiety and low positive affect comprise emotions that tend to cluster their own respective sets of symptoms. The present model adds fear with its own somewhat discrete cluster of symptoms. Some level of intercorrelation among the factors is expected in UR. A further distinction of the present model is that the low positive affect common in UR is conceived as more directly related to high physiological arousal (e.g., high cortisol and high resting heart rate) than would be the case for the depressive affects of the tripartite model.

Neurochemical Responses to Stress: High Arousal

UR in sports is caused by the imbalance between the competing demands of training and recovery. The major mood-related response to hard training is a change in the function of the hypothalamic-pituitary-adrenal axis. On this axis, Lehmann, Foster, and Keul (1993) distinguished between sympathetic and parasympathetic imbalance; the cause for either the sympathetic or parasympathetic overtraining response is chronic UR. Principal among those functions studied are catecholamine and cortisol responses, which in the sympathetic overreaching model result in fatigue with excitability, as distinct from the parasympathetic overreaching model in which they result in fatigue with depression (low positive affect) (e.g., Lehmann et al., 1993). Consistently, norepinephrine is the only variable that reliably marks the early differentiation between adequate recovery and overreaching in elite swimmers even though, as some will assert, an overreaching response is highly influenced by the athlete's mood (Mackinnon et al., 1997).

The initial response to hard training is an elevated cortisol response (Steinacker et al., 1999). For instance, at a 1996 training camp, prior to the Junior World Championships, German rowers had basal cortisol levels that were shown to be elevated by 18% after the first week of hard training, before later decreasing. As part of their literature review, the authors explained this as a common response to elevated high-intensity training that precedes later decreases in cortisol levels (the late signs of overreaching). By two weeks, an undertrained athlete may have adrenal fatigue and show relatively *low* levels of cortisol, whereas the well-trained athlete will continue to show high levels of cortisol in response to training loads (Mackinnon et al., 1997).

In sum, the first physiological step of psychological significance in UR is probably a change in cortisol levels and heightened catecholamine function. Higher arousal is the result of early adaptations to increased training. In the present model, these cortisol and catecholamine changes interact with significant cognitive and emotional events. For instance, negativity and uncertainty in thinking, especially as regards the self, has been very consistently correlated in the literature with adverse changes in physiological arousal. In 1967 Brady showed that (conditioned) response unavailability and response uncertainty were related to elevated steroid secretion in humans. Davis (1983) and others found that negativity and uncertainty in adult depressive self-description accounts for a significant portion of the variance in adrenal activity (Rogers & Craighead, 1977; Schuele & Wisenfeld, 1983). Today, for the 40 to 60% of depressives who show increased cortisol secretion, the persistent nonsuppression of adrenal hyperfunction after dexamethasone administration (the dexamethasone suppression test) reliably assists in the classification of those depressed patients who will be nonresponsive to neuroendocrine antidepressants (Heuser, 1998; Maes, Jacobs, Suy, & Minner, 1990; Wahlund, Sääf, & Wetterberg, 1995). These findings in depression research reinforce the observation that endocrine changes correlate with cognitive and emotional changes.

Thus, in the present model as shown in figure 9.1, during training stress, central importance is given to the alteration of adrenal function and to related mood alteration in the UR athlete. Basically, as an athlete fatigues, develops UR, and shifts biochemically in the early, predicted direction toward higher levels of arousal, the athlete also becomes vulnerable to showing the psychological symptoms of UR, and emotional management becomes critical. Starting from the top in figure 9.1 the athlete shows this physiological shift. This is possibly followed by changes in self-regulation and by the possible changes in mood yielding negative affect, anxiety, and fear. Eight

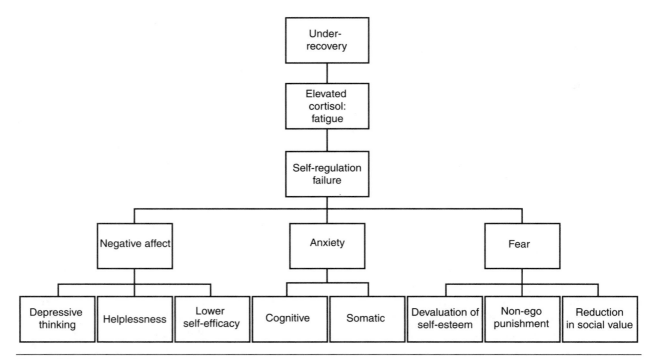

Figure 9.1 A model for underrecovery intervention.

consequences of these emotions are listed in figure 9.1 and will be discussed in detail later together with low self-regulation.

Recovery Behavior Changes Linked to Low Self-Regulation

When arousal increases beyond optimum, and when optimal, once-dominant responses become less probable, the likelihood increases for negative emotion and behavioral shifts. This high arousal of UR can precipitate poor self-regulation; recovery from training stress requires both the competence required for positive behavior as well as the self-control to use one's competency. Impaired self-regulation operates in our model as a nonspecific factor that is common to low positive affect, anxiety, and fear.

Kellmann (cf. Kellmann & Günther, 2000; Kellmann & Kallus, 1999, 2001) argues persuasively that the negative behavioral shifts that can correlate with UR may include lesser tendencies to rehydrate, eat, and sleep in a regulated way; to attend to regimens for dry-land training and stretching; and to meet one's social needs. Baumeister (1997) described this as poor self-regulation. He linked poor self-regulation (i.e., of one's recovery needs) to fatigue (Muraven & Baumeister, 2000) and emotional distress

(Baumeister, 1997). Summarizing numerous results (Isen, Nygren, & Ashby, 1988; Leith & Baumeister, 1996), Baumeister concluded that altered arousal states create a potential for self-defeating behavior and poor consideration of risks, odds, and the best path to success.

The self-control required for mood regulation is a limited-supply resource. Recently, in reviewing the evidence for this position, Muraven and Baumeister (2000) stated that self-control diminishment relates to fatiguing self-control strength. They distinguished this finding from any suggestion that NA can itself predict self-regulation breakdown. Basically, the finding that self-control emanates from a limited resource is central in the present model and helps explain how persons fail to monitor and regulate their training stress adequately when they may have already expended all self-control resources in driving through hard workouts and coping with immediate results. In other words, the athlete who works to control a bad mood and works to cope with the demands of a workout may have no self-control reserves at the end of a day with which to further self-regulate by going to bed at a reasonable time, eating a healthy meal, and socializing with friends. Repeatedly, Muraven and Baumeister (2000) asserted that repeated acts of self-control (as during training) impair performance on later tasks if these later tasks also require self-control.

Common Mood Changes Under High Arousal and High Demand on Self-Regulation

As previously stated, three forms of negative mood can arise from self-control breakdown under conditions of high arousal: (1) NA and depressive thinking (including low positive affect, low self-efficacy, and helplessness), (2) anxiety, and (3) fear. As reviewed earlier, our UR model has added to the tripartite model of depression and anxiety by including fear and self-regulation as discrete factors and by allowing that the model may apply equally to transient moods and more persistent affects. This model links generalized distress, self-regulation failures, low positive affect, and physiological hyperarousal (PH) related to anxiety states. Alternative three-factor models have left intact the central thesis of nonspecific distress and discrete, interacting moods (e.g., Zinbarg & Barlow, 1996). For instance, Zinbarg and Barlow clustered dysphoria, fear, and anxiety all under negative affect. The data of Joiner et al. (1999) suggest further support for the model demonstrating mood correlations with PH (and high cortisol) for fear and panic, subjective anxiety, and depressive thinking on the order of $r = .24$, $r = .58$, and $r = .43$, respectively. The physiological symptoms of PH include perceived overheating, dizziness, difficulty breathing, wobbly feelings, rapid heart rate, and flushing. These data are essential to an understanding of mood changes in UR.

Depressive-Toned, Negative Affect

A failure to invoke solid recovery rituals can lead to low positive affect and NA (which is not a clinical mood disorder); alternately, this can be described as a loss of positive affect. This in itself can be fatiguing (Lane & Terry, 2000). For the most part, however, fatigue is the consequence of hard training. It potentiates UR and results in activation of the hypothalamic-pituitary-adrenal axis and mood disturbance. Examples of ephemeral and typical self-reference in NA include: "I'm slow, fat, and out of shape. This whole year has been a joke. I've completely lost the respect of my teammates and I don't fit in. I'd be happier leaving to train somewhere else."

When one considers interventions for UR states, it is critically important to remember that depressive-toned self-talk is not a flag for an underlying depression in an individual who might well have been happy one week previously. The diagnosis for a Major Depressive Disorder requires that the person have generally consistent symptoms for two weeks or more. Methods for helping a UR athlete can be adapted from treatments for major depression, but it should be remembered that although intervention modalities for depression (Beck, Rush, Shaw, & Emory, 1979) have been well validated, interventions for transient moods (such as depressive-toned NA among athletes who are UR) have not (see Gross, 1998, for a conceptualization of emotion regulation that can be used in UR).

For these adaptations, we prefer the broad, three-schema triad conceptualization of depression originally proposed by Beck (1967) to the narrow self-esteem focus of Lane and Terry (2000). Beck's negative cognitive triad includes a negative view of the self, a negative view of the world, and a negative view of the future.

We also urge caution when describing negative talk in UR athletes; most elite athletes are generally positive in their outlook and might only become negative when cortisol levels increase with hard training. It is possibly better to think of "depressed" athletes as showing relatively low positive affect, and it is inappropriate to even use the term *schema* when describing negatively toned but transient negative self-referents (Davis, 1979; Davis & Unruh, 1981). With mood destabilization in UR, the athlete may show short-term negative self-reference. Davis and Unruh (1981) found that persons who had been depressed for only a short period had an unstable view of self that lacked the robust pervasiveness of negative self-views held by long-term depressives. UR athletes who have been pessimistic for a short period are highly amenable to correcting cognitive distortion when challenged because they are not depressed. Although they may engage in negative self-talk, they may not have negative self-schemas. This point is often missed in the literature on NA (Rector, Segal, & Gemar, 1998).

Low Self-Efficacy

Bandura (1977a, 1977b, 1991) was the first to propose that motivation, performance, effort, and persistence deficits and physiological stress reactions may be linked under the construct of low self-efficacy, a deficit in the judgment of one's ability to perform a desired behavior. Numerous reviews of sport research have supported this contention (e.g., Rudolph & McAuley, 1995; Schunk, 1995). Specific to the present model in which psychobiological demand is key to the development of UR, Bandura (1991), Rudolph and McAuley (1995), Weidenfeld et al. (1990), and others have shown a negative correlation between the demand response (cortisol elevation) and self-efficacy levels. The more the individual feels competent to respond to stress, the less likely the same individual is to show elevated arousal (Rudolph & McCauley, 1995). The athlete who is in a state of UR *and* showing high cortisol (postexercise) can be predicted to have compromised self-efficacy going into the next training session. Although the authors attach causal significance to self-efficacy levels, our interpretation is simply that cortisol and self-efficacy can be expected to be inversely related in UR.

This reasoning is supported by convergent sources. For example, Martin and Gill (1991) found an inverse relationship between anxiety and self-efficacy in middle- and long-distance runners. Bozoian, Rejeski, and McAuley (1994) found a positive relation between mood and self-efficacy in acute-exercise participants. Lox, McAuley, and Tucker (1995) found a positive relation between self-efficacy and subjective well-being in HIV-1 patients.

In sum, the UR athlete with high preworkout cortisol can be expected to carry low self-efficacy into the training session and can be expected to report having to work harder than usual to complete the workout (Rudolph & McAuley, 1996).

Learned Helplessness

Research in the area of learned helplessness has proliferated for 30 years largely due to the enthusiasm of M.E.P. Seligman. Learned helplessness is a significant response to uncontrollability during stress. Early reviews documented neuroendocrine depletion in states of chronic learned helplessness (Depue & Monroe, 1978). The initial studies showed deficits in learned escape and avoidance after exposure to inescapable shock (e.g., Overmier & Seligman, 1967), whereas later studies show motivational, cognitive, and emotional response deficits to uncontrollability (Abramson, Metalsky, & Alloy, 1989; Abramson, Seligman, & Teasdale, 1978). In the revised model slower response rates, slower new learning, idiosyncratic pessimism, and increased NA are attributed to learned helplessness. Notwithstanding what Charles Costello once referred to as "horrendous" conceptual problems in the theory (Costello, 1978), we propose that the treatment strategies of the reformulation have relevance to timely intervention with the UR athlete.

Arousal Changes With Learned Helplessness

Our model is based on the strong empirical association among helplessness, pessimism, and PH. When athletes perceive that training outcomes are not contingent on effort or work, this may trigger PH, or conversely, PH may lead to pessimism. UR athletes in this mode will lose the connection between training and perceived success. At this point performance suffers doubly: from the physiology of UR and from pessimism and helplessness. Although the original learned helplessness model was largely silent on neuroendocrine changes that arise from helplessness, subsequent research has clarified that an association exists between elevated cortisol and helplessness responses in controls. Empirically, the *perception* of noncontingency is not consistently essential for the *effect* of noncontingency. Thus, an athlete would not have to possess conscious thoughts about noncontingency in order to start showing helplessness.

Numerous studies have related elevated cortisol levels to uncontrollability as seen in the following examples. In nondepressed surgery patients exposed to uncontrollable stress, salivary cortisol elevated as predicted (Croes, Merz, & Netter, 1993). Dess, Linwick, Patterson, Overmier, and Levine (1983) also showed data correlating controllability with reductions in serum cortisol. Importantly, the predictability of uncontrollable stress limits the extent of the adrenocortical response. (That is, understanding and expecting the nature of an applied training stress and predicting its physiological and psychological consequences can reduce the stress response.) Uncontrollability in the form of inescapable shock has further been related to reduced responsiveness in the nucleus accumbens in studies of intracranial self-stimulation (Zacharko, Bowers, Kokkinidis, & Anisman, 1983). This finding helps connect the arousal, uncontrollability, and mood data: reduced responses in the nucleus accumbens accompany lower levels of dopaminergic activity and lower mood. More recent research suggests that although it may be the noradrenergic and not dopaminergic activity that mediates learned helplessness responses (Tejedor-Real, Costela, & Gibert-Rahala, 1997), the issue is not settled. Still, the effect on mood is hypothesized to result from central brain responses to uncontrollability. Naturalistic investigations include unemployment stress in which loss of control and perceived helplessness in the long term and urinary catecholamines in the short term have been found to increase with reactance to unemployment (Baum, Fleming, & Reddy, 1986).

Anxiety

The literature has been clear for years that PH is associated with anxiety. Martens, Vealey, and Burton (1990) and others provided ample clarification of the difference between anxious moods and anxiety disorders in sport. NA is importantly related to anxiety (Mineka, Watson, & Clark, 1998). For instance, a person who has been anxious for about six months is roughly 12 times more likely to show depression (and presumably NA before that). Anxious states precede depressive ones more than the converse, and the presence of an anxiety disorder yields a 60 to 70% lifetime risk for major depression.

Several general points shape our intervention with UR athletes who are anxious.

- Negative anxiety can result from UR, or training/competitive results can enhance the likelihood that the athlete will have high arousal and poor recovery.
- Some recovery decisions are made as a consequence of anxiety.
- Anxiety can be facilitative and positive (Burton & Naylor, 1997; Edwards & Hardy, 1996). It can moderate not only other emotions but also cognitive processes such as concentration and attention.
- Poor self-efficacy can sometimes enhance anxiety (Weiss, Wiese, & Klint, 1989).
- Anxiety is multidimensional with interactive cognitive, physical, and self-confidence dimensions (Martens, Vealey, & Burton, 1990; Smith, 1989).

Cortisol shifts reveal a constant dynamic interaction between anxiety and biochemistry (Hackfort & Schwenkmezger, 1993). In early work, Frankenhauser (1969, as cited in Hackfort & Schwenkmezger, 1993) found that the adrenaline/noradrenaline ratio reliably indicated emotional stress. We propose that depressive-toned thinking, worry, and fear can both cause and be caused by poor recovery from training stress. Adrenocortical function is influenced by general well-being, fitness, and biological rhythm. As a result, the present intervention model requires simply that the psychologist ask whether this anxiety is the consequence of physiological changes associated with poor recovery *before* exploring the meaning or the cognitive underpinnings of the anxious state.

Fear

Fear is also associated with PH. At the heart of fear is elevated activation of the amygdala, hypothalamus, and brainstem culminating in elevated corticosteroid release together with behavioral and other physical responses (Davis, 1992; Stansbury & Gunnar, 1994). Fear can be triggered simply by conditioned responses or poor self-regulation during high arousal and UR. Seligman (1971) explained that fear is easily acquired in a single trial as an adaptive response to threat when there is high arousal (a condition in which humans are biologically prepared to be wary about their safety).

Fear and anxiety are different (Hackfort & Schwenkmezger, 1993). Fear is understood as a specific reflexlike defense and protection reaction. The source of danger in anxiety is not always readily understood. Stimulus recognition in fear is key. Lazarus (1991) found that both fear and anxiety are focused on a threat of future harm, but they differ in the level of uncertainty, with fear associating more than anxiety to danger that is concrete and sudden.

Conroy, Poczwardowski, and Henschen (2001) reviewed the Lazarus cognitive-motivational-rational theory of emotion and found that emotional responses develop only when an individual perceives (and later anticipates) a change in the environment that may have an impact on goal attainment. Negative emotions, such as fear, will occur when the perceived or anticipated change is a decrease in the likelihood of achieving a goal. Birney, Burdick, and Teevan (1969) defined this decrease as failure, the nonattainment of a prescribed goal or achievement standard. Fear is associated with the potential for failure and its resultant consequences.

Birney et al. (1969) noted that when fear is generated from anticipated nonattainment, it stems from three strands of anticipated aversive experience: (1) a devaluation of one's self-estimate, (2) non-ego punishment, and (3) a reduction in one's social values.

The first experience that can generate fear, the fear of devaluation of the self-estimate, involves the risk of having to lower and thus change one's self-estimate. In a sport-achievement situation, if failure occurs, the athlete discovers that she is worse than she previously hoped or anticipated (Birney et al., 1969). The probability of failure, the attributions associated with the failure, and one's view of the consequence of failure combine to predict the magnitude of the fear.

The second experience generating fear is "non-ego punishment" related to the anticipation of a loss of rewards that go along with goal attainment. An example would be losing a spot on a team or getting injured. Birney et al. (1969) pointed out that fears are directed toward the consequences of failure, and that a form of punishment is one of the consequences. Fear increases with the size of punishment and the probability of nonattainment.

The third anticipated experience that can generate fear is social devaluation. This is the expectation that one will lose value in the estimation of one's peers and close associates. A person who fears failure may anticipate being held in negative regard by others and fear the poor opinion of others. Again, the strength of this fear is proportional to the expected magnitude of social loss that accompanies nonattainment, the importance placed on the skill to determine social value, and the regard for the person who is making the judgment.

As adapted from Conroy (2000) and shown in table 9.1, Conroy et al. (2001) found 3 higher-order fears under which 7 higher-order themes and 22 lower-order themes may be identified. Table 9.1 lists the higher-order fears and the 10 higher-order themes that were associated with Birney's failure expectation factors. Specifically, Conroy and colleagues found that the self-estimate factor

included feelings of personal diminishment, poor ability, and low control. On Birney's fear of non-ego punishment factor were appraisals related to experiencing tangible losses, wasted effort, an uncertain future, or the loss of a special opportunity. Lastly, on the reduced social values factor the Conroy group found expectations of causing important people to lose interest in oneself, disappointing or upsetting others, or experiencing an embarrassing self-presentational failure.

It is important to be aware of these anticipatory cognitions when intervening with fatigued, UR athletes. In designing interventions, the psychologist will note behaviors associated with anticipated fear such as decreasing success-oriented efforts, keeping achievement standards vague so as to render performance measurement more ambiguous, participating in very easy or very difficult tasks so that little information can be gained from performance, and making excuses for nonattainment.

Intervention With the UR Athlete

As outlined in figure 9.2, our method starts with assessing whether the athlete is underrecovered. If so, the sport psychologist promotes efforts to attain physical recovery while simultaneously assessing the psychological system along the nine lines established by the empirical base illustrated in figure 9.1 (p. 164), covering self-regulation and self-control, negative affect (NA) (with three

Table 9.1 Composite of Fear of Failure Beliefs

Higher-order fears	Appraisal
Fear of devaluing one's self-estimate	Personal diminishment
	Poor ability
	Lack of control
Fear of non-ego punishment	Wasted effort
	Tangible loss
	Crushed hope/lost opportunity
	Uncertain future
Fear of a reduction in social value	Others lose interest in me
	Others let down
	Embarrassing self-presentational failure

Adapted, by permission, from D.E. Conroy, 2000, *Using performance failure appraisals to conceptualize and assess fear of failure.* Unpublished doctoral dissertation, University of Utah, Salt Lake City, 12.

levels), anxiety (with two levels), and fear (with three levels).

With this model it is not necessary to test for elevated cortisol. By combining a knowledge of what the training template or competitive program has required with an assessment of the athlete's physical and psychosocial response to this program, it should not be difficult to determine when things are out of line.

The program is straightforward. As stated, after establishing that there is a reasonable basis for suspecting UR, promote the basics and assess the impact of UR on the psychosocial categories of UR response. Next, proceed to design an intervention based on the empirical literature that we have reviewed. The "basics" consist of encouraging sleep, hydration, eating for recovery, and attention to important social relationships. These are addressed before dealing with any psychological issues that may have arisen as a consequence of the UR state. Carefully explore deficits in physiological, psychological, and social recovery efforts. Thus, before entertaining the full spectrum of, say, sadness or fear, encourage the athlete to add a nap or bigger meals or less extra-sport demand to the recovery regimen. The sport psychologist must remember that the person with a negative bias may be *speaking* with a negative tone only because she is underrecovered.

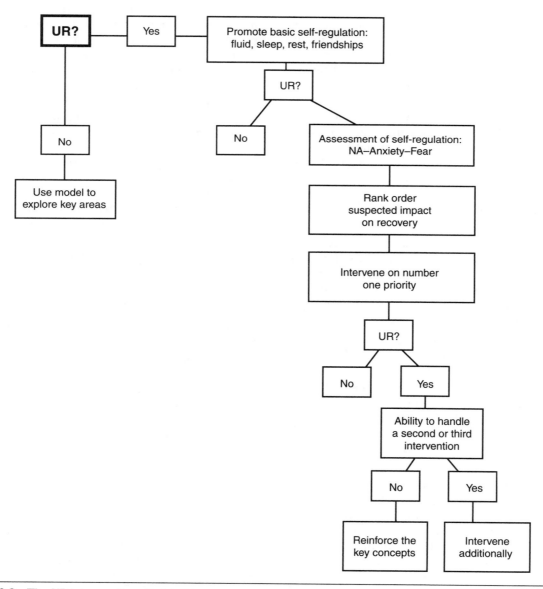

Figure 9.2 The UR intervention decision tree.

The Assessment Phase

In the assessment, within each category of UR response isolate possible questions for establishing where to intervene.

1. *Poor self-regulation.* Is the athlete missing important points in the workouts? missing significant opportunities for recovery? expressing anger inappropriately? missing deadlines? forgetting to do previously agreed tasks (such as goal setting or phoning home or rearranging academic coursework by phoning the university)? using the personal computer or TV for inordinate periods of time? having difficulty with responsible eating? unable to focus effectively when performing? showing declining/inconsistent performances?

2. *Negative affect, depressive thinking.* Is the athlete unnecessarily negative about training progress or competition results? exaggerating, overgeneralizing, self-criticizing, or showing other forms of cognitive distortion (look for the cognitive triad: self, present situation, future)? suddenly losing hope for the future? more irritable, more tearful, or showing more emotion than you think normal for him, given the circumstance? suddenly showing concentration and focusing problems? having sleep problems? not positive?

3. *Negative affect, learned helplessness.* Is the athlete expressing helplessness and saying, for instance, "I can't ever do this," or "We're weak completely because of me," or "This injury is going to affect everything from now on. It's all luck!"? feeling helpless about improving? stating that things are hopeless and unlikely to improve? unwilling to look at evidence of personal effectiveness?

4. *Negative affect, low self-efficacy.* Is the athlete saying, "I can't"? failing to set appropriate goals consistent with prior achievement? talking about quitting? not following through with set plans? showing a lack of belief that the goals are appropriate? showing poor persistence? shying away from planning? perceiving that more exertion is not possible?

5. *Anxiety-cognitive and somatic.* Is the athlete having difficulty with panic, high heart rate, or breathing control? tense and/or restless and keyed up and/or irritable? easily exhausted? fatigued? having concentration and focusing difficulty? having nausea at the time of performance? showing an inability to think clearly in key situations? yawning?

6. *Fear—three anticipation factors.* Is the athlete anxious about looking bad? losing financial support? losing parental and peer support? losing self-esteem? losing hope? losing opportunities? wasting time? any uncertainty? social expectations?

When assessing the UR responses using figure 9.2, the intervention decision tree, ask if the athlete needs to do anything on each level. Remember that, as Muraven and Baumeister (2000) have shown, calling attention to too many categories or concerns at once might exacerbate higher levels of distress and UR symptoms. Make a clinical judgment as to the areas having the greatest negative effect on training and focus there. The very nature (rapid onset and transience) of UR necessitates attention to the fact that the sport psychologist does not have several weeks to intervene; it is important to be strategic. Use both the response to training and the athlete's physiological recovery as guides for determining what to focus on with the UR athlete. Proposals by Gross (1998) are instructive relative to emotion regulation. He suggests assessing situational variables (ask if the athlete has to be in a current situation), situation modification (ask if the circumstance yielding UR mood can be altered), attention deployment (ask if the athlete could use distraction, become more focused, or direct attention differently), cognitive change (use cognitive-behavioral techniques), and response modification (ask if physiological, experiential, or behavioral responses can be altered).

The Intervention Phase

Table 9.2 lists our basic UR intervention tools. Most can be applied to several UR responses.

These basic intervention tools would generally be described as cognitive-behavioral following accepted practice in empirical research. The interventions are based on relaxation and other methods designed to alter the cognitive and behavioral responses (in this case, to UR) by correcting cognitive distortion, developing new attributions for difficulty, refocusing attention, developing coping imagery, and developing positive reflections on stressful situations. While the literature in sport psychology can be traced to interventions that were first developed for depression, learned helplessness, anxiety, panic, and fear (see Barlow & Craske, 1994; Beck, Rush, Shaw, & Emory, 1979; Seligman, 1990; and Wolpe, 1982, respectively), references exist indicating

Table 9.2   Cross-Situation Effectiveness for Interventions in UR

Intervention	Self-regulation	Depressive thinking	Learned helpless-ness	Low self-efficacy	Anxiety: cognitive and somatic	Fear: devalued self	Fear: non-ego punishment	Fear: social value
1. Physical recovery reset	x	x	x	x	x	x	x	x
2. Goal examination								
Goal reviews	x	x	x	x	x	x	x	x
Goal resetting	x		x			x	x	x
3. Relaxation promotion								
Breathing—centering	x				x	x	x	x
4. Imagery training								
Coping imagery	x	x	x	x	x	x	x	x
5. Cognitive methods promotion								
a. Attention								
Attention control training					x			
Control distraction				x	x	x	x	x
Promote reframing		x	x	x	x	x	x	x
Control procrastination	x	x	x	x	x			
Limit overthinking	x	x			x	x	x	x
b. Confidence								
Positive self-talk/affirmations	x	x	x	x	x	x	x	x
Review successes	x	x	x	x	x	x	x	x
Correct cognitive distortion		x	x	x	x	x	x	x
c. Self-reflection								
Competitive/training reflections	x	x	x	x	x	x	x	x
Review coaching plan	x	x	x	x	x			
Journals and logs	x	x	x	x	x	x	x	x
d. Balance								
Promote perspective		x	x	x	x	x	x	x
Promote social skills and interaction	x	x	x	x	x	x	x	x

X indicates potential application.

where sport psychologists have used this clinical base for applications in sport. Three fundamental sources for mental skills training are provided by Hogg (1995), Martens (1987), and Orlick (1990). Numerous others address how one might intervene in the domains we isolate for UR, although none specifically addresses the need for empirical testing of interventions, and none isolates the problem of UR (e.g., Botterill & Patrick, 1996; Van Raalte & Brewer, 1997). As suggested, the review of Gross (1998) can be a useful guide in structuring interventions for nonclinical affect alteration.

Eight UR responses are laid out in the base of figure 9.1 (p. 164). These are the principal targets for intervention and may be matched up with the five broad categories of intervention methods that are shown on the left column of table 9.2. The reader will notice that we have placed promotion of self-regulation on the top of table 9.2 as the ninth target for intervention, and we have linked it with physical recovery resetting, among the interventions. Thus, self-regulation is both a target for intervention and, when it is working well, a tool to promote recovery from UR. The intervention categories are physical recovery reset (using self-regulation), goal examination, relaxation promotion, imagery training, and cognitive methods promotion. Cognitive methods promotion is divided into four subcategories (attention, confidence, self-reflection, and balance). These intervention categories and subcategories are described in the following sections.

Self-Regulation for Promoting the Physical Recovery Reset

The most likely targets for promoting physical recovery by employing self-regulation with UR athletes will be eating, hydration, sleep, and resetting social activities. Watch that the athlete is not sabotaging his training effectiveness with low self-discipline in these areas. For instance, most athletes know that excessive sun exposure can reduce energy for training. Thus, at a training camp in a warm climate, a failure to use adequate sunscreen or a failure to go indoors for an afternoon nap can be attributed to low self-regulation. Excessive alcohol on days off from hard training can also be attributed to low self-regulation and can completely undermine the desired training effect.

As well, self-handicapping can both cause and be caused by poor recovery efforts. The athlete who is in UR may be in a compromised emotional state and may therefore need help to ensure that she does not set up distractions or extreme (excessively high or excessively low) performance goals for the training session. Self-handicapping renders failure ambiguous (Baumeister, 1997) and may make it easier for the athlete to cope with any immediate underachievement, but it ultimately must be dealt with in order to promote overall goal achievement. Misguided persistence refers to some athletes' tendency to keep working while ignoring fatigue, soreness, and injury relative to recovery. Watch for this; assist and intervene appropriately.

Athletes who are prone to binge eating or drinking patterns will be at special risk when they are in UR. Pay attention to this risk by providing support, promoting self-awareness, and providing extra structure (e.g., curfews, team meals, and coach-accompanied grocery shopping when away).

Goal Examinations

Goal setting involves establishing objectives in order to provide direction and the means for accomplishment. Goals fall on a continuum from daily/short-term goals (a more detailed plan of action that is implemented and evaluated on a short-term basis) to long-term (established objectives that may not be as detailed) to dream (what you are striving for, the overall picture) (Orlick, 1990). Goals also fall into two types: outcome and process goals. Outcome goals focus on the result, whereas process goals focus on the performance standard or the methods used to reach the desired outcome.

Goal setting can assist in increasing commitment, motivation, self-satisfaction, confidence, and optimal focus. In the case of UR athletes, identifying or reviewing goals can help them improve self-regulation and the related components that were presented earlier in the model. In order to reduce some of the demands placed on athletes, encourage them to assess and consequently reset some goals in light of new data as well as to enhance confidence and self-efficacy (see Weinberg & Gould, 1999; Williams, 1993).

Relaxation Promotion

Relaxation techniques, essential for the toolbox of the UR athlete, calm the mind and body, lessen muscle tension, lower the heart rate, and decrease subjective anxiety or perceived stress. Relaxation also helps the athlete cope with the consequences of poor self-regulation, negative affect, anxiety, and fear while facilitating recovery.

Williams (1993) divided relaxation techniques into two categories. The first involves muscle-to-mind techniques in which one trains one's sensitivity to muscle tension and learns to release that tension. Examples of this include breathing exercises and progressive relaxation, which involves contracting a specific muscle group and then relaxing it. Some of the most dramatic examples of psychological effects on performance relate to one's ability to relax. The second category of techniques involves the cognitive, or mental, approaches. These techniques work from mind to muscle, and include things like meditation and visualization. The choice may be determined by athlete preference (see Hogg, 1995; Martens, 1987; Orlick, 1990); each requires practice.

Imagery Training

Imagery can be explained as pictures that evoke sensory images and thoughts that stream through consciousness. The use of imagery involves all senses and emotions to create or re-create an experience (Weinberg & Gould, 1999; Williams, 1993). Imagery helps to provide motivation, assists with skill correction, and reminds athletes of the things that require focus. It helps to bolster flagging confidence and self-efficacy when one is struggling with UR. When using imagery, the athlete should first settle into a relaxed state before recruiting the senses and emotions.

Performance imagery, recovery imagery, and coping imagery are three techniques that may be used with UR athletes. Performance imagery involves mentally rehearsing performance skills. The UR athlete should use performance imagery away from the sport setting in order to recapture self-control and self-efficacy. Recovery imagery involves imagining the basic recovery goals being achieved or imagining oneself with the capacity to achieve goals beyond this (Botterill, Flint, & Ievleva, 1996). Coping imagery allows athletes to visualize how they would like to think and feel despite the temporary state of UR and helps to build self-confidence.

Cognitive Methods Promotion

The ability to control thinking, attention, and concentration is an important element of optimal recovery. What the UR athlete thinks can affect the way he feels and acts. This is not linear; the components interact. For example, the fatigued UR athlete may have a disappointing performance; this poor performance may, in turn, build self-defeating thoughts. This interactive cycle can be initiated by thoughts, feelings, or behaviors. Once the athlete can master the cognitive component, she can develop positive feeling states and behaviors. There are a variety of cognitive control interventions. We have divided cognitive methods into four subcategories as follows: (1) thinking, attentional, and concentration control techniques; (2) confidence building strategies; (3) self-reflection methods using journals and logbooks; and (4) maintaining balance and perspective.

Thinking, Attentional, and Concentration Control Attentional control training has roots in meditation, Eastern religious practices, and martial arts. It involves the ability to direct attention and concentration to areas that are critical for recovery, performance, and maintenance of general well-being (Nideffer & Sharpe, 1978). With attention control the UR athlete will be able to regain effective focus when distracted or when engulfed by self-defeating thoughts. Controlling attention involves two different types of focus and four different attentional styles, with width and direction dimensions. Width describes either a narrow or a broad focus of attention; direction specifies whether attention is focused internally or externally. Athletes can benefit from learning to shift attention away from low motivation or negative thoughts while in the UR state.

A variety of thought- and attention-control techniques can assist athletes to deal with the

consequences of UR. These are well covered in the ample sport psychology literature that can be found elsewhere, but it should be said that it is our opinion that these techniques apply to UR. Athletes benefit from reviewing potential distractors and engaging in problem solving relative to these possible events. When distractions occur, athletes are less anxious having already come to terms with the inevitability of distraction. Thought stopping is used to eliminate negative and counterproductive thoughts. One method involves briefly focusing on an unwanted thought, then using a trigger to interrupt or stop the thought. This would be valuable for cognitions relating to negative affect, anxiety, and fear. A second cognitive method involves reframing. This is a process that encourages the athlete to find a different way to look at a situation in order to yield an optimistic framework for understanding the consequences of UR. Countering is another cognitive-behavioral method for changing self-defeating thoughts into self-enhancing thoughts. This is done through an internal dialogue that uses facts and reason to counter the belief and assumptions that led to the negative thinking. Each of these is an example of the full cognitive-behavior treatment literature on correcting cognitive distortions.

Confidence Building Self-confidence reflects the extent to which one embraces a belief in oneself, in one's power, and in one's abilities. Confidence can easily be lost in UR and with it one's self-efficacy, assertiveness, optimism, and composure. Confidence helps to arouse positive emotions and influences the way the UR athlete perceives performance; it is also a strong determinant of recovery behaviors and actions (Weinberg & Gould, 1999; Williams, 1993). Confidence building with the UR athlete can help to solidify the belief that the athlete can overcome the present situation in addition to managing the effects of UR as depicted in the model, such as low self-efficacy, learned helplessness, and fear.

Strategies suggested for building self-confidence have been adapted from Bandura (1977a, 1977b); only a few are presented here. The first technique involves reviewing past experiences. Highlight past successes, significant events, high-pressure situations, and obstacles that the athlete has overcome that remind him of his ability to succeed, thus reinforcing the capacity to do so. Another method involves verbal persuasion, or positive self-talk. Create, and review, an affirmation list of all the positive, self-affirming comments that the athlete has received from family, friends, teammates, and coaches along with attributes that the athlete takes pride in. In addition to these two strategies you can instill a sense of confidence through vicarious experiences such as a motivational movie, video highlights, an inspirational book, or having the athlete imagine or visualize her own successful performances or those of someone she admires. These strategies may help to remind the UR athlete of what can be done despite temporary UR. Following the lead of education researchers, remember to reinforce the work ethic and the athlete's capacity to enjoy work. Some research suggests that such affirmation goes further in rebuilding persistence than does praise for the athlete's giftedness (Mueller & Dweck, 1998). If the athlete loves to compete, for instance, remember to reinforce competitive desire more than the image of being a winner.

Self-Reflection   Self-reflection involves being aware of one's thoughts and feelings in the present state along with the thoughts about that state (Goleman, 1995). In UR it can provide a concrete, current database and help to increase the athlete's awareness (Brown & Lent, 1992). There is a logical distinction between being aware of feelings and acting to change them. However, it has been suggested that the two usually go hand in hand: to recognize a negative mood is to want to get out of it (Goleman, 1995).

Self-reflection enhances awareness. Encourage the athlete to reflect on competition and training regimes, which can be accomplished by keeping logbooks (see Orlick, 1990). This can help an athlete to identify the load he is trying to maintain as well as the effectiveness of his efforts. The idea is to do more than vent; simple venting tends to even prolong negative feelings. Instead, work to promote positive thinking, feeling, and action—sometimes by addressing how to get out of the negative situation (Lightsey, 1999). If self-reflections are not pleasant, they will probably not be very useful in altering negative affect (Fichman, Koestner, Zuroff, & Gordon, 1999). Strategies to help with self-reflection include self-expressive activities such as writing thoughts and feelings into a journal; using logbooks for concrete evidence of behavior; and communicating feelings and thoughts to a support network or a professional.

Perspective and Balance   Helping an athlete to maintain balance and perspective is one of the most important aspects of any sport psychology endeavor (see Orlick, 1998). When training and competitive pressures mount while the athlete is in UR, maintaining perspective can be difficult. With the UR athlete the demands (which may be somewhat self-inflicted) usually outweigh the coping resources. Perspective helps the athlete to see the big picture and to mentally reframe what is irrationally imposed on her (Botterill & Patrick, 1996). Useful approaches for maintaining perspective include staying rational and decisive. Staying rational involves focusing on things within one's control in addition to reflecting on what is irrational (and beyond one's control). Decisiveness, on the other hand, is a form of situational goal-setting tool that can help prevent becoming overloaded with thoughts, feelings, and possibilities. Encourage the athlete to stay in the here and now rather than get preoccupied with past occurrences or future possibilities (Botterill & Patrick, 1996). Help the athlete to get through the hard parts of training successfully without becoming overloaded, fearful, or overanalytical.

When we are balanced, it is possible to find beauty and meaning in our lives. The UR athlete will have difficulty here so keep it simple; facilitate becoming optimally aware of needs for achievement *and* relaxation, work *and* play, giving *and* receiving, intimacy *and* personal space (Orlick, 1998). The UR athlete must accept these dualities at a philosophical level before he can make use of their underlying principles. The emotional and psychological payoffs can have a profound effect on physiological recovery and state. In order for an athlete to train and perform to potential, he must also be capable of finding an adequate balance in his life.

Case Examples

The following two intervention scenarios illustrate our approach. As suggested, use common sense when drawing from the list of UR interventions that have shown efficacy in clinical contexts. Before intervening with UR, make sure that the problems you address have a clear theoretical link to cortisol elevations and to the literature reviewed earlier. If they do not, then the problems are most probably not UR problems. Throughout we have repeatedly emphasized the importance of theory, but remember that without a dynamic and energized interaction between the psychologist and the athlete, the UR problems will not be resolved (Bachelor & Horvath, 1999).

Scenario A: Background and Presenting Problems

Emily is a speed skater attempting to make the Canadian Junior Team. This season she moved from her hometown to a world-class center in order to train on long-track ice and expose herself to a situation that could enhance her development. She did not know many people in either the new city or the new training center, and it was the first time that she was living away from home. In prior years Emily competed in both short-track and long-track skating. Since this was the first time that she focused her energy into the long-track discipline, and was in an environment where she could train on long-track ice every day, she expected to improve at a fast pace. However, this did not happen.

Emily was going through a lot of new experiences all at once. Within her sport she was focused on a new discipline, her training load was increased substantially, and she was working with a new coach and teammates. Outside of sport she was living in a new city, working at a new job, and had moved in with a boyfriend for the first time. With all of these new experiences, there was potential for overload.

On reflection, Emily was unhappy with her achievement in the season. She knew that she had a lot of things to work on, but she didn't feel that she had progressed. She felt that the whole first part of the season went by without her thinking about what she needed to do. She lacked direction and focus. She was often distracted by the difficult relationship that she was having with her boyfriend. They broke up early in the season, but continued to live together due to financial constraints. She felt stressed constantly at home and was always so upset that she was never able to relax or have fun. She cried often and felt self-critical. These feelings were unfamiliar to her. She had no system of social support in her new environment.

Of possibly greatest significance from an overall coping perspective, she had difficulty adapting to the new training load. She often felt tired and fatigued and never felt that she was able to recover. She had difficulty concentrating on skating, as she would come to the oval upset and unmotivated. She also had difficulties identifying the focus, techniques, and intensity that were needed for long-track skating, and this compounded her dissatisfcation and unhappiness. She did not feel that she was able to push herself in skating, which made her feel angry and agitated coming off the ice.

She developed low confidence in her skating ability together with very low self-efficacy at skating competitions.

This athlete was simply overloaded by the combination of new environment, personal stressors, and increased training volume. She was never able to relax and get away from the demands placed on her.

Indicators for UR

This athlete is fatigued, has trouble sleeping, and shows NA and/or low positive affect with an inability to relax. She cries often and is upset, agitated, frustrated, and irritable. Emily is lacking focus and direction, is discouraged, and shows low self-esteem and low self-efficacy. All of these symptoms correlate with the substantial increase in training volumes.

Interventions

Strategize on the basic recovery techniques; promote self-regulation; teach several relaxation strategies; address cognitive control, attentional control, and confidence-building methods; explore her living situation; and look at process and outcome goals to help her reestablish direction and perspective.

Scenario B: Background and Presenting Problems

Carter, a 19-year-old National Team swimmer, was happy, well-adjusted, and excited about his journey in sport. In the five years he had been swimming seriously, he had never known failure. He had set age-group records and made it to national prominence smoothly, without injury or incident.

In the year of the Olympic trials Carter was generally excited about his options and about the possibilities on the horizon. At training camps and meets, however, he would go through periods in which he would lose his extroverted, gregarious style and become withdrawn and serious—almost brooding. He would review his goals, his workout times, and his expectations to the point that they no longer energized him or helped him to focus. In fact, he would start to worry when he reviewed. After disappointing times he sometimes stopped talking altogether, withdrew from his friends, and paced on deck in an agitated, almost angry way. On one occasion he yelled at the coach and left the workout.

At other times he became argumentative and difficult to coach; he would object to doing workout sets, and he would not respond to suggestions on stroke improvement. At the conclusions of training camps or a week after competitions, regardless of the outcomes, he would return to being a positive contributor to the pool environment.

When he discussed these downturns with the sport psychologist, he seemed aware that they were predictable after about four days of exceptionally hard work or after the noise and expectations of a meet had started to take their toll. Before such a time he was happy and positive. When he began to feel stressed, he would awaken from sleep feeling not rested; the more upset he became, the more lax he was in protecting his sleep-onset ritual. He admitted to not being particularly careful, especially at training camps, about staying away from junk food dinners and snacks. Finally, he recognized that when stressed he did not smile at his friends and he became more serious about rising to the challenges before him. Carter reported some fear about letting people down (coach and parents, principally), and he said that for some reason he sometimes "just felt scared."

All of these problems lasted only a few days with peak periods of emotionality lasting a few hours.

Indicators for UR

Carter gets fatigued and then shows fear of lost social value together with agitation, some anger, resistance to authority, and argumentativeness (these fall loosely into the fear and anxiety categories of the model). Additionally, under the heading of NA and/or low positive affect with decreased self-efficacy are worry, seriousness, brooding, disappointment and self-criticism, and the urge to withdraw. Finally, under poor self-regulation he loses diligence about getting to sleep and he lets himself withdraw, argue, and eat junk food. It is possible also that he isn't showing self-control in remembering the goal to remain balanced as opposed to focusing narrowly.

Interventions

Under the heading of anxiety, teach self-awareness and anger management when in high arousal. For the sleep and eating problems, promote better self-regulation. For the NA and reduced self-efficacy, offer some cognitive strategies for maintaining rational thinking about his goals and for regaining positive self-talk and a positive attitude when he is aware of slipping into brooding

and narrow thinking. He should be taught methods for maintaining social relatedness. Self-reflection and self-acceptance methods might help him to become aware of the problems with balance when he slips into UR.

Summary

The recommended approach presented in this chapter represents basic, responsible sport psychology.

- Start with the empirical evidence that observed psychological UR problems relate in theory to the physiology of UR.

- Next, go through methods that have been reviewed in the literature and choose a set of two or three that can reliably impact on mood and self-regulation changes.

- Review the athlete's situation and decide together on a focus; this may be a short list given time and personal coping constraints. No athlete should become further overloaded by intervention, and none should risk compromising self-control by having to deal with too many strategies. This would be tantamount to complicating an injury by offering too much massage.

- Track the athlete's response to the methods used in order to intervene more effectively if UR recurs.

Remember that each person is unique and that each should be treated uniquely and patiently in the promotion of balance. By respecting the process as well as the relationship between professionals and performers, the sport psychologist can be humanly helpful instead of merely technically proficient. Make all that you can of your opportunities.

References

Abramson, L.Y., Metalsky, G.I., & Alloy, L.B. (1989). Hopelessness depression: A theory-based subtype of depression. *Psychological Review, 96,* 358-372.

Abramson, L.Y., Seligman, M.E.P., & Teasdale, J.D. (1978). Learned helplessness in humans: Critique and reformulation. *Journal of Abnormal Psychology, 87,* 49-74.

American Psychological Association. (1996). *Division 12 Task Force: An update on empirically validated therapies.* Washington, DC: Author.

Bachelor, A., & Horvath, A. (1999). The therapeutic relationship. In M.A. Hubble, B.L. Duncan, & S.D.

Miller (Eds.), *The heart and soul of change: What works in therapy* (pp. 133-178). Washington, DC: American Psychological Association.

Bandura, A. (1977a). Self-efficacy: Toward a unified theory of behavior change. *Psychological Review, 84,* 191-215.

Bandura, A. (1977b). *Social learning theory.* Englewood Cliffs, NJ: Prentice Hall.

Bandura, A. (1991). Self-efficacy mechanism in physiological activation and health promoting behavior. In J. Madden (Ed.), *Neurobiology of learning, emotion and affect* (pp. 229-269). New York: Raven Press.

Barlow, D.H., & Craske, M.G. (1994). *Mastery of your anxiety and panic, II.* New York: Graywind Publications.

Baum, A., Fleming, R., & Reddy, D.M. (1986). Unemployment stress: Loss of control, reactance, and learned helplessness. *Social Sciences and Medicine, 22,* 509-516.

Baumeister, R.F. (1997). Esteem threat, self-regulatory breakdown, and emotional distress as factors in self-defeating behavior. *Review of General Psychology, 1,* 145-174.

Beck, A.T. (1967). *Depression: Causes and treatment.* Philadelphia: University of Pennsylvania Press.

Beck, A.T., Rush, A.J., Shaw, B.F., & Emory, G. (1979). *Cognitive therapy of depression: A treatment manual.* New York: Guilford.

Birney, R.C., Burdick, H., & Teevan, R.C. (1969). *Fear of failure.* New York: Van Nostrand.

Botterill, C., Flint, F., & Ievleva, L. (1996). Psychology of the injured athlete. In J. Zachazewski, D. Magee, & W. Quillen (Eds.), *Athletic injuries and rehabilitation* (pp. 791-805). New York: W.B. Saunders.

Botterill, C., & Patrick, T. (1996). *Human potential: Perspective, passion, preparation.* Winnipeg, MB: Life Skills Inc.

Bozoian, S., Rejeski, W.J., & McAuley, E. (1994). Self-efficacy influences feeling states associated with acute exercise. *Journal of Sport and Exercise Psychology, 16,* 326-333.

Brady, J. (1967). Emotion and the sensitivity of psychoendocrine systems. In D.C. Glass (Ed.), *Neurophysiology and emotion* (pp. 70-96). New York: Rockefeller University Press.

Brown, S.D., & Lent, W. (1992). *Handbook of counseling psychology.* New York: John Wiley & Sons.

Burton, D., & Naylor, S. (1997). Is anxiety facilitative? Reaction to the myth that cognitive anxiety always impairs sport performance. *Journal of Applied Sport Psychology, 9,* 295-302.

Chambless, D.L., & Hollon, S.D. (1998). Defining empirically supported therapies. *Journal of Consulting and Clinical Psychology, 66,* 7-18.

Clark, L.A., & Watson, D. (1991). Tripartite model of anxiety and depression: Psychometric evidence and taxonomic implications. *Journal of Abnormal Psychology, 100,* 316-336.

Conroy, D.E. (2000). *Using performance failure appraisals to conceptualize and assess fear of failure.* Unpublished doctoral dissertation, University of Utah, Salt Lake City.

Conroy, D.E., Poczwardowski, A., & Henschen, K.P. (2001). Evaluation criteria and consequences associated with failure and success for elite athletes and performing athletes. *Journal of Applied Sport Psychology, 13,* 300-322.

Costello, C.G. (1978). A critical review of Seligman's laboratory experiments on learned helplessness and depression in humans. *Journal of Abnormal Psychology, 87,* 21-31.

Croes, S., Merz, P., & Netter, P. (1993). Cortisol reaction in success and failure condition in endogenous depressed patients and controls. *Psychoneuroimmunology, 18,* 23-35.

Davis, H. (1979). Self-reference and the subjective organization of personal information in depression. *Cognitive Therapy and Research, 3,* 415-425.

Davis, H. (1983). *Uncertainty in self-reference as related to 17-hydroxycorticosteroid secretion in adult depression* (Monograph). Calgary, AB: University of Calgary, Killam Archives.

Davis, H., & Unruh, W.R. (1981). The development of the self-schema in adult depression. *Journal of Abnormal Psychology, 90,* 125-133.

Davis, M. (1992). The role of the amygdala in fear and anxiety. *Annual Review of Neuroscience, 15,* 353-375.

Depue, R.A., & Monroe, S.M. (1978). Learned helplessness in the perspective of the depressive disorders: Conceptual and definitional issues. *Journal of Abnormal Psychology, 87,* 3-20.

Dess, N.K., Linwick, D., Patterson, J., Overmier, J.B., & Levine, S. (1983). Immediate and proactive effects of controllability and predictability on plasma cortisol responses to shocks in dogs. *Behavioral Neuroscience, 97,* 1005-1016.

Edwards, T., & Hardy, L. (1996). The interactive effects of intensity and direction of cognitive and somatic anxiety and self-confidence upon performance. *Journal of Sport and Exercise Psychology, 18,* 296-312.

Fichman, L., Koestner, R., Zuroff, D.C., & Gordon, L. (1999). Depressive styles and the regulation of negative affect: A daily experience study. *Cognitive Therapy and Research, 23,* 483-495.

Gaskovski, P. (1999). The clinician's art, or why science is not enough. *Canadian Psychology, 40,* 320-327.

Goleman, D. (1995). *Emotional intelligence: Why it matters more than IQ.* New York: Bantam Books.

Gross, J.J. (1998). The emerging field of emotion regulation: An integrative review. *Review of General Psychology, 2,* 271-299.

Hackfort, D., & Schwenkmezger, P. (1993). Anxiety. In R. N. Singer, M. Murphey, & L.K. Tennant (Eds.), *Handbook of research on sport psychology* (pp. 328-364). New York: Macmillan.

Heuser, I. (1998). The hypothalamic-pituitary-adrenal system in depression. *Pharmacopsychiatry, 31,* 10-13.

Hogg, J. (1995). *Mental skills for competitive swimmers.* Edmonton, AB: Art Design Printing.

Hunsley, J., Dobson, K.S., Johnston, C., & Mikail, S.F. (1999). Empirically supported treatments in psychology: Implications for Canadian professional psychology. *Canadian Psychology, 40,* 289-301.

Isen, A.M., Nygren, T.E., & Ashby, F.G. (1988). Influence of positive affect on the subjective utility of gains and losses: Is it just not worth the risk? *Journal of Personality and Social Psychology, 55,* 710-717.

Joiner, T.E., Beck, A.T., Rudd, M.D., Steer, R.A., Schmidt, N.B., & Catanzaro, S.J. (1999). Physiological hyperarousal: Construct validity of a central aspect of the tripartite model of depression and anxiety. *Journal of Abnormal Psychology, 108,* 290-298.

Kellmann, M., & Günther, K.D. (2000). Changes in stress and recovery in elite rowers during preparation for the Olympic Games. *Medicine and Science in Sports and Exercise, 32,* 676-683.

Kellmann, M., & Kallus, K.W. (1999). Mood, recovery-stress state, and regeneration. In M. Lehmann, C. Foster, U. Gastmann, H. Keizer, & J.M. Steinacker (Eds.), *Overload, fatigue, performance incompetence, and regeneration in sport* (pp. 101-117). New York: Plenum.

Kellmann, M., & Kallus, K.W. (2001). *Recovery-Stress Questionnaire for Athletes: User manual.* Champaign, IL: Human Kinetics.

Lane, A.M., & Terry, P.C. (2000). The nature of mood: Development of a conceptual model with a focus on depression. *Journal of Applied Sport Psychology, 12,* 16-33.

Lazarus, R.S. (1991). *Emotion and adaptation.* New York: Oxford University Press.

Lehmann, M., Foster, C., & Keul, J. (1993). Overtraining in endurance athletes: A brief review. *Medicine and Science in Sports and Exercise, 25,* 854-862.

Leith, K.P., & Baumeister, R.F. (1996). Why do bad moods increase self-defeating behavior? Emotion, risk taking, and self-regulation. *Journal of Personality and Social Psychology, 71,* 1250-1267.

Lightsey, O.R. (1999). Positive thoughts versus states of mind ratio as a stress moderator: Findings across four studies. *Cognitive Therapy and Research, 23,* 469-482.

Lox, C. L., McAuley, E., & Tucker, S. (1995). Exercise as an intervention for enhancing subjective well-being in an HIV-1 population. *Journal of Sport and Exercise Psychology, 17,* 345-362.

Mackinnon, L.T., Hooper, S.L., Jones S., Gordon, R.D., & Bachmann, A.W. (1997). Hormonal, immunological, and hematological responses to intensified training in elite swimmers. *Medicine and Science in Sports and Exercise, 29,* 1637-1645.

Maes, M., Jacobs, M.P., Suy, E., & Minner, B. (1990). Prediction of the DST results in depressives by means of urinary-free cortisol excretion, dexamethasone levels, and age. *Biological Psychiatry, 28,* 349-357.

Maraniss, D. (1999). *When pride still mattered: A life of Vince Lombardi.* Toronto, ON: Simon & Schuster.

Martens, R. (1987). *Coaches guide to sport psychology.* Champaign, IL: Human Kinetics.

Martens, R., Vealey, R.S., & Burton, D. (1990). *Competitive anxiety in sport.* Champaign, IL: Human Kinetics.

Martin, J.J., & Gill, D.L. (1991). The relationship among competitive orientation, sport-confidence, self-efficacy, anxiety, and performance. *Journal of Sport and Exercise Psychology, 13,* 149-159.

Mineka, S., Watson, D., & Clark, L.A. (1998). Comorbidity of anxiety and unipolar mood disorders. *Annual Review of Psychology, 49,* 377-412.

Mueller, C.M., & Dweck, C.S. (1998). Praise for intelligence can undermine children's motivation and performance. *Journal of Personality and Social Psychology, 75,* 33-52.

Muraven, M., & Baumeister, R.F. (2000). Self-regulation and depletion of limited resources: Does self-control resemble a muscle? *Psychological Bulletin, 126,* 247-259.

Nideffer, R.M., & Sharpe, R.C. (1978). *Attention control training.* New York: Wyden Books.

Orlick, T. (1990). *In pursuit of excellence.* Champaign, IL: Human Kinetics.

Orlick, T. (1998). *Embracing your potential.* Champaign, IL: Human Kinetics.

Overmier, J.B., & Seligman, M.E.P. (1967). Effects of inescapable shock upon subsequent escape and avoidance learning. *Journal of Comparative and Physiological Psychology, 63,* 28-33.

Rector, N.A., Segal, Z.V., & Gemar, M. (1998). Schema research in depression: A Canadian perspective. *Canadian Journal of Behavioural Science, 30,* 213-224.

Rogers, T., & Craighead, W.E. (1977). Physiological responses to self statements: The effects of statement valence and discrepancy. *Cognitive Therapy and Research, 1,* 99-119.

Rosenberg, E.L. (1998). Levels of analysis and organization of affect. *Review of General Psychology, 2,* 247-270.

Rudolph, D.L., & McAuley, E. (1995). Self-efficacy and salivary cortisol responses to acute exercise in physically active and less active adults. *Journal of Sport and Exercise Psychology, 17,* 206-213.

Rudolph, D.L., & McAuley, E. (1996). Self-efficacy and perceptions of effort: A reciprocal relationship. *Journal of Sport and Exercise Psychology, 18,* 216-223.

Scheule, J.G., & Wisenfeld, A.R. (1983). Autonomic response to self-critical thought. *Cognitive Therapy and Research, 7,* 189-194.

Schunk, D.H. (1995). Self-efficacy, motivation and performance. *Journal of Applied Sport Psychology, 7,* 112-137.

Seligman, M.E.P. (1971). Phobias and preparedness. *Behavior Therapy, 2,* 307-320.

Seligman, M.E.P. (1990). *Learned optimism: How to change your life.* New York: Simon and Schuster.

Smith, R.E. (1989). Conceptual and statistical issues in research involving multidimensional anxiety scales. *Journal of Sport and Exercise Psychology, 11,* 452-457.

Stansbury, K., & Gunnar, M.R. (1994). Adrenocortical activity and emotion regulation. *Monographs for the Society of Research in Child Development, 59,* 250-283.

Steinacker, J.M., Kellmann, M., Böhm, B.O., Liu, Y., Opitz-Gress, A., Kallus, K.W., Lehmann, M., Altenburg, D., & Lormes, W. (1999). Clinical findings and parameters of stress and regeneration in rowers before World Championships. In M. Lehmann, C. Foster, U. Gastmann, H. Keizer, & J.M. Steinacker (Eds.), *Overload, fatigue, performance incompetence, and regeneration in sport* (pp. 71-80). New York: Plenum.

Tejedor-Real, P., Costela, C., & Gibert-Rahala, J. (1997). Neonatal handling reduces emotional reactivity and susceptibility to learned helplessness: Involvement of catecholaminergic systems. *Life Sciences, 62,* 37-50.

Van Raalte, J.L., & Brewer, B.W. (Eds.). (1997). *Exploring sport and exercise psychology.* Washington, DC: American Psychological Association.

Wahlund, B., Sääf, J., & Wetterberg, L. (1995). Classification of patients with affective disorders using platelet monoamine oxidase activity, serum melatonin, and post-dexamethasone cortisol. *Acta Psychiatrica Scandanavia, 91,* 313-321.

Watson, D., & Clark, L.A. (1984). Negative affectivity: The disposition to experience aversive emotional states. *Psychological Bulletin, 96,* 465-490.

Weidenfeld, S.A., Bandura, A., Levine, S., O'Leary, A., Brown, S., & Raska, K. (1990). Impact of perceived self-efficacy in coping with stressors on components of the immune system. *Journal of Personality and Social Psychology, 59,* 1082-1094.

Weinberg, R. (Ed.). (1990). Training stress [Special issue]. *Journal of Applied Sport Psychology, 2* (1).

Weinberg, R.S., & Gould, D. (1999). *Foundations of sport and exercise psychology.* Champaign, IL: Human Kinetics.

Weiss, M.R., Wiese, D.M., & Klint, K.A. (1989). Head over heels with success: The relationship between self-efficacy and performance in competitive youth gymnastics. *Journal of Sport and Exercise Psychology, 11,* 444-451.

Williams, J.M. (Ed.). (1993). *Applied sport psychology: Personal growth to peak performance.* Mountain View, CA: Mayfield.

Wilson, G.T. (1996). Manual-based treatments: The clinical application of research findings. *Behavior Research and Therapy, 34,* 295-315.

Wolpe, J. (1982). *The practice of behavior therapy* (3rd ed.). New York: Pergamon Press.

Zacharko, R.M., Bowers, W.J., Kokkinidis, L., & Anisman, H. (1983). Region-specific reductions of intracranial self-stimulation after uncontrollable stress: Possible effects on reward processes. *Behavioral Brain Research, 9,* 129-141.

Zinbarg, R.E., & Barlow, D.H. (1996). Structure of anxiety and the anxiety disorders: A hierarchical model. *Journal of Abnormal Psychology, 105,* 181-193.

Hogg, J.M. (2002). Debriefing: A means to increasing recovery and subsequent performance. In M. Kellmann (Ed.), *Enhancing recovery: Preventing underperformance in athletes* (pp. 181-198). Champaign, IL: Human Kinetics.

10

Debriefing: A Means to Increasing Recovery and Subsequent Performance

John M. Hogg

Following a significant competitive event, there is need for a meaningful and exact evaluation in order to establish and share accurate performance information and to hold accountable those responsible for the results. Postperformance evaluation can be highly structured on the one hand or somewhat cursory on the other. It generally addresses both the outcome and the way the results were achieved. Debriefing is an extension of performance appraisal and involves the downloading of the information by those answerable for the event. Essentially the performance is relived to determine whether or not objectives were met as well as to determine the lessons learned. Debriefing is critical for complete mental and emotional recovery and for devising new approaches for renewed or improved subsequent performances. Performance evaluation has received adequate attention in the sport psychology literature (Hogg, in press-b; Holder, 1997) and has its roots primarily in the field of motor learning, behavior, and control (Salmoni, Schmidt, & Walter, 1984).

Debriefing is a process that has yet to be examined in applied sport psychology and likely has strong theoretical connections in attributional theory (Biddle, Hanrahan, & Sellars, 2001). It is reasonable to assume that an athlete's specific attributions are different following successful competition than they are after a negative result. Winners tend to attribute success to more stable

and internal factors, whereas losers attribute failure to unstable and external factors. Evidence of self-serving biases in postperformance attributions is present in the research (Brawley & Roberts, 1984). Because a win, a loss, or an unexpected result can elicit strong mental and emotional responses in the athlete (e.g., increased competitive anxiety), these feelings will need to be controlled or released. Performance evaluation and debriefing will vary depending on the nature of the sport, the psychological makeup of the athlete, and the performance outcome. Many coaches and athletes regard evaluation and debriefing as a critical part of the performance process and essential for optimal recovery. This chapter is written for the most part from a pragmatic perspective. For over 30 years the author was a swim coach at the club level, university level, and national level of competition. For the past 18 years the author has also been associated with both team and individual sports as an applied sport psychologist. Although debriefing protocols differ from sport to sport, and more particularly from individual to team sports, the focus here will be on debriefing individual athletes since many conclusions can be adapted to team needs. In this chapter, the process of debriefing as a means of mental and emotional recovery is addressed, a systematized and interactive debriefing model is presented, and some practical guidelines for coaches and athletes are suggested.

Definitions and Conceptual Understanding

Immediately following a major competition, athletes should reflect seriously on their performance both in terms of the process (knowledge of performance [KP]) and the outcome (knowledge of results [KR]). In the postperformance evaluative setting, information gathered from KP and KR should be integrated to allow for increased learning. When athletes win or perform especially well, they will need to celebrate their success. Alternatively, if they fail or suffer disappointment, they are more likely to rebound quickly if they can learn from their mistakes and effectively cope with their emotions. To recover from any mental and emotional stresses that accompanied the performance, athletes need to take the time to download all troubling thoughts or feelings so that the book can be firmly closed on that performance and they can move on to the next level. If they fail to take time for solitary and sincere self-reflection (Biddle, 1991; Sinclair & Sinclair, 1994) or if they lose touch with their guiding values, they will increase the likelihood of incomplete recovery states and of carrying additional baggage to the next performance. The process of *debriefing* occurs when athletes and coaches are engaged in an evaluative activity either in training or in competition, with the intended purpose of analyzing existing performance states and determining what might be improved to ensure future performance satisfaction, enjoyment, success, and fulfillment (Hogg, 1998). Debriefing also encourages the athletes to control or rid themselves of any emotional residue or perceptions of incompetence or loss of self-determination that might negatively affect their desire for success. Consequently, at a suitable time after the performance, the athletes are led through a session in which they relive all or parts of their experiences in a supportive environment and are able to draw conclusions from the experiences either by themselves (self-reflection) or with the help of significant others, such as their support staff (Boud, Keogh, & Walker, 1985). This kind of self-reflection leads to accelerated learning.

Debriefing allows athletes to discover their deepest feelings by posing some very hard questions that need to be answered accurately and honestly. The debriefing process can help athletes develop their self-knowledge and understanding and provide insights into what must be done to reach the next level of performance.

Recovery in the mental sense implies the speedy and efficient return to normal psychological and emotional states after intensive training and competition. The buildup of mental tension prior to and during competition may not have been immediately released at the conclusion of the event. Further tensions and emotional static may exist in the postperformance setting seriously affecting honest communication with the coach. Coaches can create a debriefing environment that will help to enhance recovery by (1) remaining calm and helping the athlete to remain calm in order for mind and memory to function accurately, (2) encouraging a realistic understanding of what actually occurred, and (3) inviting both internal and external feedback. Debriefing enhances mental recovery and leaves the athlete feeling excited, reenergized, and renewed.

Debriefing involves the sharing of information from both *internal* (i.e., the athlete) and *external* (i.e., the coach) sources. It provides an opportunity for athletes and coaches to share meaningful and constructive feedback relating to both performance process and outcome. Feedback can be *descriptive*, focusing on what actually happened, or *normative evaluative,* focusing on performance expectations and comparison with others or set standards (Schmidt & Wrisberg, 2000). National coaches particularly have to account for whether they reached the expected medal tally. Performances are judged not only on results associated with improved personal bests but also on whether the team won the gold medal. A careful reflection on the functioning or dysfunctioning of all performance components *(technical, physical, tactical,* and *mental/emotional)* will allow athletes to learn immediately from their experiences. However, after a debriefing session, athletes should be aware of precisely how they are progressing and where they stand relative to their performance goals.

Internal Performance Evaluation

Feedback is important if athletes are to remain in touch with what they are doing and where they are going. Since their choices need to be in tune with their belief systems, any proposed changes after the self-evaluation component of the debriefing process should be in harmony with their deepest values.

After the performance, athletes should reflect on the outcome for themselves and consider whether they did what was required. They can evaluate their feelings by asking questions such as, *Did my performance feel right?* and *Was I ready?*

Internal evaluation through self-reflection leads to self-knowledge of strengths and limitations. Athletes need to recognize their internal states before, during, and after performance; to openly acknowledge their mistakes and shortcomings; and to be aware of what they must do now to ensure optimal recovery and improve future performances. Internal evaluation allows athletes to verbalize their views about what happened and what they feel could be improved.

Once internal evaluation is completed, it is important for athletes to articulate the performance experience as part of the debriefing process. The skills required for internal evaluation are those of accurate mental recall, self-reflection, checklisting against goal states, and the ability to openly and nonjudgmentally confront and communicate with oneself. The first step in internal self-assessment is to identify what is good and what needs to be adjusted or changed. Naturally this self-examination should occur in an environment that encourages honest reflection about what really happened, as this may encourage better responses for the future. The opportunity for self-reflection in the performance review leads to accelerated learning, especially when athletes become aware of their emotional responses to their shortcomings and can exercise control over them.

External Performance Evaluation

Athletes also receive knowledge or insights about their performances from the external environment. *External evaluation* is performance feedback provided from outside sources, such as coaches, sport science observational data, statistics, video analysis, performance criteria, and so forth.

Positive and constructive feedback is vital for full physical and mental recovery (Rudawsky, Lundgren, & Grasha, 1999; Schmidt & Lee, 1999; Shea & Howell, 1999) as long as it is accurate, unbiased, and matter of fact. However, it can be open to misinterpretation if coaches focus on the wrong perspective or if the athletes' perspectives are not taken into consideration. External feedback is meaningless if it is regarded by athletes as biased and self-serving or if coaches are overly preoccupied with negative outcomes and impose guilty feelings. In this event recovery will be stalled.

External feedback should allow for two-way communication. It should be unambiguous, affording clarity rather than confusion. Evaluative feedback on aspects of mental preparation and execution should not be shrouded in mystery or guilt but should facilitate relief and provide athletes with a renewed intrinsic motivation, or inner desire, to examine their responses and to continue pursuing their dreams. If athletes are to place value on these external appraisals, they need to fully understand and trust that any constructive criticism is presented for their benefit. It shifts the power and the responsibility to them to be accountable as well as to freely take control of their efforts both in training and in competition to ensure improvements.

Some athletes intentionally seek out external evaluation and want to know how significant others perceive their performances. They are eager to listen in the search for new detail that might improve their future performances. However, it is important for athletes to realize that others' perceptions tend to be subjective. Good athletes know themselves well and are able to combine both the internal and external information to cope with their responses, accept their capabilities or shortcomings, and motivate themselves to make changes with increased self-confidence.

Developing athletes will grow in their self-knowledge provided they are open to their own insights and to the careful feedback of the support staff. The coach can help by encouraging athletes to verbalize their postperformance thoughts and feelings. A sole focus on external evaluation, in which coaches debrief athletes with excessive comments reflective of their own perceptions of the performance, would seemingly endorse the idea that coaches know best. This approach can be very protective of the coaches' own decisions and makes for easier control over athletes. The ideal approach, however, would be for both athlete and coach to share internal and external information with the goal of initiating further change, thus opening the door for optimal recovery and progression in a responsible and accountable manner.

Some Assumptions

Before considering a debriefing model, certain assumptions should be considered. The debriefing activity should always be self-enhancing rather than self-defacing. For the self-evaluative aspects of performance assessment it would be unwise to assume that athletes and coaches perceive the performance results in the same way. Individual perceptions play a critical role whether these are inflated or deflated. Both athletes and coaches may need to seek a common ground for their postperformance discussions. What an athlete may regard as a strength, the coach may judge as a limitation and vice versa. Some coaches believe that athletes tend to be irresponsible and are more likely to embellish their successes or catastrophize their failures if left to their own devices. Others believe that athletes learn best by evaluating themselves in solitary reflection, and that they eventually mature enough to do this very effectively. Regardless, it is critically important for coaches and athletes to (1) be on the same page when engaged in debriefing after performance, (2) bring a definite sense of closure to the events, and (3) recognize that even the most obvious feedback needs to be verbalized clearly, especially when athletes are seeking higher levels of performance. Younger athletes may initially prefer to avoid all forms of self-evaluation, trusting only in input from coaches. This may be a maturational limitation or reflective of a lack of self-awareness and will likely diminish in time, with experience, and with the guidance of the support staff.

Ideally, any major performance at the elite level should reflect the characteristics of quality, intensity, realism, and perfection. *Quality* suggests that the athlete is determined to make the performance count rather than simply go through the motions. The athlete is immersed in the job of performing successfully. *Intensity* implies that the athlete is committed to giving a 100% effort with emotionality and passion. The athlete is engaged in performing efficiently. *Realism* means that the athlete recognizes the demands and understands what is required. The athlete has asked the right questions and has come up with the right answers. *Perfection* reflects the successful execution of the task under conditions of automaticity and control. The athlete has processed the information and is fully engaged. All four characteristics need to be addressed seriously if debriefing is to have full meaning. Finally, a combination of subjective and objective postperformance evaluations can offer a positive opportunity to exercise resilience, leadership, trustworthiness, initiative, persuasiveness, adaptability, optimism, and emotional intelligence.

Debriefing Skills and the Role of Awareness

The successful process of performance debriefing requires athletes and coaches to develop certain skills and abilities. Competencies for the athlete include

- an ability to mentally recall all or partial aspects of the actual performance and to ask the hard questions;
- a willingness to openly acknowledge strengths and weaknesses and to be realistic about performance outcomes;
- an ability to communicate all thoughts, feelings, and actions with honesty and controlled self-criticism;
- a desire to reflect on all aspects of performance with the intention to make changes;
- an attitude of responsibility and accountability for the quality and intensity of one's effort in preparation and in execution; and most important,
- the mental skill of self-awareness, particularly to gain insights into self-perceptions and to release any feelings that will likely hinder complete mental and emotional recovery.

Competencies required by the coach are

- an awareness of personal values functioning or dysfunctioning in the postperformance setting;
- an ability to analyze the performance in an impartial and objective manner and to turn all problem-solving decisions into action;
- a willingness to allow the athletes sufficient time to reflect, learn, and recover from the performance experience;
- an ability to ask the right questions in order to challenge the status quo and to ensure the right answers;
- a readiness to offer and provide direction and to pinpoint focus for the immediate future, while encouraging leadership and responsibility in all athletes; and
- an ability to communicate in a nonjudgmental way in order to resolve any conflict and expedite purposeful change.

Obviously, a key aspect of debriefing is two-way communication that is open, honest, positive, sincere, precise, focused, forthright yet empathic, helpful, and fair. A number of sport psychologists have identified as critical the ability to communicate and listen to candid feedback by sharing knowledge and perceptions and by articulating essential and immediate needs (Anshel, 1997; Leathers, 1986; Smith & Smoll, 1996; Yukelson, 1998). There is need for heightened communication in the debriefing process for the athlete and coach to arrive at the true interpretation of events. An athlete's attributions may be affected by a win or a loss and likely it will be difficult to fully understand them without clear and precise dialogue. Both coaches and athletes need to be effective listeners and to be sure that their messages are given and received accurately. Incongruency of perceptions only causes confusion, frustration, and agitation in the recovery process.

Self-awareness on the part of athletes and coaches about their internal states, preferences, beliefs, resources, and intuitions is an important antecedent to any debriefing exercise. Self-awareness needs to be channeled particularly to those factors that can facilitate or debilitate future performances in order to recognize how emotions affect self-image and to develop strong beliefs to guide any decision making in the debriefing process. *Awareness* of any kind, including self-awareness, involves *cognitive intelligence,* that is, knowing and understanding what should be done to regain control of the performance situation (Ravizza, 1998). Awareness also involves *emotional intelligence* (Goleman, 1995, 1997), or the athlete's ability to bring together all available skills or competencies and to employ them in the execution of any performance adjustments quickly and efficiently. Developing self-awareness will help athletes to act decisively and with self-confidence.

Asking the Right Questions

In order for athletes and coaches to extract the right information from the debriefing process, they must ask themselves the *right* questions as well as the *hard* and *important* performance questions (see table 10.1) This exercise will increase self-awareness. Athletes and coaches should carefully select the kinds of questions that typically need to be asked at this time. These critical questions can be addressed with greater or lesser emphasis by athletes either immediately after the performance as part of their warm-down protocol (in the case of individual sports) or suitably distanced from the game (in the case of team sports). An athlete's honest appraisal of the performance will help her generate a productive evaluative commentary that can form the basis of a solid interaction with her coach in the postperformance setting.

Some questions directed at internal states may be hard to answer, but athletes are unlikely to

move forward if they are only looking to maintain a comfortable feeling about their performance. Athletes are unlikely to recover and improve unless they seriously attempt to assess what is good, what is wrong, and what needs to be done to make it right. When athletes are experiencing a slump and cannot fathom what is wrong, debriefing may allow them to get to their deepest feelings by addressing hard questions. This may help them find and use more effective coping responses.

Veteran athletes often regard themselves as being either too old for or beyond change. Radical change causes additional emotional upset, which further endangers performance outcome. However, experienced athletes know only too well when they are doing well versus when they are performing poorly. They need to create new performance goals for themselves along with fresh challenges that will keep their motivational and productivity levels consistently high. On a daily basis the toughest question to answer is *Does my performance actually reflect how well I did in training?*

A Suggested Debriefing Model

The choice of a debriefing procedure and how it is operationalized will depend on many factors, for example, the existing phase of training and development, the significance of the competition, the time available, the cognitive ability of the performer, and so on.

The suggested steps depicted in figure 10.1 (p. 187) are the key components for a systematized debriefing model that will both elicit new information and facilitate recovery. Athlete and coach should interpret these steps in a mutually acceptable way.

Step 1: Select the Best Time, Place, and Occasion for Debriefing

It is important to consider the options and variables accompanying the debriefing process. Debriefing may need to occur *formally* and in a semistructured way (e.g., interview or organized team meeting) or *informally* in a one-on-one situation or in contemplative time (e.g., on a long walk). It may be conducted in a *public* group format or in a *private* individual setting with each athlete. It may be arranged *immediately* after performance in an emotionally charged atmosphere or *later* after the performance when the climate is more emotionally stable. It can be carried on in a *hostile* and manipulative environment or in one

Table 10.1 Debriefing: Asking the Right Questions

Five core questions

What happened exactly? ... for you? ... for the team?

What is the impact of your performance on you? ... on the team?

How did your performance make you feel?

What did you learn—technically, physically, tactically, and mentally?

What are you encouraged to repeat or do differently for the next game/competition?

Hard questions

Who am I and where am I going?

What do I really want from my sport?

What is next for me?

How am I doing compared to my peers or other athletes?

What am I motivated to change?

Am I living up to my own expectations or other people's?

Do I have the right attitude of a champion?

How ready am I for the opportunity to perform?

Does my performance actually reflect how well I did in training?

Important performance questions

What did I do or not do to account for my performance the way it was?

Have I actually been planning for failure rather than for success?

If I know it all and consider myself so smart, why can't I create the results I truly want?

Am I using my self-protective mechanisms as an excuse for poor performance?

Which excuses after performance do I commonly rely on to justify any perceived failure?

How am I interacting (deeply or superficially) with those who can help me perform better?

Am I demanding enough of myself or am I just going through the motions?

Am I scared or threatened by upcoming performances?

What is my true direction and specific sense of purpose?

Am I continually making promises to myself that I fail to keep?

What are the filters (perceptions) through which I am currently viewing my performance?

Do I truly believe in myself in the midst of my adversity?

Am I letting others affect my thinking?

Is what I am striving to do worth the potential risk of not succeeding?

Is what I am currently doing working for me or not?

Am I effectively responding to all performance interference so that I am free to pursue my goals?

Am I threatened by my performance expectations rather than challenged?

Am I a procrastinator, and if so, why am I hesitant to take action right now?

What are my realistic payoffs for commitment and dedication to my sport?

Am I really using the latest and proven training techniques?

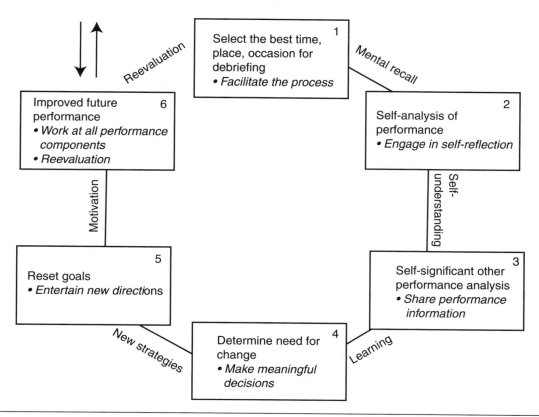

Figure 10.1   Suggested steps in the debriefing process.

that is positively constructive and *helpful*. Ideally, the coach should be psychologically present to assist with closure on a one-on-one basis, that is, fully attentive emotionally and completely involved in the process.

The debriefing process will often be influenced by the performance results. If the performance was less than stellar, athletes and coaches may feel the effects of negative mood states and a resistance to reflect on what needs to be done better. If the performance was very good, the athletes may extend their celebrations and miss reflecting on those detailed aspects of performance that might elicit more desirable behaviors. *Descriptive feedback* may best be given privately, immediately, and always constructively to ensure continued or renewed progress. *Normative evaluative feedback* is best given after due consideration and in an emotionally stable environment.

The coach and athlete should determine the most suitable time, place, and venue for brief and immediate feedback after a performance or for extensive and long-term feedback after a macrocycle (season) or significant competition. Coaches can encourage their athletes to decide

for themselves when they might best internally reflect on their performance because they need to be in a self-reflective frame of mind for maximum learning. Coaches must allocate sufficient time for the sharing of information, either deeply or superficially, in order to solve problems and create expectations around new performances. Naturally, some situations will benefit from an open debriefing environment (e.g., in a team sport), some may benefit from a closed environment (e.g., in an individual sport), and some may benefit from both. Coaches and athletes can determine and develop the optimal approach by trial and error until the best possible conditions are agreed on and alternative approaches are in place depending on the outcome.

Step 2: Indulge in Meaningful Self-Analysis Following the Performance

After competition, athletes should reflect on their performances responsibly, constructively, and accountably. Coaches should consider their own contributions to the athlete's performance as well. Because self-reflection renews learning, athletes should evaluate how they actually performed after a major competition, game, or event. They should be prepared to "look under the hood," critiquing their performances while assessing their productivity.

While the debriefing process should help athletes to face up to their disappointments, mistakes, and shortcomings, athletes must also remember to celebrate their successes. Those who do not enjoy success are usually the ones who neither acknowledge their mistakes nor choose to learn from them. Their negative attitude is a barrier to initiating the recovery process.

Once athletes have recognized their key limitations (and celebrated their successes), they should then determine what actions to take based on their own subjective findings and knowing their own inner resources, abilities, and limits. Intuitively, they may discover new performance perspectives about themselves that may motivate them to continuous learning and self-development (e.g., a greater control of mental and emotional states). Their next task will be to decide how these changes might best be integrated into training and competition. Equally, they should consider what new goals and expectations might accompany such changes.

Performance checklists, videos, self-reflective exercises, and personal journals are effective ways to mentally recall or recapture the performance in subjective detail (Hogg, 1995). Initially, athletes may require assistance and encouragement from the coach in taking such steps. Eventually, they will likely take on this responsibility for themselves.

Athletes should engage in self-reflective evaluation as close to the performance as possible or, as indicated earlier, during warm-downs to allow for accurate recall of the performance activity. In addition, they should be careful about the negative effects of either too much or too little self-criticism. Athletes who are overly self-critical risk becoming disabled by anxiety and consequently disconnected from the task of improving their performance. Such athletes would do well to maintain a sense of humor about themselves in their analyses. On the other hand, athletes who strive to maintain a comfortable feeling about their efforts and avoid constructive self-criticism will never progress to the next level of performance.

Self-awareness is only meaningful when athletes can use it to make changes. Once they have succeeded in verbalizing what they must maintain and what they must improve in order to meet a standard of excellence, they must get their achievement drive into gear. Change should never be viewed as a sign of weakness or failure. Change requires courage. There is strength to be gained from the admission of any shortcomings provided the necessary steps taken use all available resources.

Step 3: Be Open to an Exchange of Performance Feedback

While athletes are engaged in self-reflection after performance, hopefully coaches have been engaged in some self-reflection too and have unbiased information to share. Sharing experiences encourages active learning and triggers optimal recovery. If coaches and athletes are able to acknowledge and discuss the good and not-so-good aspects of performance from their own perspectives without resistance and with a view to modify or change, then athletes will be mobilized to recover fully and proceed to the next level of accomplishment. Once the environment is set up for a healthy interaction among athletes, coaches, and support staff, then the sharing of information can be prompted by the head coach or, if luxury permits, the sport psychologist. Then decisions can be negotiated about what needs to be done next. This is only realistically possible once all the emotional frustrations or disappointments associated with poor performances have been vented.

It is important when debriefing not to dwell too long on the past performance or to focus too heavily on the "should haves," "almosts," and "what ifs." Athletes and coaches should look productively into the future, but not too far ahead, as this may take concentration away from the present where it is vital to remain composed, calm, and confident rather than confused.

Any exchange of internal and external feedback must result in feelings of certainty, trust, and conscientiousness. Coaches are advised to invite athletes to relate their thoughts and feelings first while actively listening—unless athlete preferences are stated otherwise. Athletes in turn should be open to candid feedback rather than discouraging it. Neither coaches nor athletes should adopt a position that is protective against the harshness of the truth. Such a position can take different forms, including denying or not facing up to the facts of the performance, selectively filtering out key information because it might be too confrontational, simply rationalizing "good excuses," and acting as though nothing is wrong mentally. It is critical never to buy into the illusion that all is well at the cost of the truth that might open the door to improved performance. On a very practical level, athletes must be convinced of the coach's desire to improve each athlete's performance. By establishing both trust and rapport, coaches make it clear that they are willing to spend time in the debriefing process because they are totally committed to seeing the athlete *grow* and *improve*.

The shared interaction between coaches and athletes must provide for added meaning and decision making. Rationalizing the result and how it actually occurred is a meaningful exercise. If the athletes' efforts were up to expectations and justifiable, then shared feedback will lead to insightful learning and improved self-understanding. Athletes are more likely *willing* and *ready* to provide and accept evaluative feedback. Athletes who are unwilling and unprepared to commit to the debriefing process will shut down communication, and the steps to recovery will likely be stifled.

Changes for the better need to be discussed, along with the opportunities for change and their likely implications. For example, if change means more quality team practices, or the integration of mental skills into the daily training routine, or greater control of stress-recovery patterns, or a greater sense of pride and commitment, then how might these changes be best integrated, monitored, evaluated, and refined within the overall program for the future? Change will be all the more powerful if it is negotiated in harmony with the athlete's goals, sense of mission, and belief system, including the belief that self-improvement is never ending.

To summarize, athletes and coaches should attempt to concentrate on two significant questions: First, Were the performance goals attained, and if not, why? And second, How well was the performance accomplished? Sometimes it is difficult and unrealistic to answer these questions alone, but if athletes and coaches collaborate in the debriefing process, it is possible to reach desirable competencies through mutual understanding and cooperation.

Step 4: Determine the Need for Change

After listening openly, providing each other with clear and convincing messages, and focusing on what needs to be worked on technically, physically, tactically, and mentally/emotionally, athletes and coaches should devise worthwhile strategies to effect change. It is important to cope with what is actually happening in the execution of the performance rather than fixating on why it should not be happening. Athletes cannot elicit change if they fail to acknowledge what must be changed. In the face of any conflicts, it is important for those involved to negotiate and resolve all confusion and disagreement.

If the debriefing process provides athletes with the opportunity to exercise self-regulation and to grasp the meaning of what must be done, then it must also activate all the resources and means of successfully bringing about the necessary changes and their task requirements. Any new plans, routines, or strategies must be carefully thought out as to how they might best be implemented; otherwise, they will not be a part of the solution, only another problem. Eventually athletes become comfortable with critical changes and use the accompanying emotions to their advantage (Hanin, 2000). However, athletes need to be given sufficient time (which may not always be readily available) to respond to the new demands placed on them.

Step 5: Set New Goals That Are Challenging, Measurable, and Meaningful

As a result of the debriefing process, athletes and their coaches should design new or modify existing goals so that the goals reflect the new vision, trigger recovery, and act as a motivating agent to help the athletes commit to a higher level of performance. Debriefing allows athletes to check their responses, to engage in personal renewals, to revisit their dream, and to enjoy new levels of enthusiasm in the successful pursuit of the task. Much has been written about the setting and resetting of goals as a means of direction and motivation (Burton, 1992; Gould, 1998; Locke & Latham, 1985; Martin & Tesser, 1996). It is necessary to quickly reengage in the performance process, to understand the new challenges, and to mobilize all resources to meet the challenges with determined action.

Step 6: Self-Monitor for Improved Performance

This final step encourages a revised focus on all components of the performance process discussed earlier. Self-monitoring (observing and recording behaviors in response to new challenges) is a cognitive skill that will ensure a balanced approach to seeing exactly what is happening before, during, and after performances. Athletes must reengage in performance preparation and become acutely aware of any inconsistencies between what they intended to do (goal states) and what they are actually doing to ensure progress. Initially, this skill is likely conducted at the conscious level in training and can be developed with the use of select tools, such as checklists and self-reflective exercises (see figure 10.2). In time and with practice, monitoring can become fairly effortless, especially if athletes achieve a high degree of automaticity in performance execution.

Reminders of major goals should be a part of daily training, and any revised subgoals should be integrated into the practice session. For example, a competitive swimmer who decides to concentrate on purchasing and holding the water while increasing the stroke rate (turnover), strengthen the legs (using anaerobic leg kick sets), take out the first part of the swim in a faster split time (pace judgment), focus on each training repeat (attention), and be acutely aware of any negative thoughts or feelings while swimming (emotional awareness) must use every opportunity in practice leading up to competition to implement, rehearse, and monitor these goals and objectives until they become a reality.

Debriefing Tools: Monitoring Performance Evaluation and Recovery

Formal debriefing should occur as an ongoing process, allowing athletes and coaches to continually share pertinent information regarding the intensity of performance preparation as well as the quality of its execution. This should be done primarily with the objective of creating more effective ways of functioning. Although self-questioning and open-ended dialogue with coaches are purposeful ways of debriefing, there are alternatives, including writing exercises, athletic journals, art, photography, and so on. Regardless of the self-evaluative tools chosen, the coach and athlete should share in the decision-making process.

Many postperformance self-reflective tools and exercises are available for specific sports. The best tools are generally those that coaches and athletes jointly design to suit their specific needs. Tools should be simple, user friendly, adaptable,

interactive, used on a regular basis, allow for self-monitoring, and evaluated for effectiveness. Orlick (1986) provided a simple template for a post-performance self-reflection tool: Athletes should be aware of their emotional states and monitor any mood disturbances both pre- and post-performance and apply techniques to use those feelings associated with major performance factors (anxiety, confidence, concentration, and motivation) to advantage. Repeated measures using an instrument such as the Profile of Mood States (POMS; McNair, Lorr, & Droppleman, 1971, 1992), and specifically the Grove and Prapavessis (1992) abbreviated version (this version includes the scale *Self-Esteem/Confidence* and fewer items), may show pre- and postperformance mood patterns that help or hinder performance, relating to vigor, tension, anger, fatigue, depression, confusion, and self-confidence.

Checklists that focus on major performance parameters are helpful in debriefing, to avoid overloading athletes with technical information. Monitoring and evaluating optimal stress-recovery relations after major competition and leading into further competition is extremely important because one of the benefits of debriefing is the return to appropriate mental and emotional recovery states (Hogg, 2000). The use of the Recovery-Stress Questionnaire for Athletes (Kellmann & Kallus, 2001) is helpful both as a debriefing tool and to ascertain if athletes have overcome the general and specific stresses of the performance. Repeated and accurate measures of major performance constructs may provide for meaningful discussion in the debriefing process; a number of sport-specific psychometric tests are helpful provided they are interpreted accurately and used with ethical sensitivity (see Ostrow, 1996).

Figure 10.2 is an example of a self-reflective tool used by competitive swimmers and coaches to help with postperformance debriefing. Coaches can adapt this Mental States of Readiness and Satisfaction form (MSRS) to meet the needs of their own athletes/sports. It consists of a series of questions related to pre- and postperformance states.

With practice the MSRS takes a relatively short time to complete. Both coach and athlete can employ this tool separately in an individual sport, while in a team sport the coach can reflect on the team as a whole. Once completed, coaches and athletes can share their observations as outlined in step 3 of the debriefing model. The responses can be scored (See appendix 10.A on p. 198) and

For competitive swimmers   **Mental States of Readiness and Satisfaction (MSRS)**

Competition:_____   This evaluation is following: **Actual race time(s)**
Name: _____   Heats ○ _____
Event: _____   A final ○ _____
Date: _____ **Best time:**_____   B final ○ _____
                                                Long course
                                                Short course   (Please fill in the appropriate circle)

Answer the following to the best of your ability with an emphasis on your best event swum this session/competition. Use the scale: Not at all (0) – Very much (6) and blacken out ● the one response that best reflects how you feel now.

1. Overall, I am satisfied with my performance for this event.   ○ Yes ○ No
2. Purely from a mental point of view I feel that I achieved my major goals for this event.   ○ Yes ○ No ○ Partially
3. Following warm-up and immediately before my event I felt

	Not at all 0 1 2 3 4 5 6 *Very much*		*Not at all* 0 1 2 3 4 5 6 *Very much*
a. Physically warmed up	○○○○○○○	f. Healthy	○○○○○○○
b. Mentally prepared	○○○○○○○	g. Feelings of queasiness	○○○○○○○
c. Eager to race	○○○○○○○	h. In control	○○○○○○○
d. Confident	○○○○○○○	i. Focused	○○○○○○○
e. Worried about performance	○○○○○○○	j. Technically (skill wise) in tune	○○○○○○○

	Not at all 0	1	2	3	4	5	*Very much* 6
4. I was mentally ready for my race.	○	○	○	○	○	○	○
5. I was able to use my feelings/emotions to perform to my advantage.	0	1	2	3	4	5	6
a. Before racing	○	○	○	○	○	○	○
b. During racing	○	○	○	○	○	○	○

6. I had a specific race plan.   ○ Yes ○ No
7. (If yes) I was able to follow it.   ○ Yes ○ No ○ Partially
8. (If yes) it worked effectively for me.   ○ Yes ○ No ○ Partially

	0	1	2	3	4	5	6
9. Postcompetition, I was able to cope with my emotions and mood states.	○	○	○	○	○	○	○
	Very poor						*Excellent*
10. Technically my race(s) was/ (were)	○	○	○	○	○	○	○
11. Strategically my race(s) was/ (were)	○	○	○	○	○	○	○

	Not at all 0	1	2	*Very much* 3
12. During the race I found myself thinking about unrelated things.	○	○	○	○
13. My mind wandered during the race (while I was competing).	○	○	○	○
14. While racing, I found myself not paying attention to what was going on.	○	○	○	○
15. I had lapses in concentration during the race because of nervousness.	○	○	○	○
16. I became concerned because I was unable to concentrate during the race.	○	○	○	○

Complete this form 1 to 2 hours after swimming your main event(s).
Complete for both heats and finals.

Figure 10.2 Pre- and postperformance self-evaluation form.
Adapted from Hogg, in press-a.

a performance index created for future reference or comparison.

The tool, which is completed within minutes of the performance, focuses on two concerns—the athlete's perceived state of *readiness* for the performance and the athlete's perceived state of *satisfaction* and assessment of the performance. These two scores should be closely related when they are converted to percentages. In other words, the athlete's sense of readiness to perform and the athlete's degree of performance satisfaction are closely aligned. A negative difference would tend to indicate that the athlete in his own estimation has not performed up to expectation, while a positive difference would suggest that the athlete has been successful in meeting his performance expectations.

How athletes score themselves on the readiness and satisfaction scales over time and across major competitions provides further insight. For example, if athletes consistently give themselves a high readiness but low satisfaction score (a negative difference), it would indicate the need to examine more closely both their perceptions of physical and mental states of readiness and the type of attributions they customarily make after a successful or not-so-successful performance.

This monitoring and evaluative tool is an attempt at bringing consistency and realism to the performance process, providing common ground for discussing how athletes realistically think they are doing, and determining aspects of performance that need to be addressed in the immediate future. It may also help athletes reset their goals and reaffirm both their passion for the sport and any core values that guide and motivate their behavior.

Figure 10.3 illustrates the profile of a soccer player who used the MSRS across a macrocycle (16-week regular season) to plot the measures of performance readiness and satisfaction. A feature of this illustration is the player's ability both to improve the state of mental readiness and to evaluate performance efforts at a higher level of satisfaction as the season progressed.

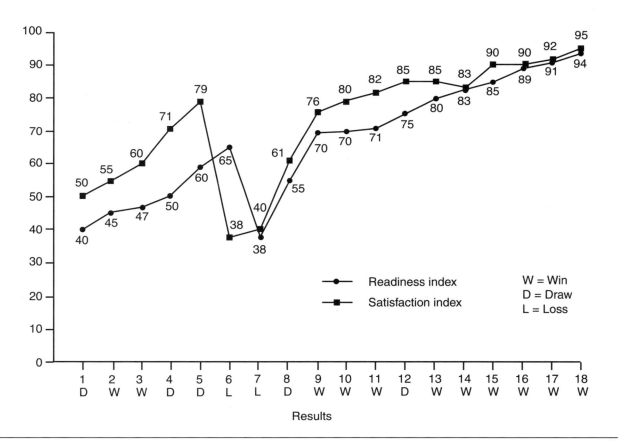

Figure 10.3 Performance readiness and satisfaction profile of a soccer player using MSRS across a regular season involving 18 league games.

Debriefing: Some Potential Problems and Issues

National team coaches need to recognize that the full-blown process of debriefing after a major competition can be quite complex, time consuming, and even expensive if carried out purposefully and effectively. But to provide athletes with an accurate feel for their performance, all four components (i.e., technical, physical, tactical, mental and emotional) should be systematically assessed as soon as possible (perhaps the day after the competition). For noninternational events, the process can be simplified to suit everyone's needs and obligations as long as the key elements of debriefing are addressed adequately.

Performance appraisal not only presents logistical difficulties but can also induce a wide range of negative emotional responses and mood disturbances, especially if the performance was disappointing or not up to expectations. Moods and emotions are likely to take time to subside, and some athletes need to return to a satisfactory homeostasis before the recovery process can begin and the debriefing process can be effectual.

Performance evaluations can be either adaptive or maladaptive, depending on their effect on the athlete being evaluated. *Adaptive* evaluations encourage the athlete to the next level, while *maladaptive* evaluations cause the athlete to plateau as a result of the athlete's resistance to self-examination or deliberate obstruction of feedback. Athletes who are resistant to or not ready for debriefing usually display little sense of inner connectedness (harmony between mind and body).

Athletes who tend to experience evaluations as maladaptive generally fall into three personality types: the *self-critic,* the *worrier,* and the *dysfunctional perfectionist.* Athletes with these personality types seem to feed off their frustrations, build up their concerns, and multiply their problems after debriefing, which deters optimal recovery. Athletes who are overly critical of their performances need guided assistance from the support staff to focus their attention in the debriefing setting on what they did well or actually accomplished relative to their clearly stated goals. They may need help to carefully consider both the internal and external information before formulating an opinion as to where blame or praise should or should not be placed.

Athletes who worry about what others think indulge in an unhealthy self-consciousness rather than simple self-awareness of their internal states. Much of the debriefing feedback can be lost if they are wrapped up in thoughts and feelings as to how their performance efforts appear to others. They invariably worry about the things that they cannot control and never quite address the tasks that are in their control. Consequently, their anxieties and fears increase to the point of causing them to choke over what they need to do in the future. The support staff should help such athletes to

- sharpen their self-awareness skills and their sense of self-efficacy,
- make positive judgments about their capacity to perform, and
- strengthen the beliefs they have about their competencies and what they can accomplish.

Athletes with high levels of self-efficacy and self-confidence, when faced with any challenge, whether as a consequence of the debriefing or not, are able to step up to the plate and take action, while those who doubt themselves often do not even try (Bandura, 1986). Finally, dysfunctional perfectionists pose problems in the debriefing process especially if they experience a need to seem perfect and cannot bear to admit their shortcomings or are enraged by criticism even if it is realistic or justifiable. They are more likely to accept responsibility for successful performances while hastily blaming themselves, others, or external conditions for perceived failures. Some dysfunctional perfectionists never admit to any mistakes, exaggerate their own competencies, close themselves off to constructive feedback, and are oblivious to their own mental lapses especially when required to focus and refocus in the debriefing setting. On the contrary, other dysfunctional perfectionists tend to dwell on their own mistakes and assume too much responsibility not only for their own errors but also those of others. The support staff can help such athletes build their courage and address their true strengths and weaknesses by asking the tough questions about their warped perceptions, by recognizing the truth of what they have done or not done to control their performance, and by helping them set a new goal-oriented course of action.

Naturally, there is always the difficulty of response accuracy in performance evaluation and debriefing communication. Athletes may be reticent to establish a rapport with the coach, especially with regard to self-evaluation, for fear that the coach may use the information for selection purposes or to predict future performances. A third party, such as a sport psychologist, might be a very helpful in establishing a sense of trust between athlete and coach.

A real issue concerns athletes who are experiencing limited performance improvement or none at all. The debriefing process should attempt to uncover some possible reasons for a decline in performance or a total lack of progress. Systematic *slumpbusting* is also an important process that is addressed and hopefully resolved with meaningful debriefing (Goldberg, 1998). Likely the slumping athlete has currently little or no investment in making the necessary changes to enhance performance. Equally, the athlete may perceive the changes as not required imminently and consequently indulges in procrastination or inertia. But very likely, the athlete, coach, and support staff failed to confront or skirted the real issues in taking the performance to the next level. It is important to address those things that sabotage the athlete's efforts to be successful.

Athletes who have poor self-confidence will require special handling in the debriefing process. They may lack the courage of their convictions; feel inadequate in terms of making adjustments; show indecision in taking the steps to mobilize their mental and emotional forces; and fail to interact by voicing their opinions, beliefs, and possibly their valuable ideas. They are often in a state of denial; that is, they are having performance problems but pretending they are not! Naturally, they will want to shy away from change or from taking any kind of calculated risk. Their debriefing should focus on the cognitive presentation of very simple, well-rehearsed plans or routines that are both familiar and successful for them. Debriefing for athletes with low self-esteem should be used as an occasion for building self-confidence so that they feel comfortable sharing their views, confronting issues without giving up easily on their opinion, and following new courses of action.

Debriefing Guidelines for Coaches

Coaches need to first recognize the crucial implications of debriefing if they are truly committed to the holistic development of their athletes. For the process to be credible, coaches are encouraged to fully understand the skills and abilities of the athlete involved and to give true value to debriefing despite its complexity. They should teach athletes the art of self-reflection after performance and show them alternative ways to approaching excellence. The debriefing process can be initially introduced in a modified format to the developing athlete. All athletes should be taught how to progressively debrief themselves responsibly and accountably using the basic mental skills and emotional competencies. Coaches need to create the debriefing environment so that it is open, respectful, nonthreatening, and nonjudgmental and leads athletes to self-discovery, learning, and optimal recovery. Coaches must accept and appreciate individual differences, always encourage input from athletes on their perspectives, and endeavor to incorporate athletes' suggestions in an effort to be proactive (Covey, 1989, 1993). Young athletes require guidance, simple routines, and coping strategies when initially experiencing the debriefing process and especially when they are overloaded with performance information.

When using debriefing tools, the coach should recognize that the tool is a positive aid to learning through interactive and articulate dialogue only if the coach's and athlete's perceptions of what happened match. It may be best to use tools sparingly if they only add confusion and possibly only following significant competitive events. The coach is very much the facilitator helping to clarify perceptions; prioritizing and operationalizing short-term goals; presenting alternative approaches or solutions; looking for trends and attributional patterns; and encouraging clear focus, self-control, and a degree of optimism.

In the initial stages of introducing the debriefing process, communication may seem a little one sided. Coaches may not be altogether clear whether the athletes have received the messages they have sent. At this stage in the process coaches should attempt to provide precise feedback in an unhurried and nonevaluative manner, listening and hearing athletes' dreams without judgment and demonstrating empathy as opposed to intolerance, indifference, or outright condemnation. In so doing, coaches engender increased feelings of self-efficacy and self-confidence in athletes. By being patient and yet persistent in preparing the ground and sowing the seeds, coaches allow their athletes to develop self-awareness and emotional intelligence as they grow in age, maturity, and competitive experience. Coaches should explain the short- and long-term benefits of the debriefing process, such as increased self-awareness, self-efficacy, and intrinsic motivation; an opportunity for mutual agreement and understanding; the application of mental skills and, in the long term, changes in direction and in attributional patterning and effective coping with specific problems.

Unquestionably, debriefing provides the occasion for coaches to enhance athletes' self-worth and feelings of competence. Coaches should nurture feelings of perceived self-efficacy, competence, self-determination, and accountability throughout the evaluative and debriefing processes, focusing equally on what was successful as well as on pertinent shortcomings (Weiss, McAuley, Ebbeck, & Weise, 1990). It is important for coaches to show the links between debriefing and improved performances if these should emerge. Adolescent athletes are occasionally preoccupied with perceived performance barriers. Both effective listening and progressive attempts at empowering athletes to control what they can control will be beneficial. Most important, coaches should help athletes to eliminate all interferences or barriers to performance potential. Coaches need to teach athletes coping solutions. Adolescent athletes particularly need to increase their levels of self-awareness and self-belief. However, with experience and maturity, athletes will become more accurate in their self-evaluations and less dependent on significant others.

Superior coaches are able, through the process of debriefing, to manage conflicts, create team synergy in the pursuit of collective goals, use interpersonal skills to get the team refocused after success, be steely-eyed without indulging in excessive positivism, and productively work with athletes after a defeat or disappointing performance outcome. They can engineer a meaningful postperformance dialogue rather than engage in heated confrontation, thereby helping athletes feel more open to change, especially if they perceive that it will make a difference in their future performances. They inspire their athletes to employ their own motivational skills and tap into their own emotional resources.

Coaches need to avoid overloading athletes with performance information, imprecise feedback, or meaningless statistics. Otherwise athletes may develop feelings of being overpowered, manipulated, and rendered helpless. Coaches should (1) avoid using guilt since it is likely to paralyze and shut down all communication, (2) refrain from an "I told you so" attitude or from using statements that are protective of their own decisions since this will only break trust, and (3) accept the fact that all athletes make mistakes. While being careful not to tolerate repeated excuses, they should factor in any unusual circumstances that may have positively or negatively contributed to the performance outcome. In the event of success and the need to celebrate, coaches should provide a socially acceptable emotional outlet in the performance evaluation setting. When commiseration is necessary in the context of a loss or poor performance, coaches need to filter all feedback in such a way that it does not destroy athletes' self-confidence. Finally, coaches should always protect those athletes who are constantly being evaluated outside of the debriefing process by those who rightly or wrongly consider themselves in a position to be judgmental, especially if performances fail to meet their own expectations.

Debriefing Guidelines for Athletes

Athletes need to experience and learn from failure as much as from success. In the formal debriefing exercise, athletes can learn to process performance results both *informationally* (by learning what to do or what not to do in the future) and *emotionally* (by learning what emotional competencies they possess that will help them to rectify their mistakes and transport them to the next level of performance). Athletes who can interpret poor performances informationally can determine why errors in performance keep recurring. Consequently, they can incorporate corrective procedures into subsequent training sessions to good effect. Athletes need to be aware of their own personal resources and develop the ability to put them to use in such a way that they can perform beyond current levels of performance. They need to learn all about the debriefing process and especially the skill of internal evaluation so that it is real, accurate, and honest.

Athletes should come to accept debriefing as a normal part of the performance environment. Awareness of accurate and honest self-assessment needs to be directed at acquiring knowledge about strengths and weaknesses and developing some idea about what the coach likes to see in the performance. As a result of regular postperformance reflection, the understanding and awareness gained from self-perceptions and from significant others will teach athletes consistency and control.

Athletes sometimes adopt a defensive attitude toward receiving constructive feedback in the debriefing setting. They may do so because they do not want to be held fully accountable for their failure. Such an attitude may be justified when athletes are discouraged from providing their input into the performance process. As a result, they might feel devoid of any responsibility for the outcome. Athletes need to refrain from hearing only the negative and from indulging in excuse making in anticipation of what needs to be done. By way of illustration, an athlete (after a poor performance) may be entertaining an excuse to avoid an intense training effort and end up exhibiting an undesirable behavior (e.g., missing an important training session). Athletes should be aware of engaging in any smoke screens or feeble excuses in the debriefing process in an attempt to deny the facts of their emotional truth. Rather than deny the truth, athletes need to accept feedback gained in debriefing and be prepared to do something constructively different by using their intuitiveness, insights, gut feelings, and emotional intelligence. They should use debriefing feedback in order to maintain or improve their performance or to redefine new challenges for themselves.

Athletes need to be aware of promoting overly ambitious or unattainable performance goals for themselves or of being unrealistic about what it takes to train more assiduously. They must also acknowledge any mental lapses that caused a shift in psychological momentum and use appropriate interventions as a means of speedily getting back on track. Finally, athletes should be prepared to respectfully confront the coach in the debriefing setting if there is a need to defend themselves in the face of any false or biased information.

Summary

Debriefing is a critical learning opportunity without which the learning process of the performance is incomplete. In the absence of debriefing, athletes are denied the opportunity to focus on the details of the task requirements. Debriefing is best conducted in a systematic and interactive manner and in a psychologically healthy environment that considers the athlete's development, maturity, and experience. Debriefing encourages self-questioning on the part of athletes and sensitive feedback from coaches and support staff who have a legitimate stake in the performance. This internal and external sharing of information encourages the building of a lasting trust and respect between athletes and coaches as well as increases the chances of improved performance. Debriefing allows athletes opportunities to exercise self-awareness and self-regulatory skills while reinforcing those aspects of performance that can be controlled. Ignorance of mental and emotional skills may result in the inability to deal effectively with debilitative performance states. Mental and physical skills tend to become dysfunctional in situations of cognitive overload, for instance, when there are time constraints, excessive levels of anxiety, and pressures in the performance environment.

Debriefing provides solutions, guidance, and feelings of certainty. The shared information allows all performance components to gradually fall into place. This creates feelings of inner peace, composure, and balance for the individual athlete and harmony for the team. Debriefing is a motivational tool that provides opportunities for athletes to safeguard and ensure continuous learning and improvement; to work cooperatively with coaches, support staff, and teammates; to absorb the fun and enjoyment of the journey to excellence; and to develop self-discipline, responsibility, and performance accountability. Recovery thrives in this positive frame.

Performance diagnoses can help coaches and athletes arrive at a balanced view of the options available. Calculated decisions about solutions or new directions can then be reflected in revised action plans fortified by the resetting of goals. All obstacles or interferences to performance potential must be addressed. Success of these plans should be monitored, evaluated, and refined for future performances in subsequent debriefing sessions. Debriefing to exchange information and to discuss what is really happening to the athlete before, during, and after performances certainly lends creativity and depth to any decisions about future performances and can build a very solid and trusting relationship between coaches and athletes. The next performance is really only as good as the lessons learned from the previous one.

References

Anshel, M.H. (1997). *Sport psychology: From theory to practice.* Scottsdale, AZ: Scarisbrick.

Bandura, A. (1986). *Social foundations of thought and action.* Englewood Cliffs, NJ: Prentice Hall.

Biddle, S.J.H. (1991). Interpreting success and failure. In S.J.Bull (Ed.), *Sport psychology: A self help guide* (pp.70-83). Marlborough,UK: Crowood Press.

Biddle, S.J.H., Hanrahan, S.J., & Sellars, C.N. (2001). Attributions: Past, present, and future. In R.N.Singer, H.A. Hausenblas, & C.M. Janelle (Eds.), *Handbook of sport psychology* (pp. 444-471). New York: John Wiley and Sons.

Boud, D., Keogh, R., & Walker, D. (1985). *Using experience for learning.* Bristol, PA: Open University Press.

Brawley, L.R., & Roberts, G.C. (1984). Attributions in sport: Research foundations, characteristics and limitations. In J.M. Silva & R.S. Weinberg (Eds.), *Psychological foundations of sport* (pp. 197-213). Champaign, IL: Human Kinetics.

Burton, D. (1992). The Jekyll/Hyde nature of goals: Reconceptualizing goalsetting in sport. In T.S. Horn (Ed.), *Advances in sport psychology* (pp. 267-297). Champaign, IL: Human Kinetics.

Covey, S.R. (1989). *The seven habits of highly effective people: Powerful lessons in personal change.* New York: Fireside.

Covey, S.R. (1993). *Principled centered leadership.* New York: Fireside.

Goldberg, A.S. (1998). *Sports slumpbusting: 10 steps to mental toughness and peak performance.* Champaign, IL: Human Kinetics.

Goleman, D. (1995). *Emotional intelligence.* New York: Bantam Books.

Goleman, D. (1997). *Working with emotional intelligence.* New York: Bantam Books.

Gould, D. (1998). Goalsetting for peak performance. In J.M. Williams (Ed.), *Applied sport psychology: Personal growth to peak performance* (pp. 182-196). Mountain View, CA: Mayfield.

Grove, R., & Prapavessis, H. (1992). Reliability and validity data for an abbreviated version of the Profile of Mood States. *International Journal of Sport Psychology, 23,* 93-109.

Hanin, Y.L. (Ed.). (2000). *Emotions in sport.* Champaign, IL: Human Kinetics.

Hogg, J.M. (1995). *Mental skills for swim coaches: A coaching text on the psychological aspects of competitive swimming.* Edmonton, AB: Sport Excel.

Hogg, J.M. (1998). The post performance debriefing process: Getting your capable track and field athletes to the next level of performance. *New Studies in Athletics, 3,* 49-56.

Hogg, J.M. (2000). *Canadian women's World Cup soccer 1999: Mental preparations.* A report for the Canadian Soccer Association. University of Alberta, Edmonton.

Hogg, J.M. (in press-a). *Mental preparation: Profiling, monitoring and evaluating swimming performance.* Edmonton, AB: Sport Excel.

Hogg, J.M. (in press-b). Postperformance evaluation: Important implications for the coach. *Proceedings of the ITFCA Conference, Edmonton, Canada, XV.*

Holder, T., (1997). A theoretical perspective of performance evaluation. In R.J.Butler (Ed.), *Sport psychology in performance* (pp. 68-86). Oxford,UK: Butterworth Heinemann.

Kellmann, M., & Kallus, K.W. (2001). *Recovery-Stress Questionnaire for Athletes: User manual.* Champaign, IL: Human Kinetics.

Leathers, D.G. (1986). *Successful non-verbal communication: Principles and applications.* New York: Macmillan.

Locke, E.A., & Latham, G.P. (1985). The application of goalsetting to sports. *Journal of Sport Psychology, 7,* 205-222.

Martin, L.L., & Tesser, A. (1996). *Striving and feeling: Interactions among goals, affect, and self-regulation.* Mahwah, NJ: Erlbaum.

McNair, D.M., Lorr, M., & Droppleman, L. (1971, 1992). *Manual for the Profile of Mood States.* San Diego: Educational and Industrial Testing Service.

Orlick, T. (1986). *Coaches training manual to psyching for sport.* Champaign, IL: Leisure Press.

Ostrow, A. (1996). *Directory of psychological tests in the sport and exercise sciences.* Morgantown, WV: Fitness Information Technology.

Ravizza, K. (1998). Increasing awareness for sport performance. In J.M. Williams (Ed.), *Applied sport psychology: Personal growth to peak performance* (pp. 171-181). Mountain View, CA: Mayfield.

Rudawsky, D.J., Lundgren, D.C., & Grasha, A.F. (1999, April). Competitive and collaborative responses to negative feedback. *International Journal of Conflict Management, 10*(2), 172-190.

Salmoni, A.W., Schmidt, R.A., & Walter, C.B. (1984). Knowledge of results and motor learning: A review and critical appraisal. *Psychological Bulletin, 95,* 355-386.

Schmidt, R.A., & Lee, T.D. (1999). *Motor control and learning.* Champaign, IL: Human Kinetics.

Schmidt, R.A., & Wrisberg, C.A. (2000). *Motor learning and performance.* Champaign, IL: Human Kinetics.

Shea, C.M., & Howell, J.M. (1999, Fall). Charismatic leadership and task feedback. A laboratory study of their effects and task performance. *Leadership Quarterly, 10*(3), 375-396.

Sinclair, G.D., & Sinclair, D.A. (1994). Developing reflective performers by integrating mental management skills with the learning process. *The Sport Psychologist, 8,* 13-27.

Smith, R.E., & Smoll, F.L. (1996). *Way to go coach: A scientifically proven approach to coaching effectiveness.* Portolla Valley, CA: Wade.

Weiss, M.R., McAuley, E., Ebbeck, V., & Weise, D.M. (1990). Self-esteem and causal attributions for children's physical and social competence in sport. *Journal of Sport and Exercise Psychology, 12,* 21-36.

Yukelson, D. (1998). Communicating effectively. In J.M. Williams (Ed.), *Applied sport psychology: Personal growth to peak performance* (pp. 142-157). Mountain View, CA: Mayfield.

APPENDIX 10.A

Instructions for Scoring Form M1-4

There are two scales of measurement to evaluate the performance. *Performance readiness* is scored out of a maximum of 77 points, and *performance satisfaction* is scored out of a total of 59 points. Intensity scores are on a scale of 0 to 6, while YES scores 5, PARTIALLY scores 3, and NO scores 0.

To determine the readiness score, add up the scores for the responses to the following questions: 3 (a-j) (but note that questions 3e and 3g are *reverse* scored), 4, 5a, and 6.

To determine the satisfaction score, add up the scores for the responses to the following questions: 1, 2, 5b, 7, 8, 9, 10, 11, 12, 13, 14, 15, and 16.

Next change the readiness and satisfaction scores to percentage scores. Then estimate the difference between the percentage satisfaction and percentage readiness scores. If the result is a negative score (i.e., the satisfaction score is less than the readiness score), the athlete may not have been totally ready (physically or mentally or both) for the performance or she is too hard on herself. If the result is a positive score (the satisfaction score is greater than the readiness score), the athlete may be performing beyond his expectations or is too easy in self-evaluation. By recording these index scores for repeated measures, the performer will become more familiar with her state of readiness and will become more accurate in the self-assessment of performance satisfaction.

Example:

Readiness score: 71/77 (71 ÷? 77 · 100) = 92%

Satisfaction score: 40/59 (40 ÷? 59 · 100) = 68%

Difference: −2

Hanin, Y.L. (2002). Individually optimal recovery in sports: An application of the IZOF model. In M. Kellmann (Ed.), *Enhancing recovery: Preventing underperformance in athletes* (pp. 199-217). Champaign, IL: Human Kinetics.

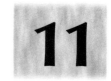

Individually Optimal Recovery in Sports: An Application of the IZOF Model

Yuri L. Hanin

Sporting activity consists of the repeated execution of motor tasks of varying complexity and intensity both in practices and in competitions. As in any demanding physical and mental work, an athlete's resources are recruited, used, and then recuperated to ensure consistently successful performance. In this "work-recovery" cycle, the need for rest (recuperation, regeneration, or recovery) is related to the fact that a healthy human gets tired. This fatigue, especially as the result of excessive work, is usually accompanied by feelings of emotional discomfort and indicates that the functional capacities of an organism are decreasing (Salmanoff, 1991). Moreover, fatigue usually accumulates over time and makes it more difficult or sometimes impossible to resume and continue work at a required level of quality and intensity, often resulting in deteriorated performance. It is important to realize that performance below one's potential and expectations ("underperformance") can happen for different reasons (weather conditions, competition site, opponents, an athlete's health status, injuries, unexpected competitive stressors, pressures outside sports, etc.). However, one of the common reasons for underperformance in different athletes across different sports is excessive work (in practices and competitions) combined with inadequate or disturbed rest (see Kellmann, this volume, chapter 1). The focus of this chapter is on the assessment and prevention of underperformance due to under-recovery after excessive work, which is reflected in an athlete's psychobiosocial states prior to, during, and after performance.

Although the importance of regaining an adequate working state for consistently successful performance is clearly recognized by athletes and their coaches, overtraining, staleness, and burnout syndromes are still among the most frequent problems encountered in competitive sports (Gould & Dieffenbach, this volume, chapter 2; Gould, Tuffey, Udrey, & Loehr, 1996; Kallus & Kellmann, 2000; Kellmann, this volume, chapter 1; Kellmann & Kallus, 1999; Morgan, 1991, 1997; Morgan, Brown, Raglin, O'Connor, & Ellickson, 1987; Raglin, 1993, 1999; Raglin & Wilson, 2000). Moreover, surprisingly little attention has been paid in sport psychology to a systematic study of individually optimal performance-recovery cycles. Most research focused mainly on preperformance (competitive) anxiety and stress (Apitzsch, 1983, 1996; Hanin, 1978, 1983, 1995, 2000b; Hardy, 1990; Hardy, Jones, & Gould, 1997; Jones, 1995; Jones & Hardy, 1990; Martens, Vealey, & Burton, 1990; Raglin & Hanin, 2000) and on monitoring postperformance mood states and mood disturbances in practices (Morgan, 1991; Morgan et al., 1987; Morgan, Costill, Flynn, Raglin, & O'Connor, 1988; Raglin, 1993, 1999; Raglin & Wilson, 2000). Recently, a more balanced approach to work-rest relationships has been advocated emphasizing the importance of an optimal match between the amount of work and recovery needed (Kallus & Kellmann, 2000; Kellmann & Günther, 2000; Kellmann & Kallus, 1999, 2000, 2001).

Apparently, the performance-emotion relationship is one of the most relevant areas of research that holds promise for accurate description, prediction, and understanding of the dynamics of optimal (and less-than-optimal) working states in practices and competitions across different athletes and sport tasks (Hanin, 1997). However, there is a growing consensus among sport psychologists that principles based on group-oriented data are less than effective when applied to individual athletes. Therefore, more individualized approaches (Bortoli, Robazza, & Nougier, 1997; Hanin, 1978, 1997, 2000a, 2000b; Morgan, 1997; Vanden Auweele, Cuyper, Mele, & Rzewnicki, 1993) have been proposed, and there is a clear trend toward a combined use of nomothetic and idiographic methodologies in sport psychology (Dunn, 1994).

One such approach is Hanin's Individual Zones of Optimal Functioning (IZOF) model (see Hanin, 1995, 1997, 2000a for a review) for understanding performance-related states in competitive sports. The IZOF model offers a framework and tools to describe, predict, and explain why and how individually optimal and dysfunctional working states can affect athletic performance. Initially, the IZOF model was applied to precompetitive anxiety (Hanin, 1978, 1986, 1989, 1995; Raglin & Hanin, 2000), but recently it was extended to pleasant and unpleasant emotions (Hanin, 1993, 1997, 2000a) and emotional-motivational (Hanin, 1999, 2000a, 2001) states.

The basic assumption of the IZOF model is that performance process and outcomes can be predicted based on the interaction effects of individually optimal and dysfunctional emotional content and intensities (zones) prior to and during performance. This notion is based on empirical findings indicating that each individual athlete has an idiosyncratic constellation of performance-related emotions and their intensities. The individualized emotional profile can be established based on an athlete's past performance history and present performance status. Furthermore, these patterns, reflecting an individual's readiness to recruit and utilize available resources, can be used as person-specific criteria to evaluate the dynamics of performance-related states in pre-, mid-, and postperformance situations. Specifically, the closer the intensity of an athlete's current state to previously established optimal zones, the higher the probability of that athlete's successful performance. In contrast, a large deviation from individually optimal intensity zones indicates a high probability of poor or below-average performance. The concept of being in or out of the zone, as well as other assumptions of the IZOF model used to describe emotion-performance relationships and predict an individual's performance, were empirically validated in different athletes and across different sports (see Hanin, 1997, 2000a, 2000c for a review).

This chapter describes how this approach can be applied to performance and recovery states as determinants of consistent excellency in elite sports. Specifically, the IZOF-based multidimensional description of individually optimal/dysfunctional states provides a constellation of sensitive person-specific and task-specific markers of an athlete's high (or low) readiness for performance. Furthermore, these markers are proposed as descriptors of optimal or dysfunctional pre- and mid-performance states and also serve as idiosyncratic indicators (and individualized criteria) of adequate (or inadequate) recovery. Thus, an athlete's failure to regain an individually optimal preperformance state resulting in subsequent underperformance, especially after excessive work, can be accurately identified and prevented. Prediction of optimal performance and prevention of underperformance, therefore, should be based on individual-oriented monitoring of pre-, mid-, and postperformance states and recovery states. The implication here is that functionally emotional dynamics reflect how athletes recruit, utilize, and recuperate their resources in a single (or/and repeated) work-recovery cycle.

The sections that follow discuss terminology and the basic assumptions of the IZOF model and describe the individual performance and recovery states that can predict optimal performance and help athletes avoid underperformance. The section ends with a discussion of the effect of individually optimal recovery skills and strategies for monitoring current emotional-motivational states related to performance and recovery.

Terminology

Working definitions of several terms used in this chapter are provided here. These terms include performance (and underperformance), recovery (and underrecovery), and optimal (and dysfunctional) psychobiosocial states related to performance and recovery.

Performance in this chapter is defined as a process of a goal-oriented task execution characterized by movement patterns and outcomes achieved (Hanin, 1995, 1997). Successful performance is defined as high-quality task execution resulting in higher-than-average (typical, customary) outcomes. Optimal performance refers to successful performance under particular conditions (athlete's readiness, weather, location, level of competition, etc.). *Underperformance* is performance below expected or customary, typical, or individually acceptable quality in a particular situation. Usually, underperformance is below the lower limit in the normal variability of an athlete's typical performance.

Recovery is an intentional self-initiated and goal-oriented activity (on-task or off-task) aimed at regaining one's level of working capacity reflected in an optimal pre- and midperformance state. Optimal (adequate, successful) recovery is a well-planned activity that matches the situational needs of an athlete in rest and results in regaining an optimal performance state. Recovery focuses on "recharging an athlete's batteries" so that recruitment and effective utilization of available (already used or overused) resources become possible again. It is a process of recuperation of different resources in order to be able to resume an interrupted activity.

Underrecovery is a special case of inadequate (incomplete or insufficient) recovery activity that does not match an athlete's needs in rest and results in a significant deviation from an athlete's optimal performance state. Usually, underrecovered athletes have problems recruiting/utilizing their resources and are not ready to resume activity or fail to perform up to their potential.

Recovery as an intentional and preplanned activity may focus on recuperating working capacity and selected (most utilized) resources: cognitive, affective, motivational, bodily-somatic, behavioral, and communicative. Thus, recovery as a process should be distinguished from rest, which is a spontaneous response to situational fatigue. Athletes usually rest during relatively short periods of inactivity (breaks) either during performance (on-task) or postperformance (off-task).

Performance states are individually optimal or dysfunctional conditions accompanying total human activity in pre-, mid-, and postperformance situations. Preperformance and midperformance emotional-motivational states are reliable predictors of successful, average, or poor performances (Hanin, 1995, 1997, 1999, 2000a). Postperformance states indicate recovery demands in an athlete and actually should be considered as transitory to prerecovery states.

Recovery state is an athlete's psychobiosocial state achieved as a result of the recovery process; it is expected to result in an enhanced ability to regain an optimal performance state. If performance is defined as a period of on-task activity in training and/or competitions, then rest is a period of spontaneous inactivity due to situational fatigue. Recovery-related states indicate how an athlete recuperates and to what extent she is ready to resume performance at an acceptable level by recruiting and utilizing available resources.

The *performance-recovery cycle* is proposed as a unit of sporting activity that emphasizes the role of a balanced interrelationship between these components and the repeated (cyclical) nature of recruitment, utilization, and recuperation of an athlete's resources. From this perspective, optimal performance states are usually the outcomes of optimal recovery process and are closely related to recovery states. In other words, the transition from optimal working states to optimal recovery states and again to optimal working states becomes of crucial importance for optimal and consistently successful performance. Moreover, idiosyncratic markers of optimal performance states and recovery states can be used to assess the quality and effectiveness of the recovery process per se. Figure 11.1 illustrates the concept of emotional dynamics in

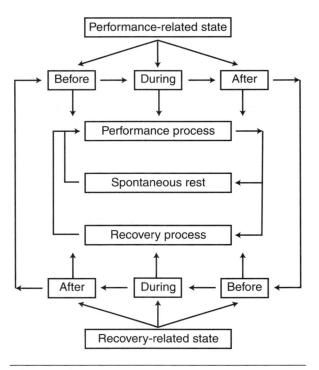

Figure 11.1 Performance-recovery unit.

the performance-recovery cycle and the notion of the transitory nature of pre-, mid-, and postperformance states and pre-, mid-, and postrecovery states.

Performance-Related and Recovery-Related States

There is a growing consensus among sport psychologists that a better understanding of overtraining, staleness, burnout syndromes, and adequate recovery processes requires more sensitive, accurate, and reliable markers of an athlete's psychobiosocial states. Most salient and important in the context of performance and recovery will be emotional, motivational, somatic, and cognitive states associated with optimal and less-than-optimal performance and recovery activity, because numerous physiological indicators are often ineffective for such purposes (Kellmann, this volume, chapter 1; Kuipers, 1998; Morgan et al., 1987, 1988; Raglin, 1993).

As a possible solution to the problem, the IZOF model proposes a multidimensional description of individually optimal performance states conceptualized as a holistic manifestation of total human functioning (Hanin, 1997, 1999, 2000a). Thus, performance states and recovery states can be identified for each athlete based on idiosyncratic descriptors (for instance, cognitive, emotional, motivational, bodily-somatic, behavioral, communicative) that reflect an individual's performance history and recovery experiences. This notion is based on the empirically established fact that skilled athletes are aware of their emotional subjective experiences related to successful performance and effective recovery. Thus, these subjective experiences might be useful in describing performance-related and recovery-related states.

Multidimensional Description of Performance-Related States

Previous IZOF-based research focused mainly on optimal and dysfunctional states related to pre-, mid-, and postperformance situations (Hanin, 1997, 2000a). It was shown that multilevel and systems descriptions of performance-related states should include at least five dimensions of emotion: form, content, intensity, context, and time. This approach, described in greater detail elsewhere (Hanin, 1997, 2000a), is recommended for the description of recovery states and recovery activity.

Form Dimension

To describe performance-related states, seven basic form components, or modalities, have been proposed in the IZOF model (Hanin, 1993, 1995, 1997). These are the already mentioned cognitive, affective, motivational, bodily-somatic, motor-behavioral, performance-operational, and communicative (interactive) components of total human functioning. All seven components are interrelated and provide a relatively complete description of a performance state. Additionally, it was shown that cognitive, affective, and motivational modalities represent psychological (mental) aspects of state, whereas bodily-somatic and motor-behavioral components represent biological or psychophysiological aspects of an individual's state. Finally, performance and communication components reflect a person's observable social interactions. Thus, all seven components constitute what was termed a person's psychobiosocial state (Hanin, 1997, 2000a). This state is used here as a framework for a complete description of total situational human functioning and factors affecting individual performance.

From this perspective, emotion is conceived as only one important component of the psychobiosocial state, which is characterized mainly by a specific constellation of subjective affective experiences. Since emotional discomfort is an important component of work-related fatigue (Salmanoff, 1991), the IZOF model focused on emotional-motivational concomitants of optimal and dysfunctional states related to successful and poor performances. It is important to note, however, that a complete description of performance states and recovery states should not be limited only to emotional content and intensity. Markers of other modalities of the state (cognitive, motivational, bodily-somatic, behavioral, communicative) are also important as indicators of specific resources that are being recruited, utilized, and recuperated. Nevertheless, the initial focus on emotion is useful from a methodological point of view, as the same approach can be used to describe other modalities of subjective experiences. The following section briefly discusses the conceptualization and assessment of person-specific and task-relevant emotional content.

Content Dimension

The content of emotions is conceptualized within the framework of four major global categories based on hedonic tone (pleasant-unpleasant) and functional impact on performance (optimal-dysfunctional) distinctions. Specifically, four global affect categories derived from the hedonic tone and emotional impact factors include pleasant and functionally optimal emotions (P+), unpleasant and functionally optimal emotions (N+), pleasant and dysfunctional emotions (P–), and unpleasant and dysfunctional emotions (N–). These four basic categories provide an initial robust and sufficiently broad structure that includes a wide range of individually relevant and task-specific emotions actually experienced by athletes prior to, during, and after performance (Hanin, 1993, 1995).

This approach is partly similar to a global dimensional perspective in emotional research emphasizing a positivity-negativity (hedonic tone) distinction (Russell, 1980; Watson & Tellegen, 1985). However, the IZOF model differs from the dimensional framework in two important aspects. First, a functional impact factor (optimal-dysfunctional influence) is added to hedonic tone, and four global emotional content categories are derived. Second, within the four global categories, a clearly individualized focus is introduced by generating idiosyncratic emotional descriptors based on each athlete's past and present experiences related to personally significant performance situations (successful and unsuccessful). Moreover, these person-specific and task-relevant emotional markers are also sensitive indicators of action tendencies and readiness to perform to one's potential. They reflect specific ways in which an individual recruits and utilizes available resources, sometimes compensates for the lack of resources, and/or is unable to recuperate immediately. Finally, idiosyncratic emotion content can be contrasted with emotional words used by other athletes (content overlap) and with the existing classifications of discrete, or "basic," emotions. For instance, table 11.1 reports top 10 pleasant and unpleasant emotions selected most often by 97 skilled male ice hockey players within each of the four global categories (Hanin, 2000a, 2000c; Hanin & Lukkarila, 1999).

These emotional descriptors characterize "typical" (aggregated) emotions experienced by skilled players in different game situations based on direct personal experiences and their awareness of these experiences. In other words, the patterns of emotional content reflecting performance-related states in ice hockey players are task specific and therefore relatively stable at the group level. It is interesting to note that the top 10 emotions in this study were nearly the same as those selected by ice hockey players in Hanin and Syrjä's earlier study (1995). However, it is also important to

Table 11.1 Top 10 Pleasant and Unpleasant Emotions in Male Ice Hockey Players (*n* = 97)

Pleasant emotions		Unpleasant emotions	
Optimal P+	Dysfunctional (P–)	Optimal (N+)	Dysfunctional (N–)
Energetic	Easy-going	Tense	Tired
Confident	Tranquil	Dissatisfied	Sluggish
Charged	Satisfied	Vehement	Unwilling
Motivated	Overjoyed	Attacking	Uncertain
Purposeful	Excited	Intense	Downhearted
Certain	Pleasant	Angry	Depressed
Enthusiastic	Comfortable	Irritated	Distressed
Willing	Calm	Nervous	Sorrowful
Cheerful	Exalted	Provoked	Afraid
Alert	Nice	Restless	Strained

Adapted from Hanin, 2000c.

realize that these group "prototype" data reflecting aggregated real-life emotional experiences of highly skilled players are still different from the emotional profiles of individual athletes.

To monitor emotional dynamics in a particular player or a particular team, the best option is to first develop individual emotional profiles using a standardized stepwise procedure described elsewhere (Hanin, 2000a). On the other hand, aggregated emotional scales are sport specific and therefore can be applied in a field setting for assessing the emotional dynamics of a team during a tournament either when individualized emotional profiles are not available or when the major focus is on group dynamics (Hanin, 1992). For instance, Hanin and associates (Hanin, Papaioannou & Lukkarila, 2001; Lukkarila & Hanin, 2000) used an aggregated emotional scale to explore the emotional dynamics in the team leaders and players during the World Junior Ice Hockey Championships. A special emphasis in these studies was on the detrimental effects of pleasant dysfunctional emotions (resulting from successful performance against weak opponents) on the team's readiness for subsequent games.

In most cases a better option would be to develop a person-oriented (or team-oriented) individualized emotional profile aimed at identifying an individual's (or team's) change, growth, and development. Only individual data will reveal to what extent partners or players performing different functions are similar or different in their emotional responses and in the ways they use their resources. On the other hand, in some cases team-aggregated emotional profiles could be useful in monitoring the team's emotional dynamics due to a change in its composition, especially in national teams in which there is a constant rotation of players (Syrjä, 2000). Moreover, team emotional profiles could be used as criteria to see how new players fit into a team and match emotional responses to practices and games. Large deviations in a team emotional profile would indicate potential problems in group or interpersonal dynamics long before working relationships may start to deteriorate.

Another example from soccer illustrates the notion of person-specific emotional content and the value of individual emotional profiles. Let us say we have two soccer players and one of them, player A, wants to develop his own emotional profile. Based on past experiences, this player selected five positive-optimal emotions (motivated, charged, brisk, resolute, active), two negative-

optimal emotions (vehement, attacking), three positive-dysfunctional emotions (calm, comfortable, pleasant), and four negative-dysfunctional emotions (tired, sad, dispirited, distressed). This individual profile is relevant for this particular athlete and is related to the game context in general (see figure 11.2a).

In contrast, player B selected quite different emotions: four positive-optimal emotions (motivated, purposeful, willing, excited), three negative-optimal emotions (irritated, dissatisfied, tense), four positive-dysfunctional emotions (good, glad, satisfied, fearless), and five negative-dysfunctional emotions (unhappy, dejected, lazy, tired, sluggish; see figure 11.2b).

Each player's emotion descriptors reflect his unique experiences in coping with successful or poor performance situations. Therefore, some of the selected emotions within the four global categories are different, whereas others are similar. However, as a first step in the analysis of emotional content, it is more important to identify specific, idiosyncratic, and functionally relevant emotions than to simply describe interindividual difference on a set of descriptors that may not be relevant to either of these two players.

It is important to note that although these examples illustrate mainly performance-related emotional experiences, they also have a direct and indirect bearing on recovery-related states. Specifically, a list of optimal pleasant emotions (category P+) helpful for players' performance (see table 11.1) reflects the ability of players to recruit and use available resources. Additionally, strong unpleasant emotions (category N+) are useful for coping with demanding situations when normal resources are not sufficient and temporary compensation is needed. On the other hand, unpleasant dysfunctional emotions (category N–) are characteristic of postperformance states experienced by the players after very intensive and typically unsuccessful work. A high intensity of these emotions clearly indicates a need for active recovery of physical, emotional, and motivational resources. Moreover, pleasant dysfunctional emotions (category P–) of high intensity, as a spontaneous response to a repeated success, can sometimes be harmful to subsequent performance due to their demobilizational and demotivational effects (Lukkarila & Hanin, 2000). Apparently, emotions in this category (such as excessive complacency) are also indicative of overrecovery.

These findings concur well with anecdotal evidence and observations of precompetition rou-

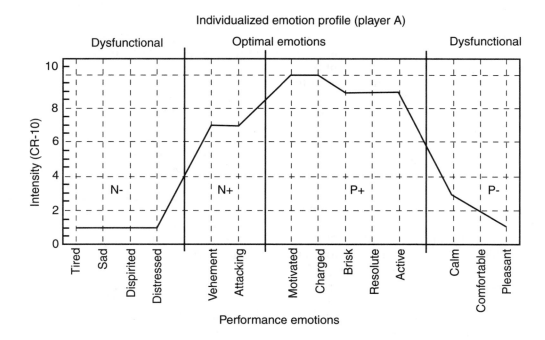

a

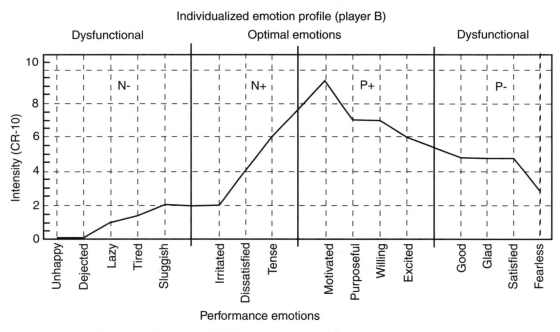

b

Figure 11.2 Individual IZOF-based emotional profiles for player A *(a)* and player B *(b).*

Reprinted, by permission, from Y.L. Hanin, 2000. Enhancing or imparing performance? In *Soccer and science—An interdisciplinary perspective,* edited by J. Bangsbo (Copenhagen: Blackwell), 76-77.

tines in the preparation of elite athletes. For instance, soccer players and track and field athletes avoid sleeping during the day before a competition. One reason is their belief and experience that having too much sleep (even an hour longer than normal) often makes you lose strength, reactivity and speed. However, additional research is clearly

needed to determine the emotional content and intensity that are optimal for the recovery process.

Intensity Dimension

The IZOF model holds that although functionally optimal emotions are important predictors of successful performance, they alone may not be sufficient: a potential detrimental effect of dysfunctional emotions should also be considered. Therefore, the notion of zone intensity, as applied to a wide range of pleasant and unpleasant emotions, has received empirical support as individualized criteria to evaluate both optimal and dysfunctional effects separately and jointly (Hanin, 1997, 2000a, 2000c, 2001). The concept of being in or out of the zone has been applied in assessments and as feedback to athletes in the form of individual emotional iceberg profiles visualizing the content and optimal intensities of individually relevant emotions as performance predictors.

As seen in figure 11.2, players A and B both have individual profiles with idiosyncratic emotional descriptors of both optimal (helpful for performance) and dysfunctional (harmful for performance) content and intensity levels. These profiles have been generated based on past repeated experiences and therefore reflect idiosyncratic patterns of emotional response prior to and during successful performance. Thus, if these athletes' current preperformance states as assessed on these descriptors are close to the previously established levels and zones of intensity, then there is a high probability of successful (or optimal) performance. If athletes' current states deviate considerably from the previously established zones (patterns), then below-average or even poor performance can be anticipated. Note that these individual profiles have different emotional items, but both are similar in shape: an elevated intensity of optimal emotions (P+N+) located in the middle and a low intensity of dysfunctional (N–P–) emotions located at the sides.

Most of the IZOF-based emotional research focused on the prediction of successful, average, or poor performances by contrasting current (pre- or midperformance) emotional states with the individual profiles and optimal intensity zones (Hanin, 1999, 2000a). Empirical findings indicate that an athlete's entering the optimal zones in a timely manner and maintaining this optimal intensity during task execution usually accompany optimal performance. As soon as the task has been completed, athletes should exit optimal (working-state) zones (reflecting an active use of available resources) and proceed to recovering their working capacity. Thus, being in the zone is equivalent to being in the state of readiness for a particular performance (availability of resources), whereas being out of the zone indicates either a decreased readiness to perform or a need for

recovery. Figure 11.3 illustrates this point by describing the dynamic of being in or out of the zone in the performance-recovery cycle.

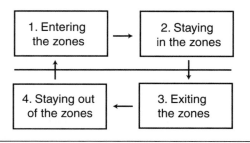

Figure 11.3 Zone dynamics (in or out) in the performance-recovery cycle.
Adapted from Hanin, 1998.

Context and Time Dimensions

Dynamic aspects of emotional states related to optimal and poor performance have been studied by contrasting emotional states in pre-, mid-, and postperformance situations in both practices and competitions. The findings obtained in soccer (Hanin & Syrjä, 1996; Pesonen, 1995; Syrjä, 2000; Syrjä, Hanin, & Pesonen, 1995), squash, badminton (Syrjä, Hanin, & Tarvonen, 1995; Tarvonen, 1995), ice hockey (Hanin, 2000c; Hanin & Lukkarila, 1999; Hanin & Syrjä, 1995; Lukkarila & Hanin, 2000), and cross-country skiing (Hanin, 2001; Hanin & Syrjä, 1997) indicate that emotional content and intensity in practices and competitions are different for the same athletes in the same sport and across different sports. Furthermore, emotional intensity usually increased after successful and unsuccessful performance situations and gradually decreased by the end of the activity. A spontaneous change in emotional content (from pleasant to unpleasant hedonic tone and vice versa) also reflected the dynamics of change in appraisal patterns (from anticipated to achieved gain and loss). Overall, the individual and group dynamics of emotional content and intensity reflected the patterns of recruitment and utilization of athletes' resources. In competitions, both the content and the intensity of emotions experienced during performance were usually different from the content and intensity of emotions experienced in pre- and postperformance situations (Hanin & Stambulova, in press). In contrast, the content of emotional response in practices was more balanced, although it was sometimes more intensive than in competitions (Hanin, 2001; Hanin & Syrjä, 1997).

Performance Emotions as Indicators of Optimal Recovery States

Until quite recently, an athlete's emotional state has been used mainly as an accurate and valid predictor of subsequent performance, especially in short-duration tasks. Moreover, optimal emotions in preperformance and midperformance situations reflect an athlete's ability to recruit and use available resources effectively. Therefore, idiosyncratic markers of optimal performance states can be used as individual criteria to evaluate the quality of the recovery process prior to individual performance. Specifically, a predominance of pleasant and functionally optimal emotions (category P+) and an absence of or low (minimum) intensity of unpleasant dysfunctional emotions (category N–) following work indicate optimal recovery outcomes. Typically, a well-recovered athlete is ready to resume task execution at an appropriate level; she is able to enter the optimal zones quickly and to maintain this state until the task has been completed.

In contrast, inadequate or disturbed recovery (underrecovery) is characterized by a moderate or high intensity of unpleasant dysfunctional emotions (N–) and a low intensity of pleasant optimal emotions (P+). Usually, underrecovered athletes are not ready to start their work again; they also need more time to enter their optimal zones and might find it difficult to stay in a working state during task execution. Actually, the first signs of insufficient recovery are (1) more than usual effort required for entering the optimal zones and (2) difficulty keeping the focus on task and staying in the optimal zones. Therefore, if an athlete enters the optimal zones more slowly than normal or experiences more difficulty in staying in the zone, it usually indicates insufficient recovery.

When an athlete's current emotional states do not perfectly match the optimal zones in pre- or midperformance situations, he may require compensatory emergency mobilization. This may include the spontaneous or preplanned use of unpleasant but functionally effective (strong) emotions, such as anger or anxiety, to cope with performance-induced fatigue. Finally, temporal emotion patterns are additional indicators of the optimality (or inadequacy) of the recovery process.

Emotional Markers of Optimal Recovery

Emotional pre- and midperformance states can serve only as indirect markers of the effective-ness (or ineffectiveness) of recovery or spontaneous rest. However, when recovery is undertaken as a specific process, emotional states should be identified that would indicate the successful or less-than-successful recuperation of the athlete's resources. Such direct markers can add to the usefulness of a detailed description of performance-related states.

As was shown earlier, several options are available for describing the emotional content and intensity that accompany the recovery process. First, we could describe emotional experiences of athletes in terms of global affect (positive and negative emotions) or as single, discrete, or primary emotions (anxiety, anger, sense of fun, self-confidence). Dozens of normative, standardized emotional or mood scales can be used to describe how athletes feel before, during, or after recovery. The most popular scales developed in nonsport settings are Spielberger, Gorsuch, and Lushene's (1970) State-Trait-Anxiety Inventory (STAI); McNair, Lorr, and Droppleman's (1971, 1992) Profile of Mood State (POMS); and Watson and Tellegen's (1985) Positive and Negative Affect Schedule (PANAS). Sport-specific scales include Martens et al.'s (1990) Competitive State Anxiety Inventory (CSAI-2) and Smith, Smoll, and Schultz's (1990) Sports Anxiety Scale (SAS).

One problem with these psychometric normative (group-oriented) scales is that they have a "fixed" content (a pool of researcher-generated items), which usually implies the same psychological meaning of emotion descriptors for all athletes. Moreover, in most cases, it is not known to what extent emotional content assessed with the normative scales reflects players' idiosyncratic subjective experiences related to successful and poor performances. Two recent studies involving 46 ice hockey players and 50 skilled soccer players (Syrjä & Hanin, 1997, 1998) provided compelling empirical evidence of the inadequacy of several standardized scales to describe the idiosyncratic emotional content of athletes' subjective emotional experiences related to performance. Specifically, based on a comparison of the content of emotional items in normative, standardized scales and individual emotional experiences as reflected in athlete-generated descriptors, these studies revealed that about 80 to 85% of emotional content (items) relevant for the individual players was not included in the standardized scales (see Hanin, 2000a, for a review). That is perhaps one reason other researchers concluded that, for instance, "the POMS may not be a sensitive indicator of staleness under all circumstances and may not necessarily differentiate between stale and intensely trained, but not stale, athletes" (Hooper, Mackinnon, & Hanrahan, 1997, p. 9).

Although more research is warranted in this area, these findings do indicate that a researcher or a practitioner using the standardized scales should be aware of the fact that more than 80% of emotional content of real performance-related subjective experiences will simply not be measured. Similar problems apparently have to be dealt with in the assessment of emotional experiences related to the recovery process itself. Moreover, in most studies monitoring the effects of overtraining in athletes, the POMS was used to assess only pre- and postperformance states but not the recovery process directly.

Another option in the description of emotional patterns in recovery is to use the individual scales with athlete-generated items that are based directly on athletes' awareness of their past recovery experiences. The IZOF framework proposes two combined principles for such individualized assessments. First, athletes select (generate) items within the framework of four global categories: positive-optimal (P+), negative-optimal (N+), negative-dysfunctional (N–), and positive-dysfunctional (P–). Thus, athletes are "forced" to report their past subjective experiences (both pleasant and unpleasant) in terms of how helpful or harmful they were for individual recovery. However, it is important that the idiosyncratic items are selected within these four categories without any restriction or limitation. As a first step in the prototype description of emotion in sport-related recovery, it seems to be the best strategy because individually generated items can then be content analyzed and classified into other content categories (*anxiety, anger, frustration, distress*, etc.).

However, in contrast to performance-related states (strong and active emotions both pleasant [P+] and unpleasant [N+]), the recovery process is apparently facilitated by such states as calm, relaxed, satisfied, content, pleasantly fatigued, and even lazy. It seems possible that strong emotions of high intensity reflecting energy or effort (pleasant and unpleasant) might be less than effective for adequate recovery. On the other hand, recovery after successful and poor performances might require different emotional experiences.

To identify emotional markers of optimal and less-than-optimal recovery, Hanin and Syrjä (1993) conducted a survey of several top Finnish cross-country skiers, highly skilled soccer players, and track and field athletes. The athletes were re-

quested, based on their past experiences, to recall recovery strategies they used after intensive training. Additionally, they identified emotions that were usually helpful or harmful for their recovery. A response from a top Finnish female track and field athlete demonstrates that pleasant, relaxing emotions are considered helpful and unpleasant, stress-related emotions are considered harmful for recovery. Specifically, this athlete thought that feeling "peaceful," "balanced," "happy," and "confident" helped her to recover more effectively and more quickly after intensive training or competition. In contrast, if she felt "nervous," "uncertain," "in a hurry," and "tense," her recovery was less than effective. Additionally, she reported that several recovery activities worked especially well for her, including optimal nutrition (specific posttraining or postcompetition food); adequate sleep/rest; being alone (privacy); taking a sauna; stretching; and listening to quiet, peaceful music. It is noteworthy that both lists of this athlete's emotions concur well with the already described top 10 emotions across four global categories (see table 11.1, p. 203). Furthermore, open-ended questions seem quite appropriate as a first step in generating person-specific and task-specific emotional markers for describing effective and less-than-effective recovery.

Optimal Recovery States

Individual emotional markers reflecting an athlete's idiosyncratic subjective experiences are sensitive and reliable indicators of optimal performance and optimal recovery. However, as mentioned earlier (Hanin, 1997, 2000a, 2000b, 2000c, 2001), a multidimensional perspective proposed by the IZOF model holds that recovery can be described using not only emotion descriptors but also markers of other modalities of psychobiosocial states such as cognitive, motivational, bodily-somatic, behavioral, and communicative markers. Extant literature and various self-report scales used in overtraining and burnout research provide numerous examples of such markers (Henschen, 2000; Kallus & Kellmann, 2000; Raglin & Wilson, 2000).

For instance, the Recovery-Stress Questionnaire (RESTQ; Kallus, 1995) is one of the few psychometric instruments addressing the issue of the need for multidimensional descriptions of recovery-stress states. This scale and one of its modifications for sport (Recovery-Stress Questionnaire for Athletes [RESTQ-Sport]; Kellmann & Kallus, 2000, 2001) actually touch on almost all components of the psychobiosocial state proposed in the IZOF model. The greatest emphasis is on emotional reactions (about 50% of all items) and somatic reactions (about 30% of all items) with somewhat less focus on communicative, motivational, cognitive, and behavioral components of a state. Performance and activity items, although important for the description of recovery-stress balance, seemed to go beyond this state-focused description.

Additionally, the frequency response format proposed in this scale (from "never" to "always") makes this instrument more traitlike and dispositional rather than situational and state oriented. Therefore, changing instructions and restructuring the subscales around state and activity components might be beneficial for future development of a more state-oriented scale. Interestingly, Kellmann (this volume, chapter 3) argues that the RESTQ-Sport is more a state-oriented than a trait-oriented instrument based on the finding that drastic changes in the recovery-stress state can be observed within three days, depending on the training athletes are undergoing. However, at the same time, Kellmann and Kallus (2001) underline the importance of temporal *stability* of the current recovery-stress state (see Kellmann & Kallus, 2001), thus implying pattern and response consistency. Apparently, more research is needed to investigate how recovery-stress balance (and imbalance) can be assessed from at least four different but closely related perspectives: as an immediate situational state, as a relatively stable condition (varying in duration), as a consistent pattern of idiosyncratic response, and as a traitlike disposition. Consequently, based on systematic research, the scale scores might be used to assess and monitor the stress-recovery relationships with a clear focus on situational dynamics or short-term stability, or a magnitude of individual differences in relatively stable patterns of stress-recovery relationships.

Individually Optimal Recovery Strategies

So far, we have discussed optimal and dysfunctional emotions related to performance and the recovery process. It is important to realize that the idiosyncratic nature of emotional response during performance suggests the existence of unique patterns in resource recruitment, utilization, and recuperation. In other words, different athletes have different preperformance routines, different preferences for performance-related skills and strategies, and apparently, different preferences in recovery methods. Of course, the sport event subculture and other environmental differences play their roles, but recovery strategies are usually specific to the individual and the task.

Based on the IZOF model, it is suggested that skilled athletes spontaneously develop and use recovery patterns, as they do performance patterns. These self-made patterns reflect their experiences and preferences as well as the resources they use to recharge themselves. Twelve (eight male and four female) elite cross-country skiers, members of the Finnish National Team preparing for the 1994 Lillehammer Olympics, were requested to list recovery methods they usually use after intensive practices (Hanin & Syrjä, 1993). The purpose of this exploratory study was not only to identify individually preferred recovery strategies but also to help athletes enhance the quality of their daily training by monitoring the work-recovery balance.

On the average, each skier reported about 10 (5-17) strategies used for recovery after intensive training. Similarity of recovery strategies across athletes was established by computing the amount of overlap in terms of shared items (worded semantically in the same way) in the lists generated by each skier. The following formula, suggested for the study of individual perception of situations (Krahé, 1986), was used with slightly modified notations to calculate interindividual overlap scores:

$$r(i, j) = \frac{nc(i, j)}{\sqrt{n(i) \times n(j)}}$$

where $nc(i, j)$ = number of shared (similar) items for an athlete i and an athlete j; $n(i)$ = number of recovery strategies used by an athlete i; $n(j)$ = number of recovery strategies used by an athlete j.

Conceptually, the overlap measure represents the similarity of recovery lists generated by individual skiers. Interindividual overlap scores vary from 0 (all items are different) to 1.0 (all items are similar). The overlap values are equal to percentages expressed in decimal form when contrasted lists have the same number of items.

As expected, the mean overlap score was low: .37 (*SD* = .14, ranging from .09 to .71), indicating a clear idiosyncratic nature of recovery strategies reported by the skiers. Even at the group level, interindividual variation of recovery strategies used by the skiers was large. A summary of their responses is reported in table 11.2.

Table 11.2 Individualized Recovery Strategies Used by Olympic-Level Finnish Cross-Country Skiers (*n* = 12)

Recovery strategies	%	Activity sample
Bodily somatic	32.2	Massage, sauna, vibration, whirlpool baths, rest, sleep
Aerobic exercise	17.0	Warming-down, stretching, swimming, jogging
Nutrition	15.2	Healthy, tasty food; carbohydrates; soft drinks
Positive emotions	14.4	Carefree, no stress, no rush, satisfied, joyful
Nonsport activity	12.7	Listening to music, reading, walking (in private)
Social activity	5.1	Staying with significant others
Past successes	3.4	Previously successful training, being in good shape
Total	100% (118 items)	

After intensive training, highly skilled cross-country skiers focus on recuperation of mainly their physical (47.4%) resources by using sauna, massage, nutrition, other physical exercise, and nonsport activity (alone or with significant others). Additionally, these skiers' recovery was greatly facilitated by positive emotional states related to their general positive well-being and previously successful performance in training.

Several replication studies in other sports (soccer, ice hockey, squash, and badminton) revealed the same trends at the group and individual levels. Specifically, clear individual preferences for recovery strategies (person specific and task specific) were prominent in all of these samples (Hanin & Syrjä, 1993). Additionally, these findings provide indirect empirical support for Kallus and Kellmann's (2000) recovery-stress balance model (see also Kellmann, this volume, chapter 1).

Barriers to Effective Recovery and Rest

The problem of underrecovery and excessive work—or rather, an imbalance between work and recovery—does exist in competitive and especially in elite and professional sport (see this volume, chapters 1, 2, 7, 8). Several barriers affect the optimal use of recovery and rest by athletes and teams in practices and competitions. First, athletes and coaches may sometimes underestimate the crucial role of systematic recovery and rest matching the work they are doing. Thus, a work-recovery balance is systematically disrupted (Kellmann, this volume, chapter 3). Second, this

underestimation is sometimes reinforced by the work-related values held by some cultures, subcultures, and athletes, with the emphasis on quantity (amount, intensity, and volume) of work rather than on its quality. In fact, most coaches and athletes focus mainly on the amount and intensity of training loads rather than on recovery methods matching this work. Third, the current performance level in practices and competitions can be an additional factor pushing an athlete to excessive work. In the case of poor performance (underperformance due to fatigue or problems with technique), an athlete continues to work intensively to eliminate uncertainty and to enhance self-confidence. However, athletes usually are unable to break this vicious circle and even do not dare to take a good break and correct this situation. In the case of successful (better-than-expected) performance, an athlete can be so overexcited with positive emotions that he does not notice the signs of fatigue and, as all perfectionists, continues to do excessive work until it is too late. Fourth, due to the reasons listed here, rest and recovery are still not considered key components of athletes' lifestyles. Therefore, fitting preplanned recovery strategies and procedures into athletes' busy schedules might be a problem both in practices and competitions unless a detailed description of an athlete's perception of these settings is provided.

Some of the barriers to effective recovery and more effective work can be partly eliminated by monitoring an athlete's practices and competitions. A typical training day and a typical racing day of a top Finnish cross-country skier (see tables 11.3 and 11.4) illustrate the idea that planning spontaneous breaks within and between practices may not be an easy task, even if the attitude toward planned rest is positive. If this skier had no race, his training week would consist of 10 sessions (twice a day for four days and once a day for two days; see table 11.3). If racing, he would have six to seven sessions (one per day; see table 11.4).

Even more illuminating could be descriptions of training and competitions of athletes in long-duration events (from hours to days and weeks) in which adding preplanned breaks of rest and recovery might require monitoring and adjusting an athlete's lifestyle.

In the previous example, as a first step to enhancing performance and recovery of this skier, the concepts of high-quality training and sufficient recovery were clarified and tailored for him considering his preparation and performance rou-

tines. Thus, to ensure high-quality training, this athlete should be rested, eat healthy food, set concrete goals, and know exactly what he is working on in each practice session. Additionally, while on the track, he should listen to his body signals and remember his previous best training experiences. His list of individual recovery strategies included 10 items: reading, listening to music, watching TV/videos, receiving a massage, taking a bath/sauna, slow swimming, walking in the streets, sitting on the balcony, sleeping, and eating good food. Based on these suggestions, this skier was able to evaluate the general quality of his work and rest for an entire week prior to his best and his less-than-successful races (Hanin, 1994).

Repeated monitoring revealed that this athlete was consistently successful in his races when he followed either of his two weekly work-recovery

Table 11.3 Typical Training Day of a Top Finnish Male Cross-Country Skier

Time	Task
8:00 A.M.	Wake up, check on weather/snow.
8:30 A.M.	Eat breakfast.
9:00 A.M.	Select and prepare skis, dress for skiing (15 min), drink sports drinks (15-20 min).
9:45 A.M. to 12:45 P.M.	First training Warm up (10-15 min), slow ski. Do aerobic training (2.5 h). Do 5 to 8 intervals at race speed (15-30 s with 1-2 min recovery after each interval). Slow ski.
12:45 to 1:30 P.M.	Eat lunch while serviceman waxes skis.
1:30 to 2:00 P.M.	Study/read.
2:00 to 2:30 or 3:00 P.M.	Sleep.
3:15 or 3:30 to 4:00 P.M.	Study/read.
4:00 P.M.	Dress for skiing.
4:15 to 4:30 P.M.	Warm up, slow ski.
4:30 to 6:30 P.M.	Second training (Do three intervals if feeling strong). Clean up skis (self or serviceman).
7:00 P.M.	Eat dinner.
7:30 to 8:00 P.M.	Read the paper, watch TV.
9:30 to 10:00 P.M.	Stretch (sometimes).
11:00 P.M.	Go to bed.

Adapted from Hanin, 1994.

Table 11.4   Typical Racing Day of a Top Finnish Male Cross-Country Skier

Time	Task
Evening before the race	Analyze track (three times, if a new track; focus on downhills, curves, uphills). Check weather forecast, starting time, starting list. Get clothing ready and go to bed by 11:00 P.M.
7:00 A.M. (4 h before the race)	Wake up, check weather forecast/snow.
8:00 A.M. (3 h before the race)	Run, stretch, shower. Eat breakfast, rest a bit, and get ready. Concentrate on the competition. Ski the track (get a feeling for the track; if 15 km race, then the entire distance plus important parts).
9:00 A.M. (2 h before the race)	Select and prepare skis, dress for skiing (15 min), and take sports drinks (15-20 min).
9:30 A.M. (1.5 h before the start)	In the skiing area, test selected skis (alone or with serviceman).
10:00 A.M.	Warm up 50 to 60 min and ski 15 km (to check any changes in the track, downhills). Slow skiing (50%) plus testing competition race—1 uphill (3-4 min).
10:45 A.M.	In the start area, dress for skiing. Serviceman brings racing skis.
12:00 P.M. (after the race)	Change clothing, have warm drink. Meet media. Warm down. Eat and drink energy drinks. Analyze and forget race.

patterns the week prior to the race (see figure 11.4). Two factors emerged as important from the athlete's perspective: (1) recovery strategies (whatever he chose to use) should match the intensity of work in practice and (2) in all cases he should try his racing speed in training prior to the competition. In all cases, when for some reason he failed to do that, his performance, especially in the first race, was less than successful. In other words, a lack of balance between work and recovery during the week prior to a competition was detrimental to this skier's performance in the race.

Optimal Recovery

Optimal recovery is a person-specific and task-specific process focused on the recuperation of an athlete's resources, which can then be recruited and used in a particular task or a series of tasks. Different *forms* (procedures, methods,

strategies) of recovery can be optimal if they are tailored to the specific needs of the athlete based on an analysis of available resources, idiosyncratic preferences, lifestyle, and sporting experiences. Optimal recovery as a process can also be described using several *quantitative* (volume, intensity), *qualitative* (specific effects), *contextual* (in or between practices and competitions), and *temporal* (duration, sequence) characteristics. Apparently, adequate recovery for one athlete might be insufficient or excessive for another. Optimal recovery results in an optimal working state and a high probability of maximal optimal effect and minimum dysfunctional effect on performance. Thus, optimal recovery usually results in a readiness for optimal performance (high achievement) under certain conditions.

In contrast, insufficient or inadequate recovery (underrecovery) fails to produce optimal preperformance states and the effective recruitment

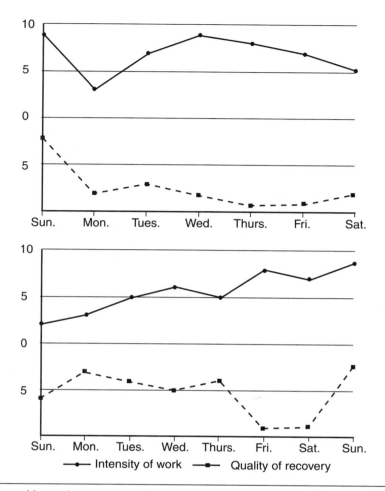

Figure 11.4 Two weekly work-recovery cycles in a top Finnish male cross-country skier.

and utilization of an athlete's resources. In an acute case, less-than-optimal recovery results in a state of complacency with clearly demotivational and demobilizational effects: an athlete in this situation is too satisfied, too relaxed, too self-confident, insufficiently alert, underaroused, and careless. In this less-than-optimal preperformance state an athlete cannot recruit her resources and might have problems resuming training, especially on the first day after such overrecovery. At such times, athletes are usually at greater risk of having unexpected injuries.

Preventing Underperformance in Athletes

Based on the previously discussed findings, observations, and assumptions, it is suggested that in order to prevent underperformance induced by underrecovery it is necessary to

- define better and below-average individual performances under different conditions;
- establish optimal and dysfunctional emotional-motivational pre-, mid-, and postperformance states;
- identify individually effective and preferred recovery strategies and recovery related states; and
- monitor pre- and postperformance states to establish optimal precompetition cycles.

These steps help to connect performance and recovery into a meaningful unit and to control an individually optimal work-rest balance. Finally, most research in overtraining and burnout emphasizes the role of optimal recovery in practices (single sessions, training cycles, etc.). However, a bigger challenge is to provide guidelines and methods for individually optimal recovery during the competitive season. Here the problem is recovery after not only each single competition but also after several competitions. Moreover, recovery should be combined with intensive training between competitions.

Finally, a special case is a situation in which an athlete has to (or is forced to) perform when he is still underrecovered. In this situation, to avoid underperformance, additional ("untapped") resources need to be recruited; this is typically reflected in high-intensity, strong, unpleasant emotions such as anger and anxiety. These strong emotions are temporal substitutes for performance-related fatigue. Such emergency situations should be followed by additional and more effective recovery to compensate for the overload of available resources.

Conclusions

This chapter focused on individual recovery patterns and strategies used in elite sports. It was emphasized that most markers of individually optimal emotional-motivational performance states are the best and most informative markers of the outcomes of effective recovery. For optimal recovery athletes must maintain individually optimal transition rhythms and a balance between intensive work and recovery. To do so, they must first identify and monitor an individually optimal balance between work and recovery by using individual emotional profiling (Hanin, 1997, 2000). Additionally, psychometric self-report scales, such as the RESTQ-Sport (see Kellmann, this volume, chapter 3; Kellmann & Kallus, 2000, 2001), Body Awareness Scale (Koltyn & Morgan, 1997; Raglin, Morgan, & Wise, 1990; Wang & Morgan, 1987), and the 24-item version of the Profile of Mood States—Adolescents (Terry, Lane, Lane, & Keohane, 1999), can assess prototype patterns and trends at the group level. In all cases, it is worthwhile to examine the dynamics of performance-related and recovery-related states and to contrast them with previously established optimal and dysfunctional patterns.

High-quality recovery has certain subjective correlates during and after recovery. Therefore, it is reasonable to suggest that an athlete's best preperformance patterns can be used as a sensitive and reliable criterion of effective recovery outcomes. Temporal dynamics of performance-related state are also important: an athlete should be able to enter an optimal zone of intensity and stay in this optimal zone until the task has been completed. Only after that, can and should an athlete exit this zone and shift to a recovery

process accompanied by other emotional states reflecting recuperation of his resources.

The findings reported in this chapter and some preliminary assumptions about the recovery process suggest that it is worthwhile to examine not only performance-related states but also emotional and motivational states related to an effective recovery process. As performance and recovery processes are interrelated, this relationship should be reflected in the dynamics of emotional-motivational states from pre-, mid-, and post-performance situations to pre-, mid-, and postrecovery situations.

Apparently, somatic and emotional components rather than cognitive components (modalities) are most important to consider in recovery-related states.

This chapter aimed to extend the application of the IZOF model to the recovery states as an important component and a prerequisite of effective reproduction of performance-related optimal states. It was shown that previously established relationships between performance and emotional-motivational states hold quite well for recovery-related states. Preperformance states can thus be used as an indirect index of recovery efficiency based on the extent to which such states are close to or within optimal intensity zones. Optimal performance states indicate that available resources can be recruited and used effectively; that is, the recovery undertaken before the present work cycle was effective (optimal). On the other hand, if preperformance states are deviating from individual optimal intensity zones, then this indicates a lack of resources, their unavailability, or situational difficulties in their utilization.

Postperformance states can be regarded as a transition to pre- and midrecovery states, facilitating active recovery of resources used during task execution. Thus, future research should focus more on the specifics of recovery-related states and their relationships with performance-related states. Moreover, athletes' and coaches' experiences in using different recovery strategies in individual and team sports (both on-task and off-task) should be systematically studied. A more holistic approach to conceptualizing preperformance and midperformance states within the context of optimal (or less-than-optimal) recovery is clearly indicated. Finally, the work-recovery cycle should be a central notion in examining the dynamics of the emotional-motivational involvement of an athlete in sporting activity.

References

Apitzsch, E. (Ed.). (1983). *Anxiety in sport.* Magglingen, Switzerland: FEPSAC.

Apitzsch, E. (1996). Psychological perspectives on overtraining. *Svensk Idrottsforskning, 12,* 7-10.

Bortoli, L., Robazza, C., & Nougier, V. (1997). Emotion in hockey and rugby. In *Innovations in Sport Psychology: Linking Theory and Practice.* Proceedings of the 9th World Congress of Sport Psychology (Part I, pp. 136-138). Wingate, Israel: ISSP.

Dunn, J.G.H. (1994). Toward the combined use of nomothetic and idiographic methodologies in sport psychology: An empirical example. *The Sport Psychologist, 8,* 376-392.

Gould, D., Tuffey, S., Udry, E., & Loehr, J. (1996). Burnout in competitive junior tennis players: II Qualitative analysis. *The Sport Psychologist, 10,* 341-366.

Hanin, Y. (1978). A study of anxiety in sports. In W.F. Straub (Ed.), *Sport psychology: An analysis of athlete behavior* (pp. 236-249). Ithaca, NY: Movement Publications.

Hanin, Y.L. (Ed.). (1983). *Stress and anxiety in sport.* Moscow: FIS.

Hanin, Y.L. (1986). The state-trait anxiety research on sports in the USSR. In C.D. Spielberger & R. Diaz-Guerrero (Eds.), *Cross-cultural anxiety* (Vol. 3, pp. 45-64). Washington, DC: Hemisphere.

Hanin, Y.L. (1989). Interpersonal and intragroup anxiety in sports. In D. Hackfort & C.D. Spielberger (Eds.), *Anxiety in sports* (pp. 19-28). Washington, DC: Hemisphere.

Hanin, Y.L. (1992). Social psychology and sport: Communication processes in top performance teams. *Sport Science Review, 1*(2), 13-28.

Hanin, Y.L. (1993). Optimal performance emotions in top athletes. In S. Serpa, J. Alves, V. Ferreira, & A. Paula-Brito (Eds.), *Sport psychology: An integrated approach.* Proceedings of the 8th World Congress of Sport Psychology (pp. 229-232). Lisbon, Portugal: ISSP.

Hanin, Y.L. (1994). Monitoring emotion dynamics and performance-recovery balance in a top Finnish cross-country skier. Unpublished data.

Hanin, Y.L. (1995). Individual Zones of Optimal Functioning (IZOF) model: An idiographic approach to performance anxiety. In K. Henschen & W. Straub (Eds.), *Sport psychology: An analysis of athlete behaviour* (pp. 103-119). Longmeadow, MA: Movement Publications.

Hanin, Y.L. (1997). Emotions and athletic performance: Individual zones of optimal functioning (IZOF) model. *European Yearbook of Sport Psychology, 1,* 29-72.

Hanin, Y.L. (1998, August). *Emotions and Enhancing Athletic Performance.* Paper presented at the 24th International Congress of Applied Psychology, San Francisco.

Hanin, Y.L. (1999). Sports-specific emotion-motivational profiling: An individualized assessment programme. In V. Hosek, P. Tilinger, & L. Bilek (Eds.), *Psychology of sport: Enhancing the quality of life.* Proceedings of the 10th European Congress of Sport Psychology (Part 1, pp. 238-240). Prague: Charles University.

Hanin Y.L. (Ed.). (2000a). *Emotions in sport.* Champaign, IL: Human Kinetics.

Hanin, Y.L. (2000b). Stress, coping & emotion in sport: A research-practice perspective. In B.A. Carlsson, U. Johnson, & F. Wetterstrand (Eds.), *Proceedings of the Sport Psychology in the New Millennium Conference* (pp. 55-61). Halmstad, Sweden: Halmstad University.

Hanin, Y.L. (2000c, May). *Emotions in hockey.* An invited paper presented at the IIHF International Coaching Symposium: Building a Hockey Base for the 21st Century. St. Petersburg, Russia.

Hanin, Y.L. (2001). Emotion-motivational profiling in skiing: An individualized assessment program. In E. Müller, H. Schwameder, C. Raschner, S. Lindinger, & E. Kornexl (Eds.), *Science and skiing II.* Schriften zur Sportwissenschaft, Band 26 (pp. 688-705). Hamburg: Verlag Dr. Kovac.

Hanin, Y.L., & Lukkarila, J. (1999). Dynamics of performance emotions in skilled junior ice-hockey players. Unpublished data.

Hanin, Y., Papaioannou, A., & Lukkarila, J. (2001). Emotion-performance relationships: A structural equation modelling analysis of the refined IZOF model. In A. Papaioannou, M. Goudas, & J. Theodorakis (Eds.), *Proceedings of the 10th World Congress of Sport Psychology,* Vol. 5 (pp. 132-134). Thessaloniki, Greece: Christodoulidi Publications.

Hanin, Y.L. & Stambulova, N.B. (in press). Metaphoric description of performance states: An application of the IZOF model. *The Sport Psychologist.*

Hanin, Y.L., & Syrjä, P. (1993). Recovery strategies in Finnish Olympic-level cross-country skiers, highly skilled soccer players and track and field athletes. Unpublished data.

Hanin, Y.L. (1994). Optimization of performance emotions: Individual scaling of performance emotions. *Top performance: Proceedings of the 1st National Congress of Elite Finish Coaches* (pp. 94-106). Jyväskylä, Finland: KIHU.

Hanin, Y.L., & Syrjä, P. (1995). Performance affect in junior ice hockey players: An application of the Individual Zones of Optimal Functioning Model. *The Sport Psychologist, 9,* 169-187.

Hanin, Y.L., & Syrjä, P. (1996). Predicted, actual and recalled affect in Olympic-level soccer players: Idiographic assessments on individualised scales. *Journal of Sport and Exercise Psychology, 18,* 325-335.

Hanin, Y.L., & Syrjä, P. (1997). Optimal emotions in elite cross-country skiers. In E. Müller, H. Schwameder, E. Kornexl, & C. Raschner (Eds.), *Science and skiing* (pp. 408-419). London: E & FN SPON.

Hardy, L. (1990). A catastrophe model of performance in sport. In J.G. Jones, & Hardy L. (Eds.), *Stress and performance in sport* (pp. 81-106). Chichester, U.K.: Wiley.

Hardy, L., Jones, G., & Gould, D. (1997). *Understanding psychological preparation in sport.* New York: Wiley.

Henschen, K. (2000). Maladaptive fatigue syndrome and emotions in sport. In Y.L. Hanin (Ed.), *Emotions in sport* (pp. 231-242). Champaign, IL: Human Kinetics.

Hooper, S.L., Mackinnon, L.T., & Hanrahan, S. (1997). Mood states as an indication of staleness and recovery. *International Journal of Sport Psychology, 28,* 1-12.

Jones, G. (1995). Competitive anxiety in sport. In S.J.H. Biddle (Ed.), *European perspectives on exercise and sport psychology* (pp. 128-153). Leeds, UK: Human Kinetics.

Jones, J.G., & Hardy, L. (Eds.). (1990). *Stress and performance in sport.* Chichester, U.K.: Wiley.

Kallus, K.W. (1995). *Der Erholungs-Belastungs-Fragebogen* [The Recovery-Stress Questionnaire]. Frankfurt, Germany: Swets & Zeitlinger.

Kallus, K.W., & Kellmann, M. (2000). Burnout in athletes and coaches. In Y.L. Hanin (Ed.), *Emotions in sport* (pp. 209-230). Champaign, IL: Human Kinetics.

Kellmann, M., & Günther, K.-D. (2000). Changes in stress and recovery in elite rowers during preparation for the Olympic Games. *Medicine and Science in Sports and Exercise, 32,* 676-683.

Kellmann, M., & Kallus, K.W. (1999). Mood, recovery-stress state, and regeneration. In M. Lehmann, C. Foster, U. Gastmann, H. Keizer, & J.M. Steinacker (Eds.), *Overload, fatigue, performance incompetence, and regeneration in sport* (pp. 101-117). New York: Plenum.

Kellmann, M., & Kallus, K.W. (2000). *Der Erholungs-Belastungs-Fragebogen für Sportler; Manual.* [The Recovery-Stress Questionnaire for Athletes, manual]. Frankfurt: Swets Test Services.

Kellmann, M., & Kallus, K.W. (2001). *Recovery-Stress Questionnaire for Athletes: User manual.* Champaign, IL: Human Kinetics.

Koltyn, K.F., & Morgan, W.P. (1997). Influence of wet suit wear on anxiety responses to underwater exercise. *Undersea and Hyperbaric Medicine, 24,* 23-28.

Krahé, B. (1986). Similar perceptions, similar reactions: An idiographic approach to cross-situational coherence. *Journal of Research in Personality, 20,* 349-361.

Kuipers, H. (1998). Training and overtraining: An introduction. *Medicine and Science in Sports and Exercise, 30,* 1137-1139.

Lukkarila, J., & Hanin, Y.L. (2000). Emotion dynamics in the winning team during the 1999 World Junior Championship. In J. Avela, P.V. Komi, & J. Komulainen (Eds.), *Proceedings of the 5th Annual Congress of the European College of Sport Science* (p. 456). Jyväskylä, Finland: University of Jyväskylä.

Martens, R., Vealey, R.S., & Burton, D. (1990). *Competitive anxiety in sport.* Champaign, IL: Human Kinetics.

McNair, D., Lorr, M., & Droppleman, L.F. (1971, 1992). *Profile of Mood States manual.* San Diego: Educational and Industrial Testing Service.

Morgan, W.P. (1991). Monitoring and prevention of the staleness syndrome. In *2nd IOC World Congress on Sport Sciences* (pp.19-23). INEFC, Barcelona, Spain.

Morgan, W.P. (1997). Mind games: The psychology of sport. In D. Lamb, & R. Murray (Eds.), *Recent advances in the science and medicine of sports* (pp. 1-31). Carmel, IN: Benchmark Press.

Morgan, W.P., Brown, D.L., Raglin, J.S., O'Connor, P.J., & Ellickson, K.A. (1987). Psychological monitoring of overtraining and staleness. *British Journal of Sports Medicine, 21,* 107-114.

Morgan, W.P., Costill, D.L., Flynn, M.G., Raglin, J.S., & O'Connor, P.J. (1988). Mood disturbance following increased training in swimmers. *Medicine and Science in Sports and Exercise, 20,* 408-414.

Pesonen, T. (1995) *Tunteiden yhteys suoritukseen juniorijalkapalloilijoilla.* (Emotion-performance relationship in junior soccer players). Unpublished Master's Thesis. Department of Psychology, Jyväskylä University, Jyväskylä, Finland.

Raglin, J.S. (1993). Overtraining and staleness: Psychometric monitoring of endurance athletes. In R.B. Singer, M. Murphy, & L.K. Tennant (Eds.), *Handbook of research on sport psychology* (pp. 840-850). New York: Macmillan.

Raglin, J.S. (1999). Psychological factors in sport performance. In R. Maughan (Ed.), *Basic and applied sciences for sports medicine* (pp. 260-289). Oxford: Butterworth-Heinemann.

Raglin J., & Hanin, Y. (2000). Competitive anxiety and athletic performance. In Y.L. Hanin (Ed.), *Emotions in sport* (pp. 93-112). Champaign, IL: Human Kinetics.

Raglin, J.S., Morgan, W.P., & Wise, K. (1990). Pre-competition anxiety in high school girls swimmers: A test of optimal function theory. *International Journal of Sports Medicine, 11,* 171-175.

Raglin, J.S., & Wilson, G.S. (2000). Overtraining in athletes. In Y.L. Hanin (Ed.), *Emotions in sport* (pp. 191-207). Champaign, IL: Human Kinetics.

Russell, J.A. (1980). A circumplex model of affect. *Journal of Personality and Social Psychology, 39,* 1161-1178.

Salmanoff, A. (1991). *Tainaja mudrost' chelovecheskogo orgamizma* (The secret wisdom of the human organism) (2nd ed.). St. Petersburg, Russia: Nauka.

Smith, R. E., Smoll, F. L., & Schultz, R. W. (1990). Measurement and correlates of sport-specific cognitive and somatic trait anxiety: The Sport Anxiety Scale. *Anxiety Research, 2,* 263-280.

Spielberger, C.D, Gorsuch, R.L., & Lushene, R.E. (1970). *Manual for the State-Trait Anxiety Inventory (STAI).* Palo Alto, CA: Consulting Psychologist Press.

Syrjä, P. (2000). Performance-related emotions in highly skilled soccer players: A longitudinal study based on the IZOF model. *Studies in Sport, Physical Education and Health, 67.* Jyväskylä, Finland: Jyväskylä University Press.

Syrjä, P., & Hanin, Y. (1997). Measurement of emotion in sport: A comparison of individualised and normative scales. In R. Lidor & M. Bar-Eli (Eds.), *ISSP 9th World Congress of Sport Psychology* (Part 2, pp. 682-684). Netanya, Israel: Wingate Institute.

Syrjä, P., & Hanin, Y. (1998). Individualized and group-oriented measures of emotion in sport: A comparative study. *Journal of Sports Sciences, 16,* 398-399.

Syrjä, P., Hanin, Y., & T. Pesonen (1995). Emotion and performance relationship in soccer players. In R. Vanfraechem-Raway & Y. Vanden Auweele (Eds.), *Proceedings of the 9th European Congress on Sport Psychology* (Part 1, pp. 191-197). Brussels, Belgium: Belgian Federation of Sport Psychology.

Syrjä, P., Hanin, Y., & Tarvonen, S. (1995). Emotion and performance relationship in squash and badminton players. In R. Vanfraechem-Raway & Y. Vanden Auweele (Eds.), *Proceedings of the 9th European Congress on Sport Psychology* (Part 1, pp. 183-190). Brussels, Belgium: Belgian Federation of Sport Psychology.

Tarvonen, S. (1995). *Suoritustunteiden ja suorituksen välinen yhteys squash- ja sulkapallopelaajilla* [Emotion-performance relationships in squash and badminton players]. Unpublished master's thesis. Department of Physical Education, Jyväskylä University, Jyväskylä, Finland.

Terry, P.C., Lane, A.M., Lane, H.J., & Keohane, L. (1999). Development and validation of a mood measure for adolescents. *Journal of Sport Sciences, 17,* 861-872.

Vanden Auweele, Y., Cuyper, B.D., Mele, V.V., & Rzewnicki, R. (1993). Elite performance and personality: From description and prediction to diagnosis and intervention. In R.N. Singer, M. Murphey, & L.K. Tennant (Eds.), *Handbook of research on sport psychology* (pp. 257-289). New York: Macmillan.

Wang, Y., & Morgan, W.P. (1987). Convergent validity of a body awareness scale. *Medicine and Science in Sports and Exercise, 19,* S579.

Watson, D., & Tellegen A. (1985). Towards a consensual structure of mood. *Psychological Bulletin, 98,* 219-235.

Kellmann, M., Patrick, T., Botterill, C., & Wilson, C. (2002). The Recovery-Cue and its use in applied settings: Practical suggestions regarding assessment and monitoring of recovery. In M. Kellmann (Ed.), *Enhancing recovery: Preventing underperformance in athletes* (pp. 219-229). Champaign, IL: Human Kinetics.

12

The Recovery-Cue and Its Use in Applied Settings: Practical Suggestions Regarding Assessment and Monitoring of Recovery

Michael Kellmann, Tom Patrick, Cal Botterill, and Clare Wilson

Much has been written about the need to prevent overtraining and burnout among athletes and coaches (Henschen, 2001; Kallus & Kellmann, 2000; Silva, 1990). In particular, it is of great importance for athletes, coaches, and relevant sport practitioners (including sport psychology consultants) to be able to monitor stress and recovery in a proactive, continual manner in order to impact positively on an athlete's situational stressors and apply necessary coping strategies and recovery suggestions when required.

Kellmann and Kallus (2001) developed the Recovery-Stress Questionnaire for Athletes (RESTQ-Sport) in order to assist with the identification of an athlete's physical and mental stress, as well as the extent of current recovery activities. Subsequent to this, Kellmann, Botterill, and Wilson (1999) developed the Recovery-Cue, a seven-item self-monitoring and evaluation instrument. The Recovery-Cue, which attempts to measure perceived exertion, perceived recovery, and recovery effort, was developed in an effort to monitor early warning signs of possible overtraining effects on a more continual basis.

The Recovery-Cue was designed not only to provide feedback regarding current stress and recovery states, but also to improve athletes' knowledge and awareness of their stress and recovery states. This would assist athletes in becoming more responsible for meeting their situational training and recovery needs. In addition, graphing the Recovery-Cue scores can assist in determining the efficacy of various interdisciplinary interventions

that have been recommended for athletes by coaches and members of the interdisciplinary sport science team (Martin, 1996).

Both the RESTQ-Sport and the Recovery-Cue can be practical and effective in the assessment and monitoring of both stress and recovery. The purpose of this chapter is to present practical suggestions and case studies regarding their use in elite training environments. Specifically, examples from triathlon, golf, track and field, and swimming will be provided.

Framework for the RESTQ-Sport and the Recovery-Cue

Researchers have recently documented various strategies for the use of both the RESTQ-Sport and the Recovery-Cue (Botterill & Wilson, this volume, chapter 8; Kellmann, Altenburg, Lormes, & Steinacker, 2001). These instruments have mostly been used during training cycles, before competitions, after time off from training, and during training camps (Kellmann et al., 2001; Kellmann & Günther, 2000; Kellmann & Kallus, 2001).

Weekly Monitoring and Evaluation

As suggested by Kellmann and Kallus (2001), the RESTQ-Sport makes it possible to determine whether changes in stress and recovery states correspond with what is expected according to the training schedule depending on the type of training, competition schedule, whether the athlete is in the middle of a "loading" week in their training cycle, and so on. Other researchers have suggested that athletes experience improved self-awareness and motivation when they consistently monitor their training and competitive performances (Hogg, 1995; Orlick, 2001; Ravizza, 2001). However, because athletes can be overwhelmed with frequent testing and paperwork, the RESTQ-Sport and the Recovery-Cue should be implemented with some degree of moderation (Halliwell, Orlick, Ravizza, & Rotella, 1999). Thus, two current approaches of the Recovery-Cue—the basic form and the Web-based Athlete Weekly Evaluation—will be outlined in the following sections.

Basic Form of the Recovery-Cue

The Recovery-Cue is a recovery protocol consisting of seven items (see appendix 12.A on pp. 227-228). Three items were developed in reference to the concepts of perceived exertion, perceived recovery, and recovery efforts developed by Kenttä and Hassmén (1998), while four items represent the scales of the RESTQ-Sport that have been shown to be crucial for recovery processes (*Physical Recovery, Sleep Quality, Social Recovery,* and *Self-Regulation*). Being aware of the problems with one-item assessments, we attempted to develop an applied tool for athletes and coaches that could be completed during training, and that would provide immediate feedback.

Athletes completing the Recovery-Cue are requested to complete the items before, during, or after their training session, and must do so on the same day and at the same time from week to week. For example, if the coach, athlete, or support staff want to receive information about the recovery effects of the past weekend, the athlete should complete the Recovery-Cue on Mondays. If they want to determine the impact training had over the current week, the athlete should complete the instrument on Friday or Saturday. Since individual differences should also be taken into account, athletes should be encouraged to choose the time and day that they feel is the most accurate reflection of their current recovery and stress states. The results are input into a computer spreadsheet so that weekly scores are graphed on a continual basis and each week's scores can be interpreted with reference to past occurrences.

Web-Based Athlete Weekly Evaluation

The Web version of the Recovery-Cue is simply an adapted weekly evaluation form that includes goal setting, debriefing, and self-monitoring. Items from the Recovery-Cue were embedded within a Web-based Athlete Weekly Evaluation form that Tom Patrick and head coach Vlastimil Cerny designed, which was already being used by members of the Manitoba National Swim Centre, in order to keep the feedback process as efficient as possible. Athletes can complete the questionnaire on their own time (from home) and the results are received as an e-mail message to the sport psychology consultant. The results are then put into the spreadsheet. Graphs are interpreted immediately and any pertinent information is shared with the athlete, coach, and/or related support staff. The Athlete Weekly Evaluation (see appendix 12.B on p. 229) was developed in an attempt to facilitate self-awareness, self-monitoring, goal setting, and performance evaluation (debriefing), and to provide an opportunity for athletes to communicate weekly with the coach and other members of the performance enhancement team (PET) through e-mail. The PET is composed of a sport psychologist, sport physiologist, nutritionist, strength and conditioning specialist, massage therapist, and athletic therapist. It was felt that by integrating the items from the Recovery-Cue into the preexisting weekly evaluation, the coaching/interdisciplinary team would obtain useful information regarding the current stress and recovery states of the athletes, while the athletes would not feel overwhelmed by having to complete yet another questionnaire. As hoped, athletes using the Athlete Weekly Evaluation have exhibited an exceptionally high acceptance and adherence rate.

Another benefit of the Web-based Athlete Weekly Evaluation is that it allows for feedback, guidance, and counseling at a distance through the use of new technologies (the Internet, e-mail, Web-cams, etc.). Although distance guidance and counseling is a very recent phenomenon, some researchers have found it to be effective (Murphy & Mitchell, 1998; Sanders & Rosenfield, 1998; Tait, 1999). The process enables the athletes, coaches, and PET to communicate even when the athletes are training and competing away from the training center. This assists the coaches and athletes by providing feedback regarding stress, recovery, and performance on a continual basis.

The Athlete Weekly Evaluation was introduced to the athletes of Manitoba National Triathlon Centre in Winnipeg, Manitoba, Canada in the fall of 2000, which coincided with the inception of the national training center in the region. Athletes were asked to complete the evaluation form either Sunday evenings or Monday mornings on a consistent basis in order for the sport psychology consultant to be able to provide feedback to the athlete, coach, and relevant support staff. The form was well received and provided the coach and interdisciplinary team with useful and timely information about the athletes' stress and recovery states.

It should be noted that in addition to the use of the Web-based Athlete Weekly Evaluation, it was felt that both the coaches and support staff would be able to use the information collected by both the Recovery-Cue and the RESTQ-Sport in collaboration with the Weekly Evaluation to aid in both the monitoring of recovery-stress states and in improving the coach and support staff's ability to individualize the training program for each athlete. The RESTQ-Sport provides more comprehensive feedback than the Weekly Evaluation form. The information gathered from the RESTQ-Sport can prove useful immediately preceding a recovery week in the training cycle or periodically throughout an athlete's taper for a major competition.

Case Study 1: Male Junior Triathlete

This 17-year-old athlete was entering his first year of competitive triathlon training. In addition to his involvement with the national triathlon center, he was actively participating in a number of other school-based sports and was attending high school on a full-time basis. Both the head coach and the support staff felt it would be important to carefully and consistently monitor recovery and stress, especially as it pertained to his physical, psychological, and social demands (e.g., the effects of the intensity and volume of physical training, expected and real demands on time, self-regulation, etc.).

In early spring, the information from the Web-based Athlete Weekly Evaluation completed on March 5 (see figure 12.1) indicated lower scores than expected in the areas of perceived exertion, perceived recovery, fun, and confidence. This was especially important, as the previous week was at

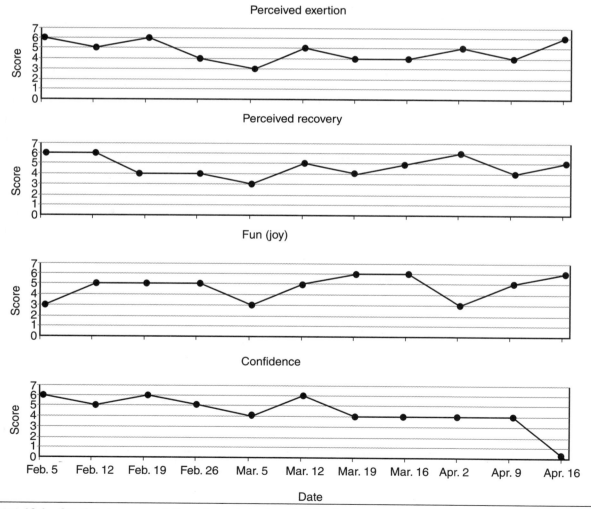

Figure 12.1 Graphical representation of a male junior triathlete's perceived exertion, perceived recovery, fun, and confidence collected using the Web-based Athlete Weekly Evaluation.

the end of a macrocycle that consisted of decreases in both volume and intensity, and it was expected that the athlete would be in a more recovered state. The other categories were stable and consistent with previous measures; therefore, only the four categories that were showing important information that differed from what was expected (according to the ongoing baseline that had been established) were reported. After the sport psychology consultant shared the information with the head coach and sport physiologist to confirm his suspicions, he and the head coach approached the athlete to inquire further. The athlete reported that he had completed a 3,000-meter race as well as participated in a basketball tournament during the previous week. Based on the results, the head coach instructed the athlete to take the next two run workouts off to rest in order to maximize his training in the week to come. As well, the athlete reported to the sport psychology consultant that the high levels of fatigue and demands on his time, coupled with his lackluster performance in training, were responsible for his feelings of apathy and lower self-efficacy.

Case Study 2: Professional Golfer

Proactive and meaningful performance feedback is difficult to obtain from athletes who travel frequently. This professional golfer sent an e-mail with a completed Athlete Weekly Evaluation to his sport psychology consultant that clearly showed unfavorable stress and recovery states (see figure 12.2). In particular, the athlete reported poor physical recovery and sleep. Low scores regarding fun and confidence prompted the sport psychology consultant to send an e-mail to the golfer in order to follow up on the athlete's information.

Based on the subsequent discussion, the consultant discovered that the golfer had not been playing well lately, and the amount of travel was starting to have a negative impact on his general level of fatigue (thus making it difficult to fall asleep). Although the discussion touched on many issues, the consultant reviewed presleep strategies, including the use of a relaxation strategy. In addition, he asked the athlete to establish a couple of process goals that he could focus on in order to direct

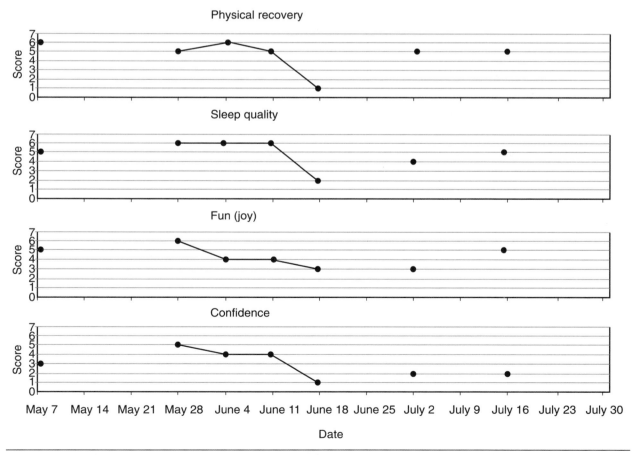

Figure 12.2 Scores regarding a golfer's physical recovery, sleep quality, fun, and confidence while on tour.

his focus away from whether he was "making the cut," and toward more process-oriented performance factors. The golfer reported some improvements in sleep, self-efficacy, and perspective over the next couple of weeks. As this is the golfer's first year on tour, however, stress and recovery states will likely continue to be inconsistent as he makes the adjustment to life as a professional golfer.

Monitoring Recovery After Training Cycles

As previously mentioned, the Recovery-Cue is most often used on a weekly basis during the training cycle (at the end of each microcycle). Support staff members collect the information for analysis and assess both individual scores and group norms. They can then plan appropriate interventions, such as changes to training intensity or work/school schedules, prompting of appropriate recovery strategies, and so on (Botterill & Wilson, this volume, chapter 8). This can prove especially useful in determining whether the athlete has achieved a recovered state after the appropriate macrocycles (macrocycles can vary from 4 to 6 or even 12 weeks depending on the sport or training program), thus facilitating optimized supercompensation. The RESTQ-Sport should also be used periodically after the end of certain macrocycles in order to provide more thorough analysis/feedback regarding the athlete's stress and recovery states.

Monitoring Recovery During the Taper

Kellmann et al. (2001) indicated that the RESTQ-Sport could be used to determine why athletes' recovery-stress states do not correspond with the expected outcomes given the respective change in training. During the taper, one would expect to find low scores in both general and sport-specific stress (with the possible exception of the *Conflicts/Pressure* scale) and high scores in general and sport-specific recovery. The RESTQ-Sport and the Recovery-Cue can provide useful information in order to assist athletes with their final preparations for competition. For example, high levels of physical stress can be met with appropriate adaptations to training, high levels of relationship stress can be met with more appropriate long-term planning (Botterill & Patrick, 1996), and low scores in self-efficacy and personal accomplishment can be mediated effectively with various brief contact interventions (Giges & Petitpas, 2000).

Case Study 3: National Track and Field Athlete

The coach of a track and field athlete approaching her national championships began to see that training was not going well; the athlete was reporting that she was under tremendous amounts of stress at work (she worked part-time as a teacher in addition to her full-time commitment as an athlete). The coach asked the sport psychology consultant to follow up with the athlete. The two decided that the RESTQ-Sport was the best instrument for assessing her current situation.

The first RESTQ-Sport assessment took place on June 14, just eight days before the athlete's upcoming competition. Results definitely confirmed the coach's observations (see figure 12.3, time 1). Together the athlete and the coach outlined a plan consisting of various recovery strategies for both the athlete and the coach in order to assist with the athlete's recovery and stress states as she approached the National Championships. In order to verify that the strategies were working, a second RESTQ-Sport was administered the day before the start of the competition. The results from the second assessment were extremely favorable (see figure 12.3, time 2), and this feedback was provided to the athlete in order to dissipate any worry that she may have been experiencing regarding her readiness to perform.

Recovery and Transition (Scheduled Breaks)

Another useful approach to monitoring stress and recovery is determining how effectively individual athletes use their time away from training/competition. Athletes must learn to use their breaks from training effectively in order to achieve physical, mental, and emotional recovery and thus achieve a desired state of readiness to return to intense training. As Kellmann and Kallus (2001) pointed out, a number of individual situations can impact the quality of "a break" from sport. Use of either the RESTQ-Sport, Recovery-Cue, or Web-Based Athlete Weekly Evaluation can again provide useful information for the coach or support staff, who can then act on it in an effective manner.

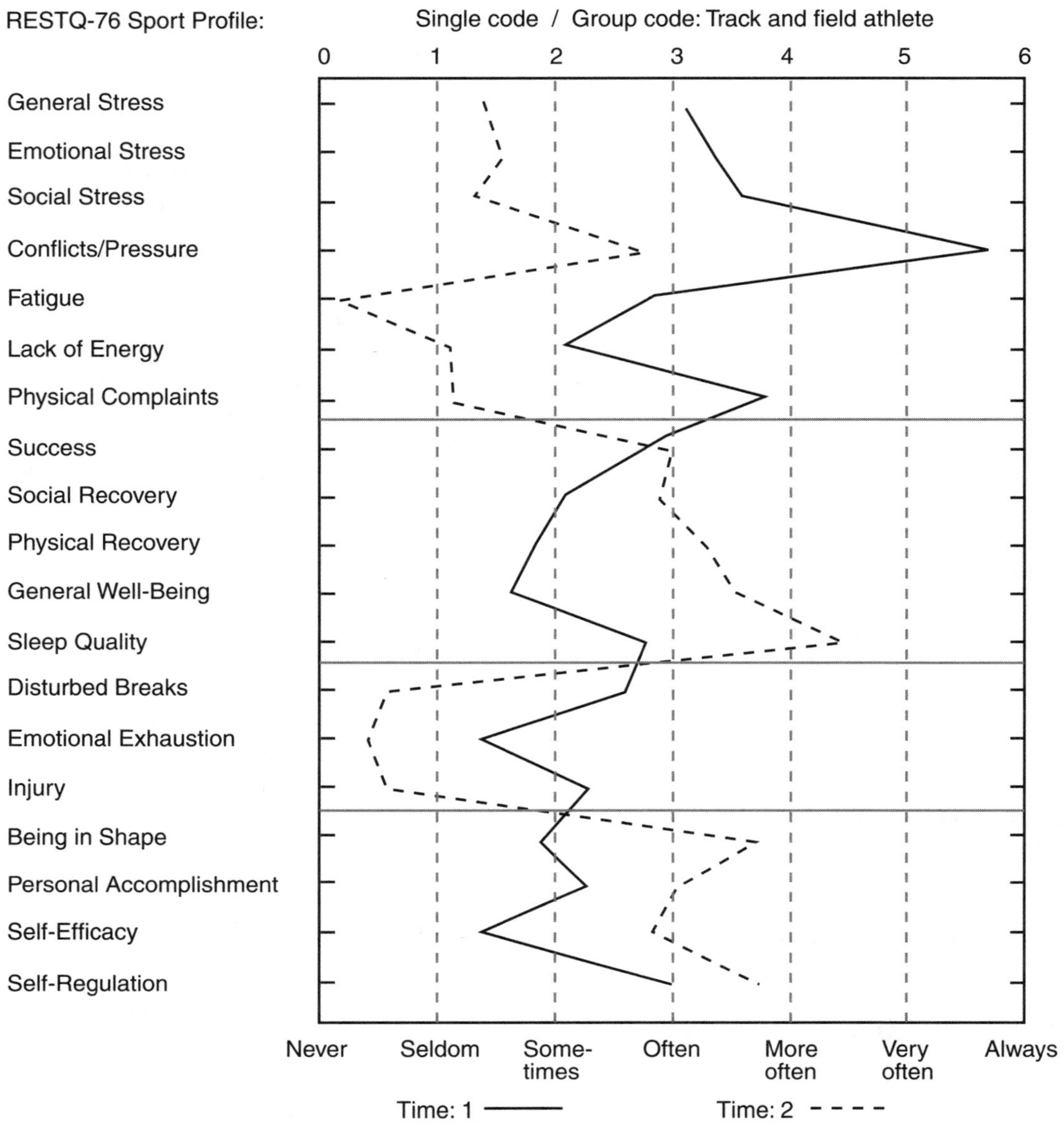

RESTQ-76 Sport Profile: Single code / Group code: Track and field athlete

Figure 12.3 RESTQ-Sport profile for a female track and field athlete at two different times during her taper.

Case Study 4: National Team Swimmers

The coach of two swimmers who had recently returned from a series of swim competitions in Europe was concerned about the level of the athletes' performance in training. The RESTQ-Sport was administered in order to get a more complete depiction of the swimmers' recovery and stress states. The results confirmed that both swimmers were experiencing high levels of fatigue and physical stress, while their recovery scores, in general, were very low (see figure 12.4). The information was communicated to both the athletes and the coach in order to determine an appropriate course

of action. In this instance, the coach adjusted levels of intensity in order to assist the athletes in making a positive transition back into training. In addition, the athletes were given the weekend off in order to catch up on sleep and attend to other personal and social roles.

Summary

Both the RESTQ-Sport and the Recovery-Cue have proved to be both useful and practical in high-performance training environments. The information that they provide has been useful to the

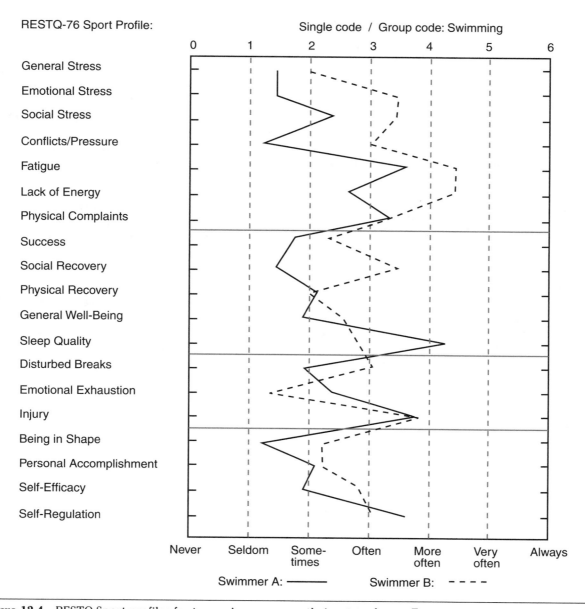

RESTQ-76 Sport Profile: Single code / Group code: Swimming

Figure 12.4   RESTQ-Sport profiles for two swimmers upon their return from a European tour.

athletes, coaches, and all members of the performance enhancement team who work on a continual basis with the athletes and coaches. However, it should be pointed out that these instruments should not be used as a replacement for effective communication. Rather, they should be seen as an important proactive tool that can aid in the creation of a more dynamic and responsive training environment. Finally, it is worth stating that the monitoring of both recovery and stress should remain the responsibility of the athletes themselves, and the tools should be used in a manner that facilitates improved levels of both self-awareness and personal responsibility.

References

Botterill, C., & Patrick, T. (1996). *Human potential: Perspective, passion, & preparation.* Winnipeg, MB: Lifeskills.

Giges, B., & Petitpas, A. (2000). Brief contact interventions in sport psychology. *The Sport Psychologist, 14,* 176-187.

Halliwell, W., Orlick, T., Ravizza, K., & Rotella, B. (1999). *Consultant's guide to excellence.* Chelsea, PQ: Baird O'Keefe.

Henschen, K. (2001). Athletic staleness and burnout: Diagnosis, prevention, and treatment. In J.M. Williams (Ed.), *Applied sport psychology: Personal growth* to peak performance (pp. 445-455). Mountain View, CA: Mayfield.

Hogg, J.M. (1995). *Mental skills for swim coaches and competitive swimmers: A text to improve mental performance.* University of Alberta, Edmonton.

Kallus, K.W., & Kellmann, M. (2000). Burnout in athletes and coaches. In Y.L. Hanin (Ed.) *Emotions in sport* (pp. 209-230). Champaign, IL: Human Kinetics.

Kellmann, M., Altenburg, D., Lormes, W., & Steinacker, J. (2001). Assessing stress and recovery during preparation for the world championships in rowing. *The Sport Psychologist, 15,* 151-167.

Kellmann, M., Botterill, C., & Wilson, C. (1999). *Recovery-Cue.* Unpublished recovery assessment instrument. Calgary: National Sport Centre.

Kellmann, M., & Günther, K.D. (2000). Changes in stress and recovery in elite rowers during preparation for the Olympic Games. *Medicine and Science in Sports and Exercise, 32,* 676-683.

Kellmann, M., & Kallus, K.W. (2001). *Recovery-Stress Questionnaire for Athletes: User manual.* Champaign, IL: Human Kinetics.

Kenttä, G., & Hassmén, P. (1998). Overtraining and recovery. *Sports Medicine, 26,* 1-16.

Martin, G.L. (1996). *Sport psychology consulting: Practical guidelines from behavior analysis.* University of Manitoba, Winnipeg.

Murphy, L.J., & Mitchell, D.L. (1998). When writing helps to heal: E-mail as therapy. *British Journal of Guidance and Counselling, 26*(1), 21-32.

Orlick, T. (2001). *In pursuit of excellence.* Champaign, IL: Human Kinetics.

Ravizza, K. (2001). Increasing awareness for sport performance. In J.M. Williams (Ed.), *Applied sport psychology: Personal growth to peak performance* (pp. 179-189). Mountain View, CA: Mayfield.

Sanders, P., & Rosenfield, M. (1998). Counselling at a distance: Challenges and new initiatives. *British Journal of Guidance & Counselling, 26*(1), 5-11.

Silva, J.M. (1990). An analysis of the training stress syndrome in competitive athletes. *Journal of Applied Sport Psychology, 2,* 5-20.

Tait, A. (1999). Face-to-face and at a distance: The mediation of guidance and counselling through the new technologies. *British Journal of Guidance & Counselling, 27*(1), 113-123.

ID Number: _____

1. How much effort was required to complete my workouts last week?

hardly any effort												
	6	6	6	6	6	6	6	6	6	6	6	6
	5	5	5	5	5	5	5	5	5	5	5	5
	4	4	4	4	4	4	4	4	4	4	4	4
	3	3	3	3	3	3	3	3	3	3	3	3
	2	2	2	2	2	2	2	2	2	2	2	2
	1	1	1	1	1	1	1	1	1	1	1	1
excessive effort	0	0	0	0	0	0	0	0	0	0	0	0
week	**1**	**2**	**3**	**4**	**5**	**6**	**7**	**8**	**9**	**10**	**11**	**12**

2. How recovered did I feel before my workouts last week?

energized and recharged												
	6	6	6	6	6	6	6	6	6	6	6	6
	5	5	5	5	5	5	5	5	5	5	5	5
	4	4	4	4	4	4	4	4	4	4	4	4
	3	3	3	3	3	3	3	3	3	3	3	3
	2	2	2	2	2	2	2	2	2	2	2	2
	1	1	1	1	1	1	1	1	1	1	1	1
still not recovered	0	0	0	0	0	0	0	0	0	0	0	0
week	**1**	**2**	**3**	**4**	**5**	**6**	**7**	**8**	**9**	**10**	**11**	**12**

3. How successful was I at rest and recovery activities last week?

successful												
	6	6	6	6	6	6	6	6	6	6	6	6
	5	5	5	5	5	5	5	5	5	5	5	5
	4	4	4	4	4	4	4	4	4	4	4	4
	3	3	3	3	3	3	3	3	3	3	3	3
	2	2	2	2	2	2	2	2	2	2	2	2
	1	1	1	1	1	1	1	1	1	1	1	1
not successful	0	0	0	0	0	0	0	0	0	0	0	0
week	**1**	**2**	**3**	**4**	**5**	**6**	**7**	**8**	**9**	**10**	**11**	**12**

4. How well did I recover physically last week?

always												
	6	6	6	6	6	6	6	6	6	6	6	6
	5	5	5	5	5	5	5	5	5	5	5	5
	4	4	4	4	4	4	4	4	4	4	4	4
	3	3	3	3	3	3	3	3	3	3	3	3
	2	2	2	2	2	2	2	2	2	2	2	2
	1	1	1	1	1	1	1	1	1	1	1	1
never	0	0	0	0	0	0	0	0	0	0	0	0
week	**1**	**2**	**3**	**4**	**5**	**6**	**7**	**8**	**9**	**10**	**11**	**12**

(continued)

5. How satisfied and relaxed was I as I fell asleep in the last week?

always	6	6	6	6	6	6	6	6	6	6	6	6
	5	5	5	5	5	5	5	5	5	5	5	5
	4	4	4	4	4	4	4	4	4	4	4	4
	3	3	3	3	3	3	3	3	3	3	3	3
	2	2	2	2	2	2	2	2	2	2	2	2
	1	1	1	1	1	1	1	1	1	1	1	1
never	0	0	0	0	0	0	0	0	0	0	0	0
week	1	2	3	4	5	6	7	8	9	10	11	12

6. How much fun did I have last week?

always	6	6	6	6	6	6	6	6	6	6	6	6
	5	5	5	5	5	5	5	5	5	5	5	5
	4	4	4	4	4	4	4	4	4	4	4	4
	3	3	3	3	3	3	3	3	3	3	3	3
	2	2	2	2	2	2	2	2	2	2	2	2
	1	1	1	1	1	1	1	1	1	1	1	1
never	0	0	0	0	0	0	0	0	0	0	0	0
week	1	2	3	4	5	6	7	8	9	10	11	12

7. How convinced was I that I could achieve my goals during performance last week?

always	6	6	6	6	6	6	6	6	6	6	6	6
	5	5	5	5	5	5	5	5	5	5	5	5
	4	4	4	4	4	4	4	4	4	4	4	4
	3	3	3	3	3	3	3	3	3	3	3	3
	2	2	2	2	2	2	2	2	2	2	2	2
	1	1	1	1	1	1	1	1	1	1	1	1
never	0	0	0	0	0	0	0	0	0	0	0	0
week	1	2	3	4	5	6	7	8	9	10	11	12

From Kellmann, Patrick, Botterill, and Wilson, 2002, The Recovery-Cue and its use in applied settings: Practical suggestions regarding assessment and monitoring of recovery. In *Enhancing Recovery: Preventing Underperformance in Athletes* edited by Michael Kellmann, Champaign, IL: Human Kinetics.

Athlete Weekly Evaluation

Week of: [   ]

What is your ID CODE? [   ]

What were your goals last week?

[   ]

Did you accomplish your goals last week?

[   ]

Did you eat well last week?

| Chips & hot dogs | 0 ○ | 1 ○ | 2 ○ | 3 ○ | 4 ○ | 5 ○ | 6 ○ | Veggies, fruit, pasta, and so on |

How was your time management last week?

| Out of control | 0 ○ | 1 ○ | 2 ○ | 3 ○ | 4 ○ | 5 ○ | 6 ○ | Planned to the second |

How much effort was required to complete your training?

| Excessive effort | 0 ○ | 1 ○ | 2 ○ | 3 ○ | 4 ○ | 5 ○ | 6 ○ | Hardly any effort |

How recovered did you feel prior to the workouts last week?

| Not recovered | 0 ○ | 1 ○ | 2 ○ | 3 ○ | 4 ○ | 5 ○ | 6 ○ | Energized and recharged |

How successful were you at rest and recovery activities?

| Not successful | 0 ○ | 1 ○ | 2 ○ | 3 ○ | 4 ○ | 5 ○ | 6 ○ | Successful |

How well did you recover physically last week?

| Never recovered | 0 ○ | 1 ○ | 2 ○ | 3 ○ | 4 ○ | 5 ○ | 6 ○ | Fully recovered |

How satisfied and relaxed were you before sleep last week?

| Restless | 0 ○ | 1 ○ | 2 ○ | 3 ○ | 4 ○ | 5 ○ | 6 ○ | No trouble getting to sleep |

How much fun did you have last week?

| None at all | 0 ○ | 1 ○ | 2 ○ | 3 ○ | 4 ○ | 5 ○ | 6 ○ | A "ton of fun" |

How confident were you regarding the achievement of your goals?

| Not confident | 0 ○ | 1 ○ | 2 ○ | 3 ○ | 4 ○ | 5 ○ | 6 ○ | Extremely confident |

How busy was school/work last week?

| Pulling my hair out! | 0 ○ | 1 ○ | 2 ○ | 3 ○ | 4 ○ | 5 ○ | 6 ○ | Lots of free time |

How busy do you expect your school/work load to be next week?

| Pulling my hair out! | 0 ○ | 1 ○ | 2 ○ | 3 ○ | 4 ○ | 5 ○ | 6 ○ | Lots of free time |

What did you do well last week?

[   ]

In what areas would you like to improve?

[   ]

What would you like more often from your coach/training sessions?

[   ]

Send   Clear

PART IV

Transfer to Related Areas

Paskevich, D.M. (2002). Recovery and health. In M. Kellmann (Ed.), *Enhancing recovery: Preventing underperformance in athletes* (pp. 233-252). Champaign, IL: Human Kinetics.

13

Recovery and Health

David M. Paskevich

What is health? How would you define it? If pressed, you might say that being healthy is feeling well and not being sick. Some say that being healthy means the absence of (1) signs that the body is not functioning properly or (2) symptoms of disease or injury (Birren & Zarit, 1985; Thoresen, 1984). However, this line of thought is overly simplistic.

More than 50 years ago, the World Health Organization (WHO; 1948) put forward a definition of health that has since been widely quoted. The definition stated that health is "a state of complete physical, mental, and social well-being and not merely the absence of disease or infirmity." Over the years, this definition has come under scrutiny and some criticism as representing an unrealistic goal. Since health and disease may coexist, and the presence of disease does not necessary reflect a loss of function and well-being, Terris (1975) suggested that the word *disease* be replaced with *illness*. Antonovsky (1979, 1987) suggested that health and illness are not entirely separate concepts and that we should consider them as ends of a continuum, stating that "We are all terminal cases. And we all are, so long as there is a breath of life in us, in some measure healthy" (1987, p. 3). Antonovsky also proposed that we refocus our attention in order to determine what enables people to stay well rather than what causes them to become ill. Nevertheless, one strength of the WHO definition was that it did emphasize the holistic nature of

health by integrating the body and spirit and including mental and physical states.

In 1988 Last elaborated and extended the WHO definition by proposing that health encompasses the following dimensions:

- Freedom from the risk of disease and untimely death
- Anatomical, physiological integrity
- The ability to fulfill personally valued family, work, and community roles
- The ability to deal with physical, biological, psychological, and social stress
- A feeling of physical well-being
- A state of dynamic balance in which an individual or group's capacity to cope with all the circumstances of living are at an optimal level

Last's contribution extends the previous WHO definition by acknowledging that how well one feels overall is as important as the estimates of disease presence. Last also extended the health concept to both individuals and groups.

Bouchard and Shephard (1994, p. 84) continued the effort to clarify the concept of health and defined health as "a human condition with physical, social, and psychological dimensions each characterized on a continuum with positive and negative poles. Positive health pertains to the capacity to enjoy life and to withstand challenges; it is not merely the absence of disease. Negative health pertains to morbidity and, in the extreme, with premature mortality."

The relationship between the mind and the body and the effect one has on the other has always been a controversial subject among philosophers, psychologists, and physiologists. However, in examining the concept of health, it is now widely recognized that several facets influence health (Bergner, 1985; Casperson, Powell, & Merritt, 1994), including the following:

- Genetic factors that govern basic health structure and other facets of health status
- Biochemical, physiological, and anatomical conditions that result in disease, disability, or handicap
- Functional factors, including the activities of daily life
- Mental factors, including moods, feelings, and affective states that are a reflection of well-being
- Health potential, which includes factors such as longevity, functional potential, and disability

Based on the previous definitions of health, one can easily understand the close connections among recovery, health, and performance/underperformance. Each of the previous conceptualizations of health included the individual's ability to deal with physical, biological, psychological, and/or social stresses. Clearly, then, researchers have embraced the viewpoint that recovery, being an active process that an individual can initiate in order to maintain or increase health, plays an integral role in helping the individual achieve optimal performance. However, research has not yet addressed many of the relationships between recovery and health in the sport context (e.g., genetic, biochemical, physiological, and mental). In this chapter I will present studies in sport when available. Otherwise, I will present research outside the realm of sport to demonstrate the potential importance of these constructs to sport, and as a possible departure point for future research in the area of health, performance, and recovery.

The purpose of this chapter is to examine the relationship between recovery and both physical and psychological health in areas not necessarily related to sport. It is not the intent of this chapter to review the literature that relates to underrecovery and *sport* performance that has been so cogently addressed in other chapters

(i.e., chapters 2, 4, 6, 7, 8, 11, and 14). I will review the research findings in exercise and health psychology in terms of the coping mechanisms, strategies, and resources that have been successful in recovery from other diseases/conditions and explore their potential use by athletes to enable successful recovery. Since little has been written about health and recovery in sport, a most useful starting point would be to examine the theoretical models previously used by exercise and health psychologists when investigating health and recovery behaviors. In doing so, future researchers may be better able to determine which theories or constructs would prove most useful for exploration in underrecovery, sport, and recovery behaviors. For example, nutrition, which may be linked to recovery, has been researched in nonsport populations from a theoretical perspective, and findings indicate a positive relationship between good nutritional habits and generally healthy behavior.

Attitudes, beliefs, and perceptions can help keep humans well. Recovery involves an interaction between the person and the environment that has important psychological and physiological effects. Within the health psychology literature, at least three traditions have been developed to aid in examining the relationship between health and recovery (Oatley & Jenkins, 1996). The first tradition, based on the psychoanalytic perspective (Alexander, 1950), asserts that unresolved conflict can produce physical problems. The second tradition is based on the premise that individuals who can share or express their feelings or experiences are less likely to develop illnesses (Pennebaker, 1995). The third tradition stems from the belief that the immune system mediates between life stresses and illness, and that being exposed to prolonged amounts of elevated stress may compromise the immune system and lead to health problems (Tessier, Fillion, Muckle, & Gendron, 1990).

In this chapter I will address the coping mechanisms, strategies, and resources that help determine the individual's responses to environmental demands, along with the relationships with other individuals that provide a major set of resources for successful recovery. When evaluating the "health" of the individual, we must move beyond the mere physical manifestations and consider biological, psychological, and/or social stresses and their relationship with performance/underperformance.

Attitudes, Beliefs, Perceptions

An individual's health behaviors are likely to be influenced by psychological factors, both emotional and cognitive. As a result, the practice of health behaviors may be a function of an individual's thoughts and beliefs. Although this line of thinking has been around since the 1950s, in recent years research has increasingly focused on individuals' attitudes and beliefs as determinants of their health practices, that is, behaviors that individuals initiate, maintain, or refrain from.

In order to convince individuals to change (e.g., their beliefs, attitudes, or behaviors), health care providers have typically relied on their professional status and the health information of the individual. Health-behavior theories and models suggest more effective methods for accomplishing individual compliance and other behavior change related to treatment regimens. Two of the major theoretical approaches to health behavior, the health belief model (Rosenstock, Derryberry, & Carriger, 1959) and the theory of planned behavior (Ajzen, 1985), emphasize be-

liefs and attitudes as determinants of individuals' health practices. Both theories argue for changes in attitudes and beliefs as a prerequisite for changes in health behaviors. However, is it reasonable to assume that we can encourage healthy living through changing individuals' attitudes and beliefs?

The Health Belief Model

Fundamental to the health belief model (HBM; see figure 13.1) is the assumption that health behaviors are more or less determined by the individual's perceived vulnerability to a health threat. Two factors, the individual's perception of susceptibility to the threat and the perceived severity of the consequences, primarily determine that individual's readiness to take health action. Thus, the model predicts that an individual will be most ready to take action when he believes that he is in danger of contracting the threat in question, and when he believes that the threat has important consequences (cf. Janz & Becker, 1984; Rosenstock, 1974).

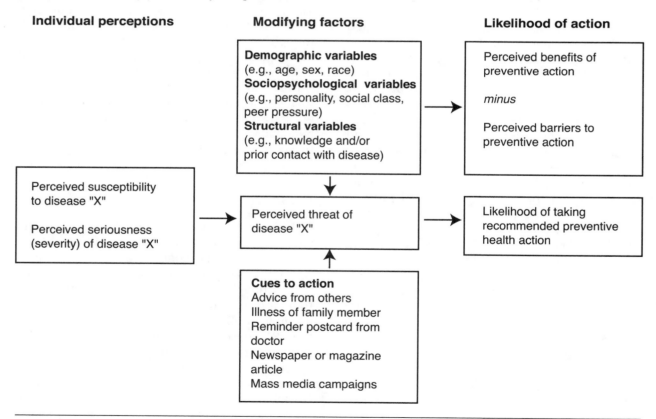

Figure 13.1 Schematic representation of the health belief model.

Two additional elements, however, also need to be included in any discussion of the HBM and its utility in predicting preventative health behavior. First, any internal or external stimulus that triggers the appropriate health behavior (i.e., cues to action) or demographic, psychological, or social factors (i.e., modifying factors) may be seen as having some potential effects on one's motivations and perceptions, although they are not viewed as direct causes of compliance. Finally, a person's evaluation of the advocated health behavior in terms of its perceived benefits versus perceived barriers (e.g., physical, psychological, and financial) must be considered (Becker & Maiman, 1975).

The HBM has generated a substantial amount of research. Studies have generally been supportive of the model in relation to health behaviors and medical compliance, finding that specific health measures are related to measures of vulnerability as well as the perceived benefits of taking action. However, in sport research, the use of the HBM is notably limited. The following studies provide examples of recent research using the HBM.

Using the HBM and the theory of reasoned action, Anshel and Russell (1997) examined the relationships between athletes' knowledge about the long-term effects of anabolic steroids and their attitudes toward this type of drug. Their primary hypothesis was that increased knowledge about the harmful effects of prolonged steroid use would be highly correlated with, and predict a negative attitude toward, ingesting steroids. However, the results obtained by Anshel and Russell revealed relatively low linear relationships between the various aspects of attitude toward and knowledge about steroid use for these athletes. Thus, greater knowledge about steroids and their effects on physical and mental health was not significantly related to athletes' attitudes about the use of steroids in sport.

In nonsport-related research, Chew, Palmer, and Kim (1998) tested the influence of the HBM by having participants in the study view a television program related to nutritional behavior. They proposed to identify relevant factors of the HBM that would provide the motivation for people to engage in healthy dietary behavior. The impact of the television program was assessed using a longitudinal study with 300 participants (35-54 years old) that measured the influence of path coefficients in the HBM that predicted salience, motivation, and healthful eating behavior. Their findings

suggested that nutrition behavior was influenced by susceptibility and efficacy mediated through health motivation and salience. Viewing the television program boosted salience regardless of age, education, or household size by significantly increasing the participants' confidence in their nutrition base knowledge.

Sapp and Jensen (1998) conducted an evaluation of the HBM for predicting perceived and actual dietary quality. Their assessment relied on data collected from 1,502 respondents by the U.S. Department of Agriculture in its 1991 Continuing Survey of Food Intakes by Individuals and the Diet and Health Knowledge Survey. The HBM provided a good prediction of perceived dietary quality, but provided weak-to-moderate predictions of seven measures of actual dietary quality that were calculated from food intake records.

The HBM has been widely used as a theoretical framework for the study of disease prevention. The model has been used to study a variety of preventative health behaviors, including those related to HIV. Soo Hoo (1999), in evaluating the HBM as a predictor of HIV self-protective behavior in college students, used structural equation modeling to examine construct variables. Although aspects of model fit were found, an insufficient degree of fit between the hypothesized model and the data prevented full model analysis. However, in regression-based path analysis used to test the model, several of the relationships expressed in the HBM were confirmed, including benefits and barriers, and psychosocial structural variables, which were found to be significant predictors of safer sex intentions.

Concerns

Although the previously described studies provide favorable results for the HBM, significant questions about the model have been raised. Theorists such as Wallston and Wallston (1984) argued that although the HBM seems highly plausible, there are several concerns about the model. For example, Wallston and Wallston suggested that the HBM represented more a catalog of variables than a testable model because of its imprecise specification of the exact relationships between its variables and health behaviors. Additionally, the model has tended to operationalize the various components in different ways, thereby affecting the consistency in variable measurement.

In relation to the application of the HBM to behaviors other than health and medical compliance (e.g., exercise), the strongest support for the HBM has been found for components of the model related to other theories. The perceived barriers component, which relates to self-efficacy, has stronger support than other components in the model, and a self-efficacy component has been added to the model (Rosenstock, Strecher, & Becker, 1988). Research by Kelly, Zyzanski, and Alemagno (1991) and Zimmerman and Conner (1989) suggested that social support, which related to social norms, should also be added as a component of the model. Finally, Quah (1985) questioned whether the HBM is applicable cross-culturally, as her study in preventative health behavior in three ethnic groups in Singapore found that the usefulness of the HBM in predicting behavior differed considerably among different groups.

The Theory of Planned Behavior

The attitude-based theory of planned behavior (TPB; Ajzen, 1985) has received considerable recent attention in the psychological literature. The TPB (see figure 13.2) is an extension of the theory of reasoned action (Ajzen & Fishbein, 1980; Fishbein & Ajzen, 1975), which states that many social behaviors are voluntarily controlled and that intention is the immediate determinant of behavior (Ajzen & Fishbein, 1980).

The primary goals of the theory of reasoned action (Fishbein & Ajzen, 1975) were to understand and predict social behaviors. In the theory of reasoned action, behavioral intentions are the product of two basic determinants: (1) attitude toward the behavior and (2) social norms. Attitudes toward a behavior are based on an individual's positive or negative evaluation of performing the behavior, and social norms has to do with how an individual perceives social pressures to perform or not perform specific behaviors. Consequently, attitudes and subjective norms influence the individual's intention to carry out (or not carry out) the behavior(s) in question. Finally, an individual's intention to perform the behavior determines actual behavior. Depending on the situation, the individual, and the behavior in question, it is thought that the relative importance of one's attitudes and social norms will vary.

The TPB moves beyond the theory of reasoned action by adding the concept of perceived behavioral control. Perceived behavioral control, similar to self-efficacy (Ajzen & Madden, 1986), involves the perceptions about how easy or difficult adoption of the behavior will be and whether one has the resources and opportunities to carry out the required behavior(s). Perceived behavioral control, as defined by Ajzen in 1991, is determined by the perceived presence or absence of required resources and opportunities and of anticipated obstacles (i.e., the control belief), and by the perceived power of control factors to facilitate or inhibit the behavior.

Perceived behavioral control, in contrast to attitude and subjective norm, is seen as having both a direct effect on behavior (which attitude and subjective norm do not), as well as an indirect effect on behavior through intentions. Therefore, the TPB predicts two possible effects of perceived behavioral control on behavior. In the first case, perceived behavioral control reflects motivational factors that indirectly affect behavior through intentions. In the second case, perceived behavioral control is not mediated by intentions and thus has a direct link to behavior (Madden, Ellen, & Ajzen, 1992).

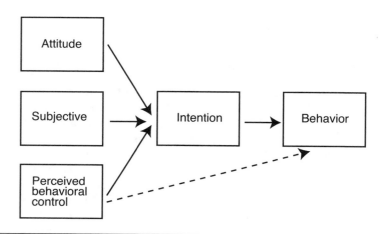

Figure 13.2   Schematic representation of the theory of planned behavior.

At a preliminary stage, the TPB shows promise for explaining and predicting a variety of health and exercise behaviors. The TPB was developed as a deliberate attempt to broaden the applicability of the theory of reasoned action to include nonvolitional behaviors by incorporating explicit considerations of perceptions of control over performance of the behavior as an additional predictor of behavior (Conner & Sparks, 1996). As a result, published studies using the TPB have been mounting. However, the use of the theory in sport settings is again quite limited.

Godin and Kok (1997) reviewed the literature for application of the TPB in the domain of health and verified the efficiency of the theory to explain and predict related behaviors. From 1985 to 1997, 56 studies were identified, and findings indicate that the theory performs very well for the explanation of intent. Attitude toward the behavior and perceived behavioral control were most often the significant variables for the explained variation in intention. Intention remained the most important predictor, however, in half the studies reviewed; perceived behavioral control added significantly to the prediction. The following studies highlight some of the current research in health and exercise behaviors using the TPB.

Mummery and Wankel (1999) studied the utility of the TPB to predict training adherence in a sample of adolescent competitive swimmers. Results indicated that training intention was significantly related to training behavior, and that the direct measures of the TPB (i.e., attitude, subjective norm, and perceived behavioral control) predicted a significant portion of the variance in the measure of training intention. Thus, Mummery and Wankel's findings suggest that the TPB offers insight into training behaviors and may aid in predicting training intention.

Preliminary evidence indicates that physical exercise may help cancer patients cope with the negative side effects of their treatment. Courneya and Friedenreich (1999) examined the utility of using the TPB for understanding cancer patients' motivation to exercise during treatment for breast cancer. One hundred sixty-four women who had been diagnosed with breast cancer within the previous two years participated in the retrospective study. These women were asked to recall their beliefs and exercise behavior during cancer treatment using a self-administered, mailed questionnaire. Findings indicated that (1) the salient beliefs of breast cancer patients concerning exercise were different from those of the healthy popu-lation, (2) intention and perceived behavioral control were significant determinants of exercise during cancer treatment, and (3) attitude and subjective norm were significant determinants of intention. The results of this study are preliminary, but they suggest that the TPB may be a viable framework on which to base interventions designed to promote exercise during cancer treatment.

Hillhouse, Adler, Drinnon, and Turrisi (1997), in investigating health protective behaviors, examined the application of the TPB to the prediction of sunbathing, tanning salon use, and sunscreen use intentions and behavior. Investigating the psychological determinants of high-risk UV radiation exposure-related behaviors, undergraduates from a midsized southeastern university were assessed on their psychological and behavioral tendencies toward such behaviors. The results generally supported the TPB as an explanatory model for high-risk behavior. Attitudes were strongly associated with high-risk intentions (e.g., the decision not to use sunscreen, or the use of tanning salons), whereas subjective norms were less associated with those same behaviors. Perceived behavioral control was found to moderate the relationship among attitudes, norms, and intentions to sunbathe and tan at a salon.

On a final note, one strength of the TPB is that there is heavy emphasis in that the measurement of the behaviors in question is specific to the context and the goal in question (i.e., specificity of the behaviors and situation(s) under consideration; Maddux, 1993). However, as with the HBM model previously discussed, researchers have raised some conceptualization and measurement issues with the TPB. Wallston (1992) argued that perceived control has been more or less operationalized as self-efficacy, and that because of this conceptual similarity, the measurement protocol set out by Bandura (1986) for self-efficacy should be used, rather than perceived behavioral control, as the primary construct. Brawley (1993) also pointed out that the measurement protocol of self-efficacy is better developed than that of perceived control at this time. Other researchers such as Courneya and McAuley (1995) examined the role social support plays in mediating the relationship between the cognitive constructs from the TPB and adherence to health behaviors. It is clear that future research using the TPB will have to examine the role(s) played by self-efficacy and social support. If they are conceptually simi-lar to the role of perceived behavioral control and social norms, they should be integrated into the theory.

Summary

The importance of using the HBM and TPB in underrecovery and sport is that the tenets of both theories are constructs that may be related to healthy living and recovery (e.g., perceptions of susceptibility and perceived severity, attitudes, normative beliefs, and perceived behavioral control). It is also possible, by using theory to measure or gauge what individuals' cognitions and feelings are—thus making them amenable to change—we can intervene in a systematic and controlled manner to enhance recovery behaviors. Because attitudes, subjective norms, and perceived behavioral control influence the athlete's intention to carry out (or not carry out) the behavior(s) in question, in order to change or modify an athlete's thoughts and beliefs, we must understand her attitudes, beliefs, and the role social norms and perceived behavioral control play in her current behavior or the target behavior. For example, in the TPB, if an athlete's attitude is that she needs to do more work (thus predisposing her to overtraining/underrecovery), and the social norms (i.e., social support) around her support the behavior, the athlete may, in fact, believe that it is natural or healthy to train at a level that will ultimately lead to staleness or burnout.

Thus, any internal or external stimulus that triggers the appropriate health behavior (e.g., cues to action such as reminders from coaches, advice from other athletes, or educational awareness through magazine or newspaper articles) or demographic, psychological, or social factors (e.g., age, personality, or knowledge about overtraining/underresting) should be seen as having some potential effects on an athlete's motivations and perceptions. The athlete's evaluation of the advocated health behavior in terms of its perceived benefits versus perceived barriers (e.g., physical, psychological, and financial) must be considered and addressed. Like health behaviors, performance behaviors are influenced by psychological factors, both cognitive and emotional.

Correlates of Health and Recovery

The evolving understanding of how psychosocial and behavioral factors affect health and disease processes has been marked by the investigation of specific relationships and the mechanisms underlying them. Stress and other emotional responses are components of complex interactions of genetic, physiological, behavioral, and environmental factors that affect the body's ability to remain or become healthy and/or to resist or overcome disease. Regulated by nervous, endocrine, and immune systems, and exerting powerful influence on other bodily systems and other health-relevant behaviors, stress and emotion appear to have important implications for the initiation, prevention, promotion, or treatment of cancer, HIV, cardiovascular disease, and other illnesses. Health-enhancing or health-impairing behaviors, including diet and exercise, can compromise or benefit health and are directed by a number of influences as well. Finally, health behaviors related to being ill or trying to avoid disease or its severest consequences are important. Seeking care and adhering to medical regimens and recommendations for disease surveillance allow for earlier identification of health threats and more effective treatment and recovery. The following studies examine correlates of the health-recovery relationship, which include health preventative, maintenance, or recovery constructs or behaviors.

According to Leung, Waller, and Thomas (1999), research evidence suggests that people with anorexia nervosa and bulimia nervosa exhibit dysfunctional cognitions not related to food, weight, or shape. Leung and colleagues assessed the impact of unhealthy core beliefs among females (aged 17-50 years) regarding eating disorders and their symptoms. Twenty restricting anorexics, 10 bulimic anorexics, 27 bulimics, and 23 controls completed Young's (1994) Schema Questionnaire, which included measurements of eating behaviors and attitudes. The results indicated that both anorexic and bulimic women had significantly higher levels of unhealthy core beliefs than comparison women did. Additionally, different patterns of association existed between core beliefs and eating psychopathology in anorexic and bulimic women. Thus, it is suggested that future clinical practice incorporate core beliefs as a potential element in the assessment and treatment of eating disorders.

Some researchers have identified athletes as a population at risk for the development of eating disorders (Greskoo & Karlsen, 1994). Anorexia and bulimia now rank among the major health problems in the United States (Taub & Blinde, 1992), and an even greater variety of disordered eating patterns among athletes pose potential health problems (Yeager, Agostini, Nattiv, & Drinkwater, 1993). Picard (1999) examined the level of competition as a factor for the development of eating disorders in female collegiate athletes. Picard's study examined eating attitudes among a sample of female NCAA Division I and Division III collegiate athletes and nonathlete controls. Results indicated that collegiate athletes at higher levels of competition showed greater signs of pathological eating and were at an increased risk for developing eating disorders. Although educational programs geared to the specific needs of collegiate athletes will be helpful, some argue that efforts should be directed toward helping younger athletes develop healthy attitudes and behavioral practices.

Jorgenson, Frankowski, and Carey (1999) examined the stress-buffering effects of the "sense of coherence" (psychological well-being) among 116 undergraduates (70 females and 46 males; mean age = 18.6 years). Self-reported physical well-being and psychological distress were assessed on two occasions separated by two months. Assessment of sense of coherence occurred at time 1, whereas assessment of negative life events for the past year occurred at time 2. Sense of coherence correlated negatively with negative life events and reported psychological symptoms on both occasions (time 1 and time 2). Negative life events correlated positively with assessments of psychological distress from time 1 and time 2. Negative life events correlated positively with physical ailments reported on both occasions only among students who had a low sense of coherence. This significant correlation persisted after accounting for the relationship between psychological and physical symptoms.

Plante (1999), in his review of the literature concerning the positive emotional effects associated with attempting to become physically fit and the belief in one's physical fitness, suggested that biological mechanisms cannot fully explain the well-known relationship between physical exercise and emotional health and well-being. The correlation between physical exercise and emotional health and well-being may be due in part to the fact that exercise serves as (1) a type of meditation, distraction, or biofeedback; (2) a psychological buffer from stress; or (3) a method to obtain social support and an increased sense of mastery, control, and self-efficacy. Plante, however, suggested that conceivably exercise is beneficial simply because those who exercise think it

is. Thus, exercise may act as a placebo, with suggestion playing a major role. Therefore, a connection between perceived fitness and purely physical health outcomes may exist.

Ai, Dunkle, Peterson, and Bolling (1998) addressed multifactorial determinants of postoperative psychological recovery and the effects of private prayer, a form of spiritual coping, on the recovery of 151 older patients (aged 40-80 years). Psychological adjustment via the Symptom Checklist-90-R (Derogatis & Cleary, 1977), health conditions, social support, and spiritual coping were measured after coronary artery bypass graft (CABG) surgery. Results indicated that most subjects prayed about their postoperative problems and that private prayer appears to significantly decrease depression and general distress one year post-CABG.

In summary, on the basis of the research conducted to date, it is reasonable to conclude that many factors are positively related to health improvement, maintenance, and recovery. Stress, emotional responses, diet, exercise, cognitions, seeking care, and so forth have all been shown to affect the health-recovery relationship. Additionally, even though relationships between health and other variables were presented in an independent or unrelated fashion, it is important to bear in mind the dynamic, multifaceted nature of these psychosocial and behavioral factors, and the fact that they are often interwoven.

The Stress Relationship

What is stress? To different people it may mean different things. Some individuals may define stress as the amount of pressure or tension they feel, whereas others may define stress as unpleasant external forces or an emotional response. Throughout the 20th century, various models of stress have differed in terms of their definition and emphasis (i.e., either psychological or physiological factors) and their description of the relationship between individuals and their environment. However, most contemporary definitions of stress agree on the following points:

- The external environment acts as a stressor.

- The response to the stressor is stress or distress.

- The stress response involves biochemical, physiological, behavioral, and psychological changes.

Lazarus and Launier (1978), who regarded stress as a transaction between people and their environment, developed the most commonly used conceptualization of stress: Stress involves an interaction between the stressor and distress.

Lazarus's work in the 1970s on stress introduced a new understanding of the stress response to the field of psychology (Lazarus, 1975; Lazarus & Cohen, 1973, 1977). Unlike Cannon's (1932) and Seyle's (1956) early models, in which stress was conceptualized as an automatic response to an external stressor, Lazarus argued that stress involved a transaction between individuals and their external world. He believed that a stress response was evoked if an individual appraised a potentially stressful event as actually being stressful. Thus, Lazarus's appraisal model described individuals as psychological beings who appraise the outside world and are not simply passively responding to it.

The main premise of Lazarus and Folkman's (1984) transactional model of stress is that stress cannot be defined solely by situations, since much of the stress reaction depends on the characteristics of the individual: "The important role of personality factors in producing stress reactions requires that we define stress in terms of the transactions between individuals and situations, rather than either one in isolation" (Lazarus, 1966, p. 5). Thus, individuals' reactions to a stressor depend on the way they appraise the situation. Lazarus (1966) emphasized a sequence of appraisals.

Lazarus (1966) identified two forms of stress appraisal, (1) primary and (2) secondary. Primary appraisal, according to Lazarus, occurs when the individual initially appraises the event itself as being either irrelevant, benign and positive, or harmful and negative. Secondary stress appraisal occurs when the individual evaluates the pros and cons of the coping strategies at his disposal. Primary appraisal involves an appraisal of the outside world, whereas secondary appraisal involves an appraisal of the individual himself.

Folkman and Lazarus (1985) described stress as a "disturbed person-environment relationship that coping is meant to change" (p. 150). Minimal stress may be inferred either due to no threat being perceived (from primary appraisal) or due to the person's belief that her resources are sufficient to deal with the perceived threat (dependent on secondary appraisal). When a situation is perceived as highly stressful, an individual may feel anxious and benefit from some form of learned coping strategy. Coping can be defined as "constantly changing cognitive and behavioral efforts to manage specific external and/or internal demands that are appraised as taxing or exceeding the resources of the person" (Lazarus & Folkman, 1984, p. 141). Coping is a form of dealing with a threat by altering the perception of stress in a situation.

Lazarus and Folkman (1984) distinguished two main types of coping: (1) problem-focused coping (PFC) and (2) emotion-focused coping (EFC). PFC occurs when one believes that one can do something to remove or manage the problem causing the distress, in this way treating or dealing with the situation itself. Examples of PFC include problem solving, planning, and increasing effort. EFC is used in situations when one thinks that little can be done to actually remove the threat; the individual must therefore regulate her symptoms or emotions in relation to the perceived threat. Wishful thinking and self-blame are examples of EFC. Both forms of coping are usually evident in stressful encounters (Folkman & Lazarus, 1980, 1985), and they will either facilitate or impede each other (Lazarus & Folkman, 1984).

Stress and Psychological Appraisal

Stress is a significant part of today's world. We all have stress in our daily lives, and it is only realistic to recognize that these stress levels will fluctuate depending on our circumstances and our responses to these stresses over time. For example, Baltzell (1999) examined psychological factors and resources related to rowers' coping in elite competition. The purpose of the study was to further understand the coping in elite sport by determining the predictive powers of coping based on hardiness, optimism, social support, psychological well-being, and athletic coping skills. Results from 61 elite rowers showed that 64% of the coping variance was explained by three independent variables: (1) goal setting and mental preparation, (2) social support of friends, and (3) psychological well-being. Differences were also found in the coping strategies used in the most and least effective coping experiences. Overall, the findings indicate that it is possible to develop the habit of effectively coping with competitive pressures and expectations to perform, but doing so depends on the athlete's willingness to reflect and learn from the rowing experiences.

Over the past 25 years researchers have tried to determine whether psychological variables predispose athletes to, or buffer athletes from, injury (Williams, 1996). Results from this line of inquiry seem to indicate that athletes experiencing many recent stressors who do not have the resources and skills to cope with the stress seem most at risk for injury. In 1992 Hanson, McCullagh, and Tonymon examined the relationship of personality characteristics, life stress, and coping resources to athletic injury. Personality characteristics (i.e., locus of control and sport competition anxiety), history of stressors (i.e., life stress, daily hassles, and past injury), and moderating variables (coping variables and social support) were assessed preseason for 181 track and field athletes from four Division I and II universities. In terms of injury severity, the four variables of coping resources, negative life stress, social support, and competitive anxiety differentiated severity groups. In terms of injury frequency, coping resources and positive life stress differentiated the groups.

The ability of the athlete to cope with injury is obviously a significant determinant in rehabilitation. A number of researchers have investigated coping resources. Udry (1997) reported that the use of instrumental (problem-focused) coping was a significant predictor in rehabilitation adherence. Quinn and Fallon (1999) reported that the elite athletes in their study tended to use active coping strategies rather than alternative coping strategies such as denial. They found that the coping strategies tended to remain stable and consistent throughout the recovery process. Murray (1999) examined stress and coping in 31 male collegiate football players on a Division IA championship team and 40 male recreational athletes in terms of emotional adjustment to sport injury. Murray found that emotional adjustment to sport injury was determined by appraisals of both personal and situational factors. Some researchers have suggested that proper identification and teaching of coping skills to injured athletes would greatly enhance their ability to return to competition (Heil, 1993; Petitpas & Danish, 1995; Smith, Scott, & Wiese, 1990; Williams, Rotella, & Heyman, 1998).

Bernier (1998) investigated the situational determinants of coping with severe reactions to work-related stress, including burnout, and the processes and strategies involved in the successful resolution of the crisis caused by an incapacity to work due to physical and emotional exhaus-

tion. A comparative analysis of the accounts of 20 human service workers and 16 other professionals led to the identification of common processes. Of interest to researchers who wish to intervene, Bernier found that the recovery process was long and could take from one to three years, and that various strategies such as objectively changing one's work environment, seeking reassurance, understanding causes, and seeking support were all used in successful recovery.

It has long been recognized that 40% or more of all patients who walk into a medical facility suffer from psychosomatic symptomology alone or physical disease that has strong emotional or situational overtones (Collings, Jr., 1984). In the past, health care workers tended to treat the presenting symptomology and not examine the true cause if it was not obviously organic. However, this situation is changing. As more medical programs are becoming preventative in nature, the relationship between life's stressors and the occurrence of organic disease is becoming more widely accepted. Behavioral and attitudinal opportunities for intervention have set the stage for new approaches in health care (Collings, Jr., 1984).

Because psychological stress responses result from a perceived imbalance between demands and psychosocial resources, researchers have identified a multitude of factors relevant to this transaction, including the chronicity and predictability of stimulation, opportunities for control, psychological coping responses, and the availability of social support. The mechanisms through which stress responses may increase the risk of illness are poorly understood, however, and researchers are often required to fall back on a poorly defined "biological predisposition" to account for individual differences in susceptibility to disease (Steptoe, 1992). However, with more recent developments in the study of the impact of stress on psychological and physiological functioning, researchers are examining the utility of cognitive-behavioral stress management interventions, biofeedback, relaxation, guided imagery, hypnosis, individual and group psychotherapy, and aerobic exercise as possible treatment mechanisms that may affect immune function and promote quality of life.

The evolving understanding of how psychosocial and behavioral factors affect health and disease processes has been marked by investigation into the specific relationships and mechanisms underlying them. Stress and other emotional responses are components of complex interactions of genetic, physiological, behavioral, and environmental factors that affect the body's ability to remain healthy or to resist or overcome disease. Thus, stress and emotion appear to have important implications for disease surveillance and may allow for earlier identification of health threats and more effective treatment of cancer, HIV, cardiovascular disease, and other illnesses (Baum & Posluszny, 1999). Baum, Herberman, and Cohen (1996) suggested that the application of such behavioral techniques to reduce distress and enhance coping skills has great promise in reducing the costs associated with chronic disease and in enhancing quality of life among those afflicted.

Ingledew, Hardy, Cooper, and Jemal (1996) examined the relationships between health behaviors that participants reported using as coping strategies and other, more documented coping strategies. Items reflecting the use of health behaviors (including relaxation, eating and weight control, preventative medicine, exercise and fitness, safety, sleep, caffeine use, alcohol use, smoking, and general self-care) as ways of coping with stressful situations were developed. These 30 items were interspersed with COPE (Coping Orientation to Problems Experienced) items. COPE is a multidimensional coping inventory that assesses the different ways in which people respond to stress. Five scales measure conceptually distinct aspects of problem-focused coping (active coping, planning, suppression of competing activities, restraint coping, seeking of instrumental social support); five scales measure aspects of what might be viewed as emotion-focused coping (seeking of emotional social support, positive reinterpretation, acceptance, denial, turning to religion); and three scales measure coping responses that arguably are less useful (focus on and venting of emotions, behavioral disengagement, mental disengagement). The entire questionnaire was administered with COPE instructions to 256 adults (aged 16-74 years). Factor analysis of the health behavior items along with the 13 COPE scales eventuated in a six-factor solution, explaining 48% of the variance. Three factors reflected problem-focused coping, emotion-focused coping, and avoidance; and three distinct factors reflected exercise, eating, and self-care. Women tended more toward emotion-focused coping and eating than did men. Older participants tended more toward problem-focused coping and self-care, and less toward eating compared with younger participants. Because the health behaviors formed quite distinct factors, it is suggested

that health behaviors may serve coping functions other than the previously well-documented functions of problem-focused coping, emotion-focused coping, or avoidance.

Osteoarthritis is one of the most prevalent chronic illnesses in older women in the United States. Along with limitations in physical functioning, osteoarthritis creates numerous sources of physical and emotional stress in daily life. Greater understanding of the mechanisms of stress, coping, and adaptation can assist women in improving their ability to cope with ongoing health problems. Tak (1998) conducted a study to identify the relationships among physical functioning, chronic daily stress, coping strategies, beliefs about personal control, perceived social support, and life satisfaction among older women with osteoarthritis. The sample included 107 women aged 60 or older who were diagnosed by a physician as having osteoarthritis. Six survey questionnaires and a personal information form were used for data collection. Using an adaptation of Lazarus and Folkman's theory of stress and coping, Tak found the following:

- Physical functioning was significantly related to chronic daily stress.

- Individuals with poorer functional ability experienced greater chronic daily stress and reported more use of emotion-focused coping strategies.

- A positive relationship existed between problem-focused coping strategies and perceived support.

- An internal health locus of control was positively related to perceived social support.

- The independent variables of comorbidity, financial status, chronic daily stress, perceived social support, and health locus of control accounted for 48% of the variance in the life satisfaction total scores.

- In particular, perceived social support and internal health locus of control significantly predicted life satisfaction.

In today's world, individuals may perceive themselves as having a less secure future and may experience greater anxieties about their abilities to meet future demands, more competitive pressures, and many other real and perceived stresses. It should not be surprising, therefore, that these influences are reflected in the individual's performance (e.g., in terms of success or failure) and the body's performance (e.g., in terms of sickness or health). If stress and other emotional responses are components of this complex interaction between the individual and the environment, understanding how psychosocial and behavioral factors affect health-enhancing or health-impairing behaviors will aid individuals in optimizing recovery.

Since differences have been found in the coping strategies used in the most and least effective coping experiences, findings indicate that it is possible to teach athletes to develop the habit of effectively coping with competitive pressures and expectations to perform. The learning of this habit, however, will depend on the athlete's willingness to reflect and learn from previous experiences. Hardiness, optimism, psychological well-being, and athletic coping skills will all serve to enhance health, recovery, and performance.

Health and Social Support

In Alameda County, California, a group of researchers gathered data on more than 7,000 people over a nine-year period. They found that the common denominator that most often led to good health and a long life was the amount of social support a person enjoyed (Haffen, Jarren, Frandsen, & Smith, 1996). The researchers concluded that individuals with social ties, regardless of their source, lived longer than people who were isolated (Minkler, 1986). After controlling for factors such as obesity, cigarette smoking, alcohol consumption, lack of exercise, harmful health practices, and poor health at the beginning of the study, their results indicated that people who had been classified as lonely and isolated were dying at three times the rate of those who had stronger social ties (Locke & Colligan, 1986; Syme, 1987). As part of the follow-up to the initial Alameda study, health and death records were monitored for an additional 8 years (bringing to 17 years the length of the study). Later analyses of the data revealed the same results: Individuals with the strongest social ties had the lowest mortality rates, even after controlling for age, sex, race, health status at the beginning of the study, depression, health practices, and the manner in which people viewed their own health (Seeman, Kaplan, Knudsen, Cohen, & Guralnik, 1987).

In a study similar to the Alameda County study, another group of researchers studied 2,754 adults in the small community of Tecumseh, Michigan. After undergoing thorough medical and psychological assessments, individuals were rated according to their personal relationships, with researchers taking special care to record the number of friends, degree of closeness to relatives, participation in group activities, and choice of activity (Locke & Colligan, 1986). The researchers followed this group of adults carefully for a 10-year period (from the early 1970s to the early 1980s) and found that individuals who had the strongest social ties and were most socially involved had the best health. Individuals identified as being more socially isolated had four times the mortality rate of those who were more socially involved.

Various competing ideas of why or how social support may influence health across the life span have been put forth. Numerous researchers have emphasized the role social support provides through informal social networks in potentially mitigating the health-damaging consequences of life stress (Cohen & Wills, 1985; Kessler & McLeod, 1985; Vaux, 1988), whereas others have emphasized the role of controlling or regulatory actions by one's social network in promoting healthy, and deterring unhealthy, activities and behaviors (e.g., Hughes & Gove, 1981; Umberson, 1987). Although many social scientists believe that the health benefits afforded by social support are attributable to the positive, supportive, affirming aspects of relationships with others (Sarason, Shearin, Pierce, & Sarason, 1987), researchers have yet to come up with definitive reasons why social support affects health. However, it is apparent that social support does affect physical health in terms of both mortality and the onset of disease (Cohen, 1990).

If social support does influence or mediate the stress-illness relationship, then one must try and determine what the possible mechanisms are. Two theories have been put forth to explain the role of social support in health status (Ogden, 1996). The main effect hypothesis suggests that social support is itself beneficial and that the absence of social support is itself stressful. The very presence or absence of social support may reduce the effect of the stressor or act as a stressor, respectively. Thus, social support may have effects independent of stress. Belonging to a large social network may provide the person with positive experiences and an ongoing set of socially rewarding roles. In doing so, social support could enhance well-being by promoting positive affect as well as giving a person an increased sense of self-esteem and belonging. If this is the case, then such positive effects would be helpful in dealing with stress; however, these effects are important regardless of whether one is experiencing stress. Conversely, not being associated with a strong social network (i.e., being isolated) may have deleterious effects on well-being (e.g., self-esteem) and cause an increase in stress independent of physical illness.

The second theory that suggests that social support helps individuals to cope with stress is the stress buffering hypothesis. According to this view, individuals who are experiencing stress receive the support of others, which provides the needed resources for dealing with the situation and thus "buffers" the individual against possible ill effects.

Of the two theories, which one best describes the effects of social support on an individual's health? The answer to this question depends on the research question being asked and a great deal on how one conceptualizes and operationalizes social support. Social support has been defined in a number of ways. Initially, it was defined according to the number of friends available to an individual. However, this definition has been amended to include not only the number of friends supplying the social support, but also the satisfaction with that support (Sarason, Levine, Basham, & Sarason, 1983). Social support, as defined by Wallston, Alagna, De Vellis, and De Vellis (1983, p. 369) "describes the comfort, assistance, and/or information one receives through formal or informal contacts with individuals or groups." The underlying assumption of social support is that supported individuals are physically and emotionally healthier than nonsupported individuals. A broad range of interpersonal behaviors by members of a person's social network may help the person successfully cope with a number of trying life events and circumstances. Much of the research on social support has implied that it is the primary factor in the maintenance of health-promoting regimens (Duncan, 1993). However, little research has directly addressed the psychological needs associated with different kinds of events (Cohen & Hoberman, 1983), and it is still unclear whether certain forms of social support are maximally beneficial in the context of specific domains of functioning (e.g., physical activity and dieting) (Russell & Cutrona, 1987).

The influence of social support on health behaviors has been examined from a number of multidimensional perspectives, and in each of these models varying types or components of support appear to converge on a similar set of dimensions. In 1974 Weiss developed a theoretical framework that described six different social functions, or provisions, that may be obtained from social relationships: attachment, social integration, reassurance of worth, reliable alliance, guidance, and opportunity for nurturance. Attachment represents emotional support, or the ability to turn to others for comfort and security during times of stress. Social integration (network support) reflects a sense of belonging to a group of people who share common goals or interests. Reassurance of worth (esteem support) represents the bolstering of a person's sense of self-esteem by providing the individual with positive feedback regarding her skills and abilities in a particular situation. Reliable alliance (material support), or tangible aid, refers to the assurance that the individual can count on concrete instrumental assistance from others, regardless of circumstances. Guidance (instrumental support, or informational support in the form of advice and information) provides the individual with possible solutions or courses of action in dealing with the stressful life situations she faces. The last provision, opportunity for nurturance (active support), is the belief that individuals need to feel that others need them.

In a manner similar to Weiss's (1974) theoretical framework, Amick and Ockene (1994) studied the effect of social support on heart disease. They believe five components make up effective social support: (1) being cared for and loved with the opportunity for shared intimacy; (2) being esteemed and valued, thus having a sense of personal worth; (3) having a sense of belonging by sharing companionship, communication, and mutual obligations with others; (4) having "informational" support such as access to information, appraisal, advice, as well as guidance; and (5) having access to physical and/or material assistance.

A number of studies have examined whether social support influences the health status of the individual. From a sport injury perspective, the amount of support an athlete receives from family, friends, teammates, coaches, and the community will greatly influence injury recovery (see Hardy & Crace, 1993, for a full review). Certainly the establishment of support groups for individuals such as cancer patients (Taylor, Falke, Shoptaw, & Lichtman, 1986), persons with disabilities (Suarez de Balcazar, Seekins, Paine, Fawcett, & Mathews, 1989), and AIDS patients (Kelly et al., 1993) shows, overwhelmingly, the valuable role social support can play in effective rehabilitation programs. In addition to the coping resource that social support can provide, it can also provide what Heil (1993) described as "secondary gain," referring to the favorable consequences such as increased attention and sympathy from significant others.

Mainwaring (1999) examined the psychosocial impact of athletic injury and rehabilitation on athletes in a holistic model that incorporated the psychological, physical, and social domains emphasized by severely injured athletes. Mainwaring's focus was to determine the "restoration of self," which reflected a persistent, underlying motivation to overcome disability (i.e., severe knee injuries). This "restoration of self" was influenced by perceived rehabilitation gains, perceived social support, coping strategies, affective state, expectations about the roles of the physiotherapist and physician, attitude toward disability, and the information the athlete received about the injury and recovery process.

Ryska and Yin (1999) used the buffering hypothesis (in which social support is seen to moderate, or "buffer," the impact of stress on the individual and thus indirectly affect emotional well-being) in a competitive sport environment. They examined perceptions of coach support and precompetitive anxiety among male and female high school tennis athletes. Their analysis of the data revealed a significant support-anxiety effect in the high-trait anxious athletes only. Results suggest that perceived coach support represents an important mediating factor in the sport stress process among highly anxious athletes.

In 1998 Vlahos examined interpersonal, individual, and situational factors associated with burnout in student-athletes. Vlahos's aim was to develop a model concerned with the relationships between athletes' experiences of burnout and individual, interpersonal, and sport-specific factors. The model proposed that athlete burnout would be related to athletes' personality traits (e.g., level of neuroticism and extroversion), experiences of competitive stress, level of confidence in athletic abilities, and perceptions of social support. Results suggest a complex interaction between athletes' individual, interpersonal, and situational variables and their experience of burnout. Athletes' perceptions of support from significant adults were found to directly affect their experience of burnout, whereas it indirectly affected their experience of burnout through its impact on levels of neuroticism and extroversion.

The athletes' levels of neuroticism and competitive anxiety were found to directly affect their experience of burnout. Additionally, further analyses indicated that the athletes' levels of extroversion had an indirect effect on their experiences of burnout (based on the athletes' reported levels of sport self-confidence) and sport self-confidence had an indirect effect on their experiences with competitive trait anxiety.

Yates (1996) explored the extent to which social support from a spouse and a health care provider was associated with short- and long-term recovery outcomes in 93 patients (aged 30-80 years) two months after a cardiac illness. Seventy-three subjects responded to a follow-up questionnaire one year later. Tangible aid from the spouse was associated with better short-term psychological recovery. Satisfaction with and more emotional support from the spouse were associated with better short- and long-term psychological recovery outcomes. Greater satisfaction with health care provider support was associated with short- and long-term physical recoveries. Results highlight the value of different sources and types of support as having differential effects on physical and psychological recovery outcomes.

Recent research indicates that middle-aged exercisers have reported that exercising with friends and social groups has been one of the key motivating factors in general practitioner referral for exercise schemes (Fox, Biddle, Edmunds, Killoran, & Bowler, 1997). Roberto (1992) examined the strategies used by 101 older women (aged 65-94 years) to cope with their hip fractures. Roberto interviewed the participants, who described their health, income, ability to perform tasks of daily living, cognitive functioning, locus of control, level of depression, informal network, and use of coping strategies. Results indicated that participants used a variety of different coping strategies, with "seeking social support" being the most frequent. A strong belief in external control was the only resource predictive of the coping strategies employed. The use of several emotion-focused coping strategies was associated with poorer functional recovery.

Measuring social support is not easy, and many of the social support measures used in health psychology reflect similar dimensions. However, the literature in health psychology and related areas (Cohen, 1988; Cohen & Wills, 1985; Shumaker & Brownell, 1984; Wallston et al., 1983) has indicated that social support plays a role in stress reduction and health promotion. It is suggested that social support may play a similar role in many other health-related behaviors, such as rehabilitation and compliance behaviors.

Summary and Recommendations

The research advances in health and recovery are proceeding in many new directions, including health behaviors and medical compliance and, more recently, exercise, physical activity, and sport. The advances have been illustrated in this chapter with examples from the most recently published studies. At the center of these advances is a common conceptual belief that attitudes, beliefs, and perceptions have the ability to affect an individual's health and recovery behaviors (i.e., the coping mechanisms, strategies, and resources that have resulted in successful recovery from other diseases/conditions). The theoretical models of health belief and the theory of planned behavior, along with constructs such as coping styles and social support, were used to outline the perspectives relevant to definitional, conceptual, and measurement considerations for current and future research. In order to provide a perspective for future research, a summary of past and present correlates of health and recovery were presented in theoretical models that use attitudes and beliefs as determinant of individuals' health practices and psychosocial and behavioral factors that affect health and disease processes.

Also discussed were the issues important to making research advances, such as (1) the multidimensional nature of the health-recovery process, (2) correlates of the health-recovery process, such as health-enhancing or health-impairing behaviors including diet and exercise, and (3) the social context in which the recovery takes place. As a starting point, relevant links using theories from the fields of exercise and health psychology provide conceptual overviews to operational definitions necessary for research to be advanced in the area of underrecovery and sport. Thus, if one were to summarize what the potential lessons for guiding practice in the area of health and recovery are, they might include the following:

- When evaluating the "health" of the individual, we must move beyond the mere physical and consider biological, psychological, and/or social stresses and their relationships to performance/underperformance.

- Any internal or external stimulus that triggers the appropriate health behavior (e.g., cues to action such as reminders from coaches, advice from other athletes, or educational awareness through magazine or newspaper articles) or demographic, psychological, or social factors (e.g., age, personality, or knowledge about overtraining/ underresting) should be identified for each athlete. These may affect motivations and perceptions.

- The athlete's evaluation of the advocated health behavior in terms of its perceived benefits versus perceived barriers (e.g., physical, psychological, and financial) must be considered and addressed.

- Like health behaviors, performance behaviors are influenced by psychological factors, both cognitive and emotional.

- Because attitudes, subjective norms, and perceived behavioral control influence athletes' intention to carry out (or not carry out) the behavior(s) in question, in order to change or modify athletes' thoughts and beliefs, we must understand their attitudes and beliefs and the role social norms and perceived behavioral control play in their current behavior or the target behavior.

- Stress and other emotional responses are components of complex interactions between the individual and the environment. Understanding how psychosocial and behavioral factors affect health-enhancing or health-impairing behaviors will aid individuals in optimizing recovery.

- Hardiness, optimism, psychological well-being, and athletic coping skills can all serve to enhance health, recovery, and performance.

- Since differences have been found in the coping strategies used in the most and least effective coping experiences, findings indicate that it is possible to teach athletes to develop the habit of effectively coping with competitive pressures and expectations to perform. The learning of this habit, however, depends on the athlete's willingness to reflect and learn from previous experiences.

- Social support, which has been shown to potentially mitigate the health-damaging consequences of life stress, may play an important role in mediating the sport-stress process, particularly among highly anxious athletes or athletes that are injured and/or returning from injury.

- If the underlying assumption of social support is that supported individuals are physically and emotionally healthier than nonsupported individuals, then we must ensure that the athletes under our direction not only perceive that they are supported, but also are satisfied with the support. Since much of the research on social support has implied that it is the primary factor in the maintenance of health-promoting regimens, we must try and create positive, supportive, and affirming relationships with athletes within the sport and encourage the development of the same types of relationships with others outside the sport.

Future Research on Recovery and Health

A useful starting point for future research may be to examine, review, and reflect critically on the research findings in the exercise and health psychology literature in relation to the coping mechanisms, strategies, and resources that have resulted in successful recovery from other diseases and conditions. If research is done properly, we may eliminate "borrowing" the problems of past research while at the same time not having to reinvent the wheel in trying to determine which behaviors may be used by athletes to enable them to recover successfully.

For research to advance in sport, the simple description of the correlates of health and recovery processes will not suffice. Health behaviors related to prevention as well as recovering from training and illness must include psychosocial interventions based on theory to set the stage for new initiatives in the research community. Recovery is a manifestation of many processes that may moderate desirable personal outcomes of being healthy, avoiding disease, or overcoming its severest consequences. However, these outcomes will not be fully understood without research that focuses on these processes. Without such research advances, interventions that are designed to manipulate recovery processes and enhance, retain, or regain health will have a reduced chance of success. This chapter describes new directions with clear paths for investigators to either challenge or follow. In 5 to 10 years, reviews of the health-recovery research will determine if these paths have been well traveled and if new advances in health-recovery research have been made.

References

Ai, A.L., Dunkle, R.E., Peterson, C., & Bolling, S.E. (1998). The role of private prayer in psychological recovery among midlife and aged patients following cardiac surgery. *Gerontologist, 38* (5), 591-601.

Ajzen, I. (1985). From intention to actions: A theory of planned behavior. In J. Kuhl & J. Beckman (Eds.), *Action-control: From cognition to behavior* (pp. 11-39). Heidelberg, Germany: Springer-Verlag.

Ajzen, I. (1991). The theory of planned behavior. *Organizational Behavior and Human Decision Processing, 50,* 179-211.

Ajzen, I., & Fishbein, M. (1980). *Understanding attitudes and predicting social behavior.* Englewood Cliffs, NJ: Prentice Hall.

Ajzen, I., & Madden, T.J. (1986). Prediction of proficient technique and successful lesion detection in breast self-examination. *Health Psychology, 3,* 113-127.

Alexander, F. (1950). *Psychosomatic medicine: Its principles and applications.* New York: Norton.

Amick, T.L., & Ockene, J.K. (1994). The role of social support in the modification of risk factors for cardiovascular disease. In S.A. Shumaker & S.M. Czajkowski (Eds.), *Social support and cardiovascular disease* (pp. 260-261). New York: Plenum Press.

Anshel, M.H., & Russell, K.G. (1997). Examining athletes' attitudes toward using anabolic steroids and their knowledge of the possible effects. *Journal of Drug Education, 27* (2), 121-145.

Antonovsky, A. (1979). *Health, stress, and coping.* San Francisco: Jossey-Bass.

Antonovsky, A. (1987). *Unraveling the mystery of health: How people manage stress and stay healthy.* San Francisco: Jossey-Bass.

Baltzell, A. (1999). *Psychological factors and resources related to rowers' coping in elite competition.* Unpublished doctoral dissertation, Boston University.

Bandura, A. (1986). *Social foundations of thought and action: A social cognitive theory.* Englewood Cliffs, NJ: Prentice Hall.

Baum, A., Herberman, H., & Cohen, L. (1996). Managing stress and managing illness: Survival and quality of life in chronic disease. *Journal of Clinical Psychology in Medical Settings, 2* (4), 309-333.

Baum, A., & Posluszny, D.M. (1999). Health psychology: Mapping biobehavioral contributions to health and illness. *Annual Review of Psychology, 50,* 137-163.

Becker, M.H., & Maiman, L.A. (1975). Sociobehavioral determinants of compliance with health and medical care recommendations. *Medical Care, 13,* 10-24.

Bergner, M. (1985). Measurement of health status. *Medical Care, 23,* 696-704.

Bernier, D. (1998). A study of coping: Successful recovery from severe burnout and other reactions to severe work-related stress. *Work & Stress, 12* (1), 50-65.

Birren, J.E., & Zarit, J.M. (1985). Concepts of health behavior and aging. In J.E. Birren & J. Livingston (Eds.), *Cognition, stress, and aging.* Englewood Cliffs, NJ: Prentice Hall.

Bouchard, C., & Shephard, R.J. (1994). Physical activity, fitness, and health: The model and key concepts. In C. Bouchard, R.J. Shephard, & T. Stephens (Eds.), *Physical activity, fitness, and health: Consensus statement* (pp. 77-89). Champaign, IL: Human Kinetics.

Brawley, L.R. (1993). The practicality of using social psychological theories for exercise and health research intervention. *Journal of Applied Sport Psychology, 5,* 99-115.

Cannon, W.B. (1932). *The wisdom of the body.* New York: Norton.

Casperson, C.J., Powell, K.E., & Merritt, R.K. (1994). Measurement of health status and well-being. In C. Bouchard, R.J. Shephard, & T. Stephens (Eds.), *Physical activity, fitness, and health: Consensus statement* (pp. 180-202). Champaign, IL: Human Kinetics.

Chew, F., Palmer, S., & Kim, S. (1998). Testing the influence of the health belief model and a television program on nutrition behavior. *Health Communication, 10* (3), 227-245.

Cohen, S. (1988). Psychosocial models of the role of social support in the etiology of physical disease. *Health Psychology, 7,* 269-297.

Cohen, S. (1990). Social support and physical illness. *Advances, 7* (1), 35-48.

Cohen, S., & Hoberman, H.M. (1983). Positive events and social supports as buffers of life change stress. *Journal of Applied Social Psychology, 13,* 99.

Cohen, S., & Wills, T.A. (1985). Stress, social support and the buffering hypothesis. *Psychological Bulletin, 98,* 310-357.

Collings, Jr., G.H. (1984). Stress and the workplace. In J.D. Matarazzo, S.M. Weiss, J.A. Herd, N.E. Miller, & S.M. Weiss (Eds.), *Behavioral health: A handbook of health enhancement and disease prevention* (pp. 1079-1086). New York: Wiley.

Conner, M., & Sparks, P. (1996). The theory of planned behaviour and health behaviours. *Predicting health behaviour: Research and practice with social cognition models* (pp. 121-162). Buckingham, UK: Open University Press.

Courneya, K.S., & Friedenreich, C.M. (1999). Utility of the theory of planned behavior of understanding exercise during breast cancer treatment. *Psycho-Oncology, 8* (2), 112-122.

Courneya, K.S., & McAuley, E. (1995). Cognitive mediators of the social influence adherence relationship: A test of the theory of planned behavior. *Journal of Behavioral Medicine, 18* (5), 499-515.

Derogatis, L.R., & Cleary, P.A. (1977). Confirmation of the dimensional structure of the SCL-90: A study in construct validation. *Journal of Clinical Psychology, 33* (4), 981-989.

Duncan, S.C. (1993). The role of cognitive appraisal and friendship provisions in adolescents' affect and motivation toward activity in physical education. *Research Quarterly for Exercise and Sport, 64,* 314-323.

Fishbein, M., & Ajzen, I. (1975). *Beliefs, attitudes, intention, and behavior: An introduction to theory and research.* Reading, MA: Addison-Wesley.

Folkman, S., & Lazarus, R.S. (1980). An analysis of coping in a middle-aged community sample. *Journal of Health and Social Behavior, 21,* 219-239.

Folkman, S., & Lazarus, R.S. (1985). If it changes it must be a process: Study of emotion and coping during three stages of a college examination. *Journal of Personality and Social Psychology, 48,* 150-170.

Fox, K.R., Biddle, S.J.H., Edmunds, L.E., Killoran, A., & Bowler, I. (1997). Physical activity promotion through primary health care in England. *British Journal of General Practice, 47,* 367-369.

Godin, G., & Kok, G. (1997). The theory of planned behavior: A review of its applications to health-related behaviors. *American Journal of Health Promotion, 11* (2), 87-98.

Greskoo, R.B., & Karlsen, A. (1994). The Norwegian program for primary, secondary, and tertiary prevention of eating disorders. *Eating Disorder Journal Treatment Prevention, 2,* 57-63.

Haffen, B.Q., Jarren, K.J., Frandsen, K.J., & Smith, N.L. (1996). *Mind/body health: The effects of attitudes, emotions, and relationships.* Boston: Allyn & Bacon.

Hanson, S.J., McCullagh, P., & Tonymon, P. (1992). The relationship of personality characteristics, life stress, and coping resources to athletic injury. *Journal of Sport & Exercise Psychology, 14*(3), 262-272.

Hardy, C., & Crace, K. (1993). Dimensions of social support in dealing with sport injuries. In D. Pargman (Ed.), *Psychological bases of sport injuries* (pp. 121-144). Morgantown, WV: Fitness Information Technology.

Heil, J. (1993). *Psychology of sport injury.* Champaign, IL: Human Kinetics.

Hillhouse, J.J., Adler, C.M., Drinnon, J., & Turrisi, R. (1997). Application of Ajzen's theory of planned behavior to predict sunbathing, tanning salon use, and sunscreen use intentions and behaviors. *Journal of Behavioral Medicine, 20* (4), 365-378.

Hughes, M., & Gove, W.R. (1981). Living alone, social integration, and mental health. *American Journal of Sociology, 87,* 48-74.

Ingledew, D.K., Hardy, L., Cooper, C.L., & Jemal, H. (1996). Health behaviours reported as coping strategies: A factor analytical study. *British Journal of Health Psychology, 1,* 263-281.

Janz, N.K., & Becker, M.H. (1984). The health belief model: A decade late. *Health Education Quarterly, 11,* 1-47.

Jorgensen, R.S., Frankowski, J.J., & Carey, M.P. (1999). Sense of coherence, negative life events and appraisal of physical health among university students. *Personality & Individual Differences, 27* (6), 1079-1089.

Kelly, J.A., Murphy, D.A., Bahr, G.R., Kalichman, S.C., Morgan, M.G., & Stevenson, L.Y. (1993). Outcome of cognitive-behavioral and support group brief therapies for depressed, HIV-infected persons. *American Journal of Psychiatry, 11,* 1679-1686.

Kelly, R.B., Zyzanski, S.J., & Alemagno, S.A. (1991). Prediction of motivation and behavior change following health promotion: Role of health beliefs, social support, and self-efficacy. *Social Science and Medicine, 32,* 311-320.

Kessler, R.C., & McLeod, J.A. (1985). Social support and mental health in community psychology. In S. Cohen & L. Syme (Eds.), *Social support and health* (pp. 219-240). Orlando, FL: Academic Press.

Last, J.M. (1988). *A dictionary of epidemiology.* New York: Oxford University Press.

Lazarus, R.S. (1966). *Psychological stress and the coping process.* New York: McGraw-Hill.

Lazarus, R.S. (1975). A cognitively oriented psychologist looks at biofeedback. *American Psychologist, 30,* 553-561.

Lazarus, R.S., & Cohen, F. (1973). Active coping processes, coping dispositions, and recovery from surgery. *Psychosomatic Medicine, 35,* 375-389.

Lazarus, R.S., & Cohen, J.B. (1977). Environmental stress. In I. Altman & J.F. Wohlwill (Eds.), *Human behavior and the environment: Current theory and research* (pp. 90-127). New York: Plenum Press.

Lazarus, R.S., & Folkman, S. (1984). *Stress, appraisal, and coping.* New York: Springer.

Lazarus, R.S., & Launier, R. (1978). Stress-related transactions between person and environment. In L.A. Pervin & M. Lewis (Eds.), *Perspectives in interactional psychology* (pp. 287-327). New York: Plenum Press.

Leung, N., Waller, G., & Thomas, G. (1999). Core beliefs in anorexic and bulimic women. *Journal of Nervous & Mental Disease, 187* (2), 736-741.

Locke, S., & Colligan, D. (1986). *The healer within.* New York: Dutton.

Madden, T.J., Ellen, P., & Ajzen, I. (1992). A comparison of the theory of planned behaviour and the theory of reasoned action. *Personality & Social Psychology Bulletin, 18* (1), 3-9.

Maddux, J.E. (1993). Social cognitive models of health and exercise behavior: An introduction and review of conceptual issues. *Journal of Applied Sport Psychology, 5,* 116-140.

Mainwaring, L.M. (1999). Restoration of self: A model for the psychological response of athletes to severe knee injuries. *Canadian Journal of Rehabilitation, 12* (3), 145-154.

Minkler, M. (1986). The social component of health. *American Journal of Health Promotion, 1* (2), 33-38.

Mummery, W.K., & Wankel, L.M. (1999). Training adherence in adolescent competitive swimmers: An application of the theory of planned behavior. *Journal of Sport & Exercise Psychology, 21* (4), 313-328.

Murray, J.F. (1999). *Emotional adjustment to sport injury: Effects of injury severity, social support and athletic identity.* Unpublished doctoral dissertation, University of Florida.

Oatley, K., & Jenkins, J.M. (1996). *Understanding emotions.* Cambridge, MA: Blackwell Scientific.

Ogden, J. (1996). *Health psychology: A textbook.* Philadelphia: Open University Press.

Pennebaker, J.W. (Ed.). (1995). *Emotion, disclosure, and health.* Washington, DC: American Psychological Association.

Petitpas, A., & Danish, S.J. (1995). Caring for injured athletes. In S.M. Murphy (Ed.), *Sport psychology interventions* (pp. 255-281). Champaign, IL: Human Kinetics.

Picard, C.L. (1999). The level of competition as a factor for the development of eating disorders in female collegiate athletes. *Journal of Youth and Adolescence, 28* (5), 583-594.

Plante, T.G. (1999). Could the perception of fitness account for many of the mental and physical health benefits of exercise? *Advances in Mind-Body Medicine, 15* (4), 291-295.

Quah, R.S. (1985). The health belief model and preventative health behavior in Singapore. *Social Science and Medicine, 21,* 351-363.

Quinn, A.M., & Fallon, B.J. (1999). The changes in psychological characteristics and reactions of elite athletes from injury onset until full recovery. *Journal of Applied Sport Psychology, 11* (2), 210-229.

Roberto, K.A. (1992). Coping strategies of older women with hip fractures: Resources and outcomes. *Journals of Gerontology, 47* (1), 21-26.

Rosenstock, I.M. (1974). Historical origins of the health belief model. *Health Education Monograph, 2,* 409-419.

Rosenstock, I.M., Derryberry, M., & Carriger, B. (1959). Why people fail to seek poliomyelitis vaccination. *Public Health Reports, 74,* 98-103.

Rosenstock, I.M., Strecher, V.J., & Becker, M.H. (1988). Social learning theory and the health belief model. *Health Education Quarterly, 15,* 175-183.

Russell, D., & Cutrona, C.E. (1987). The provisions of social relationships and adaptation to stress. In W.H. Jones & D. Perleman (Eds.), *Advances in personal relationships* (Vol. 1, pp. 37-67). Greenwich, CT: JAI Press.

Ryska, T., & Yin, Z. (1999). Testing the buffering hypothesis: Perceptions of coach support and pre-competitive anxiety among male and female high school athletes. *Current Psychology: Developmental, Learning, Personality, Social, 18* (4), 381-393.

Sapp, S.G., & Jensen, H.H. (1998). An evaluation of the health belief model for predicting perceived and actual dietary quality. *Journal of Applied Social Psychology, 28* (3), 235-248.

Sarason, B.R., Shearin, E.N., Pierce, G.R., & Sarason, I.G. (1987). Helping police officers cope with stress: A cognitive-behavioral approach. *American Journal of Community Psychology, 7,* 593-603.

Sarason, I.G., Levine, H.M., Bashan, R.B., & Sarason, B.R. (1983). Assessing social support: The Social Support Questionnaire. *Journal of Personality and Social Psychology, 44,* 127-139.

Seeman, T.E., Kaplan, G.A., Knudsen, L., Cohen, R.D., & Guralnik, J.M. (1987). Social network ties and mortality among the elderly in the Alameda County study. *American Journal of Epidemiology, 126* (4), 714-723.

Seyle, H. (1956). *The stress of life.* New York: McGraw-Hill.

Shumaker, S.A., & Brownell, K. (1984). Toward a theory of social support: Closing conceptual gaps. *Journal of Social Issues, 40,* 11-36.

Smith, A.M., Scott, S.G., & Wiese, D.M. (1990). The psychological effects of sports injuries: Coping. *Sports Medicine, 9,* 352-369.

Soo Hoo, W.E. (1999). *Evaluation of the health belief model as a predictor of HIV self- protective behavior.* Unpublished doctoral dissertation, University of Southern California.

Steptoe, A. (1992). The links between stress and illness. *Journal of Psychosomatic Research, 35* (6), 633-644.

Suarez de Balcazar, Y., Seekins, T., Paine, A., Fawcett, S.B., & Mathews, R.M. (1989). Self-help and social support groups for people with disabilities: A descriptive report. *Rehabilitation Counseling Bulletin, 33* (2), 151-158.

Syme, L.S. (1987). Coronary artery disease: A sociocultural perspective. *Circulation 76* (Supplement I), I-II2.

Tak, S.H. (1998). *Chronic daily stress, coping strategies and resources, and life satisfaction among older women with osteoarthritis.* Unpublished doctoral dissertation, University of Texas at Austin.

Taub, D.E., & Blinde, E.M. (1992). Eating disorders among adolescent female athletes: Influence of ath-letic participation and sport team membership. *Adolescence, 27,* 833-848.

Taylor, S.E., Falke, R.L., Shoptaw, S.J., & Lichtman, R.R. (1986). Social support, support groups, and the cancer patient. *Journal of Consulting and Clinical Psychology, 54* (5), 608-615.

Terris, M. (1975). Approaches to an epidemiology of health. *American Journal of Public Health, 65,* 1037-1045.

Tessier, R., Fillion, L., Muckle, G., & Gendron, M. (1990). Quelques mesures-criteres de stress et la prediction de l'etat de sante physique. Une etude longitudinale [Some criterion-measures of stress and the prediction of physical health. A longitudinal study]. *Canadian Journal of Behavioral Science, 22,* 271-281.

Thoresen, C.E. (1984). Overview. In J.D. Matarazzo, S.M. Weiss, J.A. Herd, N.E. Miller, & S.M. Weiss (Eds.), *Behavioral health: A handbook of health enhancement and disease prevention* (pp. 297-307). New York: Wiley.

Udry, E. (1997). Coping and social support among injured athletes following surgery. *Journal of Sport & Exercise Psychology, 19,* 71-90.

Umberson, D. (1987). Family status and health behaviors: Social control as a dimension of social integration. *Journal of Health & Social Behavior, 28* (3), 306-319.

Vaux, A. (1988). *Social support: Theory, research, and intervention.* New York: Praeger Publishers.

Vlahos, A.J. (1998). *Interpersonal, individual, and situational factors associated with burnout in student-athletes.* Unpublished doctoral dissertation, Michigan State University.

Wallston, B.S., & Wallston, K.A. (1984). Social psychological models of health behavior. An examination and integration. In A. Baum, S.E. Taylor, & J.E. Singer (Eds.), *Handbook of psychology and health (Vol. 4): Social psychological aspects of health.* Hillsdale, NJ: Erlbaum.

Wallston, K. (1992). Hocus-pocus, the focus isn't strictly on locus: Rotter's social learning theory modified for health. *Cognitive Therapy and Research, 16,* 183-199.

Wallston, K.A., Alagna, S.W., De Vellis, B.M., & De Vellis, R.F. (1983). Social support and physical illness. *Health Psychology, 2,* 367-391.

Weiss, M.R. (1974). The provision of social relationships. In Z. Rubin (Ed.), *Doing unto others* (pp. 17-26). Englewood Cliffs, NJ: Prentice Hall.

Williams, J.M. (1996). Stress, coping resources and injury risk. *International Journal of Stress Management, 3* (4), 209-221.

Williams, J.M., Rotella, R.J., & Heyman, S.R. (1998). Stress, injury, and the psychological rehabilitation of athletes. In J.M. Williams (Ed.), *Applied sport psychology: Personal growth to peak performance* (pp. 409-428). Mountain View, CA: Mayfield.

World Health Organization. (1948). *Constitution of the World Health Organization.* Geneva: World Health Organization.

Yates, B.C. (1996). The relationship among social support and short- and long-term recovery outcomes in men with coronary heart disease. *Research in Nursing & Health, 18* (3), 193-203.

Yeager, K.K., Agostini, R., Nattiv, A., & Drinkwater, B. (1993). The female athlete triad: Disordered eating, amenorrhea, osteoporosis. *Medicine and Science in Sports and Exercise, 25,* 775-777.

Young, J.E. (1994). *Cognitive therapy for personality disorders: A schema-focused approach.* Sarasota, FL: Professional Resource Press/Professional Resource Exchange, Inc.

Zimmerman, R.S., & Conner, C. (1989). Health promotion in context: The effects of significant others on health behavior change. *Health Education Quarterly, 16,* 57-75.

Wrisberg, C.A., & Johnson, M.S. (2002). Quality of life. In M. Kellmann (Ed.), *Enhancing recovery: Preventing underperformance in athletes* (pp. 253-267). Champaign, IL: Human Kinetics.

14

Quality of Life

Craig A. Wrisberg and Matthew S. Johnson

You just get tired of the same old routine and having to deal with it.

National champion, NCAA Division I springboard diver

When you do it [train, condition, compete] every day it gets boring and you begin to think "God, this is terrible—if I don't get a break soon I'm going to go nuts!"

NCAA Division I tennis player

The primary theme of this book is that optimal recovery is an important, yet frequently overlooked, element of successful performance. In the opening chapter, Michael Kellmann suggests that athletes rarely monitor their levels of stress in a systematic fashion. As a result, they may find themselves experiencing staleness and even burnout without knowing why. To reduce the probability of such occurrences, Kellmann suggests that athletes be encouraged to assess their stress and recovery activities periodically to be sure that they are maintaining an optimal recovery-stress balance.

In this chapter the concept of quality of life (QOL) and its possible relationship to the recovery-stress balance is discussed. More specifically, attention is devoted to aspects of athletes' lives that have the potential to either enhance or diminish their ability to maintain an optimal balance. The literature that is cited in this chapter is representative of studies that have examined the life experiences of athletes within the context of training and competition. Particular emphasis is given to qualitative research involving interviews with a variety of performers. Thus, in this chapter the reader will encounter the "voices" of athletes who regularly experience the struggle of maintaining an optimal recovery-stress balance and preserving their QOL in the midst of intense demands.

The chapter begins with a brief description of the most prominent definitions of QOL that have been proposed in the scientific literature and a discussion of the methods used by researchers attempting to measure life quality. Separate sections are then devoted to a synthesis of the findings from quantitative and qualitative studies that suggest ways athletes' QOL is enhanced or compromised by life events they experience on a regular basis. The chapter concludes with suggestions for optimizing athletes' recovery-stress balance and QOL.

Defining and Measuring Quality of Life

Quality of life is a term common to a number of disciplines ranging from economics to nursing (Dijkers, 1999). Not surprisingly, QOL has been broadly defined and conceptualized. Generally speaking, it is presumed to be an abstract concept composed of a constellation of factors. At any point in time a person's overall QOL can range from low to high, depending on the level of quality of the composite of QOL factors. Components of QOL contained in most existing definitions include the degree of physical, mental, emotional, and/or spiritual health, life satisfaction, the possession of socially desirable characteristics, and positive affect (Dijkers, 1999).

Although considerable philosophical differences exist among the numerous definitions and conceptualizations of QOL (Farquhar, 1995; Mor & Guadagnoli, 1988), most seem to emphasize the *perception of the individual* in question. For example, Dalkey, Lewis, and Snyder (1972) and Pflaum (1973), respectively, define QOL as the *degree* of satisfaction of an individual's *perceived* psychophysiologic needs and the *degree* to which individuals *perceive* the environment as facilitating or retarding their essential functioning.

To date, most researchers have used a quantitative approach to measure QOL. In the majority of studies, respondents are asked to complete a questionnaire containing a variety of QOL components. Such questionnaires are classified as either objective or subjective (Dijkers, 1999). Objective questionnaires are based on the assumption that all people share similar opinions about the components that constitute life quality. These types of questionnaires contain components that are usually determined by the person(s) developing the instrument, with little or no input from the prospective respondents. Subjective questionnaires, on the other hand, are based on the assumption that individuals themselves are the best judge of the components and level of their own QOL. There-

fore, subjective instruments begin with a section in which respondents are asked to list the components *they feel* are most salient to their own QOL. Having done this, respondents are then instructed to rate the *current level* of their QOL for each component listed. (For a more comprehensive review of methodological issues surrounding the development and use of objective and subjective questionnaires, see Dijkers, 1999.)

In recent years, there has been a growing debate over whether quantitative approaches—even those of a subjective nature—are the best means of evaluating QOL. As Dijkers (1999) pointed out:

The debate as to whether QOL should be measured and whether it can be measured clearly is based on value judgments and epistemological assumptions. (For instance, "The multidimensionality of life can be summarized into a single judgment without losing essential information," "People have given thought to their quality of life and, upon request, can rate their satisfaction with specific domains of life.") Beyond that, even the basic step of selection of a measurement approach reflects assumptions that may not be shared by everyone (Dijkers, 1999, p. 291).

As an alternative to quantitative measurement, Dijkers (1999) suggested that qualitative methods be employed by researchers who wish to (1) accurately identify the domains of QOL for a particular individual, (2) determine the standards the person uses to evaluate each domain, and (3) identify ways the individual calibrates those standards.

A primary vehicle of qualitative research studies is the interview. The purpose of qualitative interviews is to obtain as rich a description as possible of some aspect of a person's life experience (e.g., the athlete's experience of training and competing)—in the person's own words. Depending on the purpose of the study, the researcher selects the most appropriate interview format and data analysis procedure (see Berg, 1995, for an overview of possible interview formats). Once the interview is completed, the researcher transcribes the individual's audiotaped comments, then organizes them into thematic categories. Each category, or *theme,* presumably represents an essential component of the person's experience.

The key criterion of validity in qualitative research is that a reader adopting the same viewpoint as the researcher be able to see the same things the researcher saw, regardless of whether the reader agrees with the researcher's interpretation (Giorgi, 1970). To achieve this criterion, the qualitative researcher typically uses an interpretive group to obtain consensus regarding the themes that seem to characterize participants' experiences. In addition, the researcher maintains a dialogue with participants to assure that the thematic structure identified by the researcher and the interpretive group represents an accurate depiction of the participant's life experience.

In the following two sections, discussion is devoted to some of the research that has examined aspects of athletes' life experiences that enhance or diminish their QOL. In the first section a brief overview of the results of quantitative studies is presented. Then a considerably longer section is offered that contains examples of qualitative research examining the experiences of athletes.

Quantitative Studies of QOL

To date, quantitative investigations of QOL have primarily been conducted on clinical populations. Participants in these studies have usually been individuals who have experienced one or more of a variety of physical and mental threats to QOL. Examples of such clinical studies include those that have assessed the QOL of language-disabled adults (Lomas, Pickard, & Mohide, 1987), individuals with long-term mental illness (Fabian, 1990), patients undergoing hip replacement (O'Boyle, McGee, Hickey, O'Malley, & Joyce, 1992), patients with closed-head injury (Klonoff, Costa, & Snow, 1986), cancer patients (Kreitler, Chaitchik, Rapoport, Kreitler, & Algor, 1993), and patients with chronic illnesses (Adang, Kootstra, Baeten, & Engel, 1997).

Very little quantitative research has examined the QOL of athletes. One exception is a study conducted in 1982 by Morris, Lussier, Vaccaro, and Clarke. The purpose of this investigation was to determine the levels of various components of QOL of 10 nationally ranked female distance runners compared to those of a group of nonathletes. To achieve this objective, the researchers administered Pflaum's (1973) Life Quality Inventory to all participants. The inventory is an objective questionnaire that addresses four fundamental categories of QOL:

1. Biophysical functioning (e.g., physical well-being)
2. Self-development and personal growth (e.g., self-acceptance)

3. Primary social functioning (e.g., in face-to-face relationships)
4. Secondary social functioning (e.g., within a group or in an institutional context)

The results of the Morris et al. (1982) study revealed no differences between the groups for any of the individual QOL components. However, the total QOL score of the elite athlete group was found to be significantly higher than that of the nonathletes. Thus, it appears that the experience of competitive running may have contributed in a generally positive fashion to the QOL of these women athletes. However, the authors offered no discussion of possible reasons for this advantage. Moreover, it should be noted that the instrument used in this study was one that was validated on a population of individuals that included disabled persons, university professors, clinical psychologists, and university administrators. Thus, it is possible that at least some of the items participants responded to were not particularly appropriate for assessing the QOL of elite athletes.

In contrast, the possibility that QOL may not be as high for athletes as for a comparison group of nonathletes was suggested by the results of a more recent and extensive quantitative investigation conducted by the American Institutes for Research (1988a, 1988b). This study was sponsored by the Presidents' Commission of the National Collegiate Athletic Association (NCAA) and represented an attempt to assess the effect of participation in intercollegiate athletics on the lives of more than 4,000 student-athletes from Division I universities. The comparison group consisted of individuals who were involved in nonathletic extracurricular activities (e.g., drama, marching band) involving a time commitment similar to that required of student-athletes. All participants completed a questionnaire that assessed their personal experiences (i.e., social experiences, educational experiences) and self-descriptions (e.g., self-esteem, locus of control).

The results of this study suggested that several aspects of the lives of student-athletes from "big-time" athletic programs contribute to heightened levels of stress and lowered levels of recovery (see Wrisberg, 1996, for a more detailed discussion). For example, athletes reported spending more time per week in their sport, missing more classes, and spending less time participating in outside extracurricular activities than did individuals in the comparison group. Moreover, athletes, particularly those participating in high-visibility, revenue-generating sports (i.e., football, basketball), performed at a lower level academically, experienced "intense" or "extremely intense" pressure to ignore physical injury and pain, and were "bothered" or "greatly bothered" by extreme tiredness or exhaustion. Compared to the control participants, athletes perceived that their actions were controlled to a greater extent by "chance" or "powerful others." Although the athletes indicated that they found it easier to travel to new places and to obtain summer jobs, they expressed a lower level of overall satisfaction with their performance than did individuals in the control group. Taken together, the findings of this study offered little support for the notion that scholarship collegiate student-athletes experience high levels of QOL.

Of relevance to this chapter, the results of this large-scale investigation suggest that NCAA Division I student-athletes spend most of their time doing, witnessing, or talking about activities related to their sport and have little additional time for recovery activities. Moreover, it appears that many of these individuals experience several sources of stress that might be expected to affect their recovery-stress balance and QOL. For example, athletes who demonstrated deficient academic performance possibly experienced increased stress because of a fear of being academically disqualified from competing, or perhaps of being dismissed from the university altogether. In addition, athletes who felt pressured to perform while injured could have experienced an increase in stress level because of a worry that their impaired physical condition would reduce their capability of meeting the demands of training and competition or increase their risk of an even more serious injury.

To summarize, the results of the limited available quantitative research seem to indicate that athletes experience unique sources of stress that diminish their QOL. Less clear are the specific aspects of life quality that are compromised as a result of participation in high-performance sport.

Table 14.1 Summary of Qualitative Research Assessing Experiences of Athletes

Authors	Participants/sport(s)	Purpose
Gould, Guinan, Greenleaf, et al. (1999)	U.S. Olympic athletes from more and less successful teams (12 females, 11 males)	Positive and negative factors influencing performance
Gould, Jackson, & Finch (1993a)	U.S. national champion figure skaters (10 females, 7 males)	Positive and negative aspects of being a national champion
Gould, Jackson, & Finch (1993b)	U.S. national champion figure skaters (10 females, 7 males)	Sources of stress
Gould, Tuffey, Udry, & Loehr (1996)	Former U.S. junior national tennis players (6 females, 4 males)	Sources of burnout
Gould, Tuffey, Udry, & Loehr (1997)	Former U.S. junior national tennis players (2 females, 1 male)	Sources of burnout
Scanlan, Stein, & Ravizza (1989)	Former U.S. national champion figure skating competitors (11 females, 15 males)	Sources of enjoyment
Scanlan, Stein, & Ravizza (1991)	Former U.S. national champion figure skating competitors (11 females, 15 males)	Sources of stress
Wrisberg (1996)	Inductive analysis of published literature containing quotes from a wide variety of athletes representing different sports	Factors influencing life quality
Wrisberg, Johnson, & Brooks (2000)	NCAA Division I student-athletes from a variety of sports (6 females, 6 males)	Experience of life as a university student

Qualitative Studies of QOL

As mentioned earlier, there is a growing feeling that qualitative approaches may offer a more effective means of assessing individuals' QOL than quantitative approaches do. For one thing, qualitative methods allow researchers considerably more flexibility in obtaining information about the exact nature of people's life experiences.

During the 1990s, a number of qualitative studies were conducted to determine salient aspects of the competitive experiences of elite athletes. A representative sample of this research is presented in table 14.1. The purpose of qualitative research is to identify prominent themes that, taken together, characterize the unified whole of participants' experiences. Different themes may be more or less salient to different participants. The objective of qualitative research is not to generalize findings to a larger population but rather to accurately describe the experiences of a qualified subgroup of individuals who have experienced the phenomenon in question (in this case, athletes who have experienced sources of stress and enjoyment). Therefore, sample size is not such a critical issue for qualitative researchers. The pattern of results arising from interviews with athletes suggests that they experience a wide variety of sources of stress and enjoyment that have the potential to affect not only their recovery-stress balance but also their QOL.

In this section, themes that have emerged from the studies listed in table 14.1 are discussed in relationship to the four categories of QOL identified by Pflaum (1973). As mentioned previously, those categories are: (1) biophysical functioning (e.g., physical well-being), (2) self-development and personal growth (e.g., self-acceptance), (3) primary social functioning (i.e., in face-to-face relationships), and (4) secondary social functioning (i.e., within a group or in an institutional context). A graphic depiction of the contribution of Pflaum's four categories of QOL to overall QOL is presented in figure 14.1.

The following discussion also contains numerous quotes from the participants of the selected studies listed in table 14.1. The majority of these quotes come from a recent interview study with NCAA Division I student-athletes representing a variety of sports (Wrisberg, Johnson, & Brooks, 2000). Participants in the Wrisberg et al. (2000) study were asked to respond to the following open-ended question: *As you reflect on your experiences as a university student, what kinds of things stand out for you?* It is important to note that participants were asked to talk about their experiences as college students rather than as college athletes. That all participants spoke almost exclusively about their experiences as student-athletes suggests that their sport participation was a prominent activity for them during their years at the university.

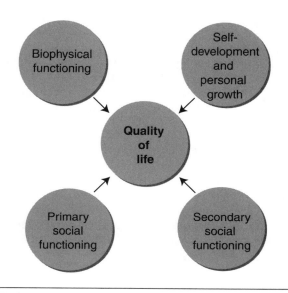

Figure 14.1 Four categories of quality of life that contribute to overall quality of life.

Adapted from Pflaum, 1973.

Biophysical Functioning

Health and fitness are essential ingredients for elite athletes who aspire to perform at near-peak levels on a consistent basis. Feeling strong and capable is one aspect of biophysical functioning that minimizes athletes' stress and enhances their QOL. Simply put, athletes enjoy feeling fit. The comment of a former elite figure skater suggests that she enjoyed the feeling of training hard.

—I think the biggest thrill I had was the actual performance and training. . . . I felt real good like if I'd worked real hard and I was exhausted. And I'd come home and go to bed and my legs would ache and I just felt like I could hardly be alive. And I liked that. (Scanlan, Stein, & Ravizza, 1989, p. 79)

In some cases, athletes derive pleasure from strength and conditioning activities associated with their sport. The following quote from a college softball player suggests that she and her teammates had fun during strength and conditioning workouts because of the type of atmosphere created by the conditioning coach.

— We had fun in the weight room 'cause we had a trainer who was just really silly. She'd play music during our cardiovascular workout, and then we'd dance a little bit. Weights were fun. We got to talking, you know, and really enjoyed the workout. (Wrisberg et al., 2000)

Obviously, the demands of training are not always pleasurable, but, as the following comment of a collegiate springboard diver suggests, such demands are accepted by athletes as necessary aspects of their lives.

— In my sport we have a 6 A.M. practice, so there's no like staying out really late at night . . . like at a place that's really hopping on Wednesday night. Hmm, I wonder how many times I've gone out on Wednesday night! Alright, maybe I've been in the library, but I haven't been out playing or partying or whatever. So, that's what I mean I guess about being an athlete. (Wrisberg et al., 2000)

Unfortunately, many athletes succumb to the notion that more training is better. As the following comments suggest, some performers are aware of this tendency, whereas others are not. One athlete felt that the tendency to overtrain might have been a reason his team underachieved during the 1996 Olympic Games.

— Sometimes you go a little overboard on [training]). . . . I think the last weeks that we did. (Gould, Guinan, Greenleaf, Medberry, & Peterson, 1999, p. 389)

A similar sentiment was expressed by the following U.S. junior national tennis player who had suffered from burnout.

— I was almost too motivated . . . trying to do too much, more than my body can handle. (Gould, Tuffey, Udry, & Loehr, 1997, p. 269)

Occasionally, athletes observe overtraining tendencies on the part of their teammates. One college tennis player said he worried about a teammate who perpetually placed himself at risk of injury by long-term overtraining.

— One guy on the team doesn't know when to stop with his training. He's a great guy but he works too hard and now he has a stress fracture in his back. Last year he broke a foot. He goes too much. He wants it too bad. (Wrisberg et al., 2000)

Some athletes long-term overtrain because they have been socialized to believe that rest and recovery is a sign of weakness. One college distance runner said he felt guilty for taking a day off.

— I feel like I'm weak if I decide to take a day off. It's like, I'm not, you know—I set pretty high standards, you know—if you can't get out there and run, then what are you doing running (NCAA) Division I track? (Wrisberg et al., 2000)

A common end product of long-term overtraining is injury, which is perhaps the biggest threat to the biophysical functioning of athletes. As the comments of the following individuals suggest, injury is something they accept and endure on a regular basis. One college football player said this:

— When I had that groin injury (the coaches) made me scrimmage anyway. . . . I mean, I had no business being out there. (Wrisberg et al., 2000)

The following college track and field performer spoke of her frustration with foot injuries and the ongoing experience of rehabilitation and treatment needed for her to be able to return to competition in as short a time as possible.

— It just always seems to be the feet . . . different parts of the feet . . . now they are saying that it is arthritis so it'll be just . . . I'll always have some kind of injury, some kind of problem. It's just a matter of getting it well so that I can compete again later or the next day. (Wrisberg et al., 2000)

A serious threat to the quality of biophysical functioning mentioned by some athletes is weight control. This is particularly the case for individuals who compete in sports that have an aesthetic component (e.g., gymnastics, figure skating, diving) or that favor leaner people. As the following comment of a figure skater suggests, the pressure of maintaining body weight continually bombards such athletes.

— You should do a whole story on weight in figure skating; it is such an appearance sport. You have to go up there with barely anything on. . . . It's not like I'm really skinny or anything, but I'm defi-

nitely aware of it. I mean I have dreams about it sometimes. So it's hard having people look at my thigh and saying, "Oops, she's an eighth of an inch bigger," or something. It's hard . . . . Weight is continually on my mind. I am never, never allowed to be on a vacation. Weight is always on my mind. (Gould, Jackson, & Finch, 1993a, p. 149)

One source of stress for some athletes is travel, particularly when trips are long and buses are the mode of transportation. The following remark by a college soccer player indicates how exhausting this form of travel was for her.

— Travel (by bus) is physically draining. I would rather play two games at home than take an entire weekend to travel somewhere to play one game. You can go home and sleep in your own bed. Your books are there. You can study. (Wrisberg et al., 2000)

In summary, several aspects of athletes' life experiences appear to represent threats to the quality of their biophysical functioning. Although the comments of individuals presented in this section suggest that intense, short-term overtraining can be a source of enjoyment and contribute to an athlete's improved self-efficacy, they also illustrate how long-term overtraining can threaten QOL when the athlete succumbs to the notion that more is better, chronically overtrains to the point of injury, and worries excessively about body weight.

Self-Development and Personal Growth

Another component of life quality identified by Pflaum (1973) is self-development and personal growth. Like everyone else, athletes experience a higher level of QOL when they are able to engage in the kinds of activities that allow them to grow as human beings. Unfortunately, interview data suggest that several factors may prevent athletes from achieving the type of personal growth they long for.

For some athletes the biggest deterrent to self-development is their own perfectionist tendencies. Sadly, people who refuse to accept anything less than perfection are unable to experience the satisfaction that comes from improved performance (Henschen, 1998). The following comment by an elite figure skater illustrates the frustration that can accompany an athlete's expectations of perfection.

— I was a perfectionist . . . that's probably the hardest thing; I was just a perfectionist all the time. . . . I would never accept myself not doing it perfectly. (Scanlan, Stein, & Ravizza, 1991, p. 115)

Without exception, the most pervasive deterrent to athletes' personal improvement and self-development seems to be the virtual absence of discretionary time. In practically every study listed in table 14.1 (p. 256), athletes expressed frustration over the limited amount of time they had to pursue activities outside their sports. Indeed, athletes' lives appear to be continuously occupied by events and people competing for their time (e.g., physical training, schoolwork, family, friends, coaches, teammates, support staff, intimate relationships).

Routine demands on athletes' time include a long training season, travel, and other sport-related activities. The accumulated effect of such multiple demands is often a feeling of powerlessness. The following comment by a college basketball player indicates that her competitive experience included a reluctant acceptance of a high level of tedium.

—At this level, the season is so long. And then there's the traveling and schoolwork and everything. It's really hard balancing basketball with your personal time . . . which basically you don't have any of. (Wrisberg et al., 2000)

A junior national tennis player who had suffered burnout described the demands of high-level competitive sport participation in a more succinct fashion:

— I completely had no social life whatsoever. I wouldn't do anything except tennis and study. (Gould, Tuffey, Udry, & Loehr, 1997, p. 264)

Athletes who compete at the university level often experience a lockstep schedule necessitated by the competing demands of academic and athletic activities. The following comments by a college distance runner are representative of the daily experience of many scholarship student-athletes.

— Well, it's like, the way it is now, everything is set in a routine. It's almost like I go through the day like a zombie. I wake up at 6 A.M. to go for a morning run, run a few miles, and come back. I've got to eat breakfast in like 30 minutes and get a

shower, drive to campus for class from like 8 to 12 or so, get home, get lunch, sometimes get a nap, then go to track practice from 3 to 6, come back home, watch TV, study, and fall asleep. Next day, you get up and it's pretty much the same thing. So, if you want to go out and be social, you have to sacrifice something, you know. If I go out tonight, I won't be able to get up early tomorrow morning, or it'll be really hard. So, it's almost like you can't do things because of that. That's what really bums you, that schedule you have to keep. (Wrisberg et al., 2000)

Another college track and field athlete described the pressure he felt from having to juggle all of his required activities in a limited time frame.

— Right now is a really tough week. I've got a few tests and I've got a big race coming up. I feel like I have a lot of expectations—people expecting a lot of me. It's almost like everyone that expects one thing of me doesn't realize that I have other things going on, too. You've got one class and the teacher is assigning all kinds of stuff, so she doesn't think I could have other things and have a life and have other classes. And with track, it's the same story. (Wrisberg et al., 2000)

A college golfer expressed how the quality of his sport performance suffered when he was distracted by problems in the classroom.

— When I was struggling with a class, I found myself regretting going to the golf course. I couldn't concentrate on what I was doing. At practice I just tended to go through the motions. (Wrisberg et al., 2000)

When athletes feel overburdened by their routine activities, even the slightest additional demand can elicit a high level of stress and frustration. The following comment by a college tennis player illustrates how an additional inconvenience was particularly irritating.

— (The university) provided me with housing, but soon after I moved in I found out there was a leak in the ceiling . . . so I had to move out. They wanted to assign me to another place but it was noisy. Finally, I got a place I liked. But it was all such a hassle. Here I have to move all my stuff into one place and then five days later I have to move everything out of there and into another place. It was all such a waste of time and a real irritation. (Wrisberg et al., 2000)

On rare occasions athletes have the opportunity to protest additional impositions on their personal time. One college springboard diver described an experience she had in a meeting with athletic officials who were trying to implement more informational seminars for athletes.

— They're (athletic officials) talking about implementing more programs for athletes— more seminars that take about two hours each. So I speak up and say "Hey guys, we don't have any more time!" And they're like "Well wait, you need to know about this and you need to know about that." So I say, "That's great but there comes a point in time when you are putting too much on athletes. I mean we reach a point where we don't even care anymore." We just have to have some time for ourselves and I'm afraid they don't understand that. (Wrisberg et al., 2000)

Family members, friends, coaches, roommates, and others can also occupy athletes' discretionary time. Such interactions may serve to facilitate or diminish the quality of athletes' personal growth and self-development. A college volleyball player spoke of the stress imposed by a demanding roommate.

— My roommate is one of those people who seem to need some sort of chaos in her life all the time. I've just become a victim of the chaos she needs in her life. I dread going home at night. (Wrisberg et al., 2000)

In some cases athletes are able to find the time to engage in activities that promote recovery. The following college softball player spoke of several outside activities that she enjoyed with a supportive teammate.

— Outside of practice we'll go to the movies or we'll talk, go to Bible study or something together. She [teammate] is there for me and I'm there for her. (Wrisberg et al., 2000)

Some athletes seem to be aware of the importance of recovery activities and of maintaining balance in their lives. Such was the case for the following college tennis player.

— I like to do a little bit of everything. I like to watch old Western movies. I like to read the newspaper. I like to shop. I like to play tennis. I like to write. When I have good balance in my life, I feel like I'm on top of the world. (Wrisberg et al., 2000)

A highlight of the competitive experience of many athletes is the opportunity for travel. A number of individuals mentioned how much they enjoyed the times they had when competing at faraway locations. For some individuals, travel represented a temporary escape from the demands of their everyday lives. Travel was clearly a highlight in the experience of the following track and field athlete.

> *— Traveling is like my favorite thing. It's like a big vacation every weekend. You travel with the guys that you know real well and you have a good time. They give you meal money and you get whatever you want to eat. It's so nice to just get away from the grind for a while. (Wrisberg et al., 2000)*

A college tennis player related a particularly enjoyable experience he had during his conference's indoor championship tournament.

> *— We had the conference championships in New Orleans one year. It was the best week of my life. The amount of resources available to us is just amazing. I mean, we had our own plane. We stayed at the Hilton. The courts are right inside the hotel. We got a lot of meal money. Coach just said, you know, "Enjoy yourself. Go look around." We practiced at certain hours. It was great. (Wrisberg et al., 2000)*

Many athletes realize that their participation in sport affords them opportunities to go places and see things they might otherwise never experience. Such was the case for the following college golfer and springboard diver, respectively.

> *— Traveling is unbelievable . . . the opportunities they give us here . . . going to places like Mexico, Las Vegas, San Francisco . . . just experiences like that I would have never got to do if I wasn't a collegiate athlete. (Wrisberg et al., 2000)*

> *— One of my teammates and I both qualified for the World Championships in Rome. After competition on the last night, I said to him, "Let's walk around the old city." So here we are walking around Rome in the early hours of the morning. What an awesome experience that was! It might never have happened if I wasn't an athlete. (Wrisberg et al., 2000)*

In summary, the comments of athletes obtained from qualitative interviews suggest that sport participation can retard their personal growth and self-development in several ways. The most prominent appears to be the lack of time available to engage in recovery activities outside the sporting environment. Athletes are keenly aware of the demands placed on them by sport-related activi-

ties and, for student-athletes, school-related expectations. When all of the required time demands are added up, there is very little time left for anything else; and this is frustrating for athletes. A few individuals find ways to engage in occasional outside activities, either by themselves or with a friend, whereas others experience additional drains on their discretionary time as a result of other demands (e.g., a "high maintenance" roommate). One aspect of athletes' lives that contributes to their personal growth is travel. Athletes appreciate the opportunities they have to experience new places and to enjoy a break from their everyday routines. Unfortunately, it appears that, for the most part, the recovery-stress balance of high-performance athletes may be compromised by the relative lack of opportunity to engage in active recovery activities.

Primary Social Functioning

Another component of athletes' lives that affects their stress and recovery levels is the quality of their primary social functioning. Relationships with family members and significant others have the potential to enhance or diminish athletes' overall QOL.

A concern for some athletes is the financial pressure that their sport participation places on their family's resources. One figure skater commented that the monetary costs of her sport were a source of stress for her family that created considerable tension.

> *— My family was always under financial burdens, sacrificing everything so I could skate. We didn't have the money, and things were going really bad, and it was like . . . caused a lot of tension, you know. We haven't got the money. How else are you gonna make your house payment? Or, you don't know how you're going to pay for the coach or lessons or whatever. (Scanlan, Stein, & Ravizza, 1991, p. 114)*

Occasionally, athletes attempt to relieve some of their family's financial responsibilities by seeking employment during the off-season. However, such well-intentioned gestures can exact their own toll on the athlete. One college track and field athlete expressed the frustration he felt as a result of adding summer employment to his already busy schedule.

> *— During the summer I wanted to help Dad pay for things so I got a job serving at a restaurant and pretty much worked double shifts*

every day. I was running in between shifts and then running again at night . . . sometimes after midnight. I tried to take a class but had to drop it. I think I wore down and wasn't ready when classes resumed. . . . I didn't have the drive I needed. (Wrisberg et al., 2000)

Family members can also be an important source of support and encouragement for athletes. When that's the case, visits home can help individuals recover from the demands of their sport. Such was the experience of the following college softball player.

— Winter vacation I just spent it mostly with my family . . . most of the time just soaking up love from my family. (Wrisberg et al., 2000)

For other athletes, trips home represent an additional source of stress rather than recovery. A college distance runner spoke of the difficulty he faced when returning home to visit his divorced parents.

— My parents are divorced so it's sort of a soap opera when I go back home. I don't look forward to it and I don't like to deal with it. (Wrisberg et al., 2000)

Athletes often find themselves struggling to meet the demands of their sport when they are experiencing problems with their families. One college football player described the problems his father was facing and how this situation created considerable concern for him and his family.

— My father had gotten laid off, you know, from his job and everything and that was really tough on my family and all that. . . . That's when he started his drug use, he started experimenting with the "crack."

He and my mother weren't getting along and my sister was just a teenager and had no guidance from my folks at all. It was just awful. (Wrisberg et al., 2000)

Of all family members, fathers exert perhaps the biggest influence on athletes' lives. Unfortunately, for many athletes, their fathers represent a serious source of stress. The following comment by a junior national tennis player who had experienced burnout illustrates this phenomenon.

— My biggest problem was there was no separation between the role of the father and the coach. So we wouldn't talk about anything else but tennis whether we were eating or if there was a match on television. Everyone had to watch it and

he'd comment, and whether or not you agreed with him, it didn't matter 'cause, you know, he was always right. You had to do it this way and, you know, he always made us do certain exercises when he wanted and was very strict on getting things done the way he thought, and he didn't leave any room for like personal feelings. (Gould, Tuffey, Udry, & Loehr, 1997, p. 265)

Relationships with significant others can also represent sources of support or stress for athletes, depending on the nature of the relationship. Several athletes stated that their lives were made easier by intimate relationships. As one college volleyball player put it:

— He (boyfriend) makes me feel so good about myself. He is so, just affectionate and sweet, and so loving and caring. I don't know if I'd make it without all of his support. (Wrisberg et al., 2000)

A college tennis player who was a native of Scandinavia and attending school in the United States conveyed a similar experience.

— My second year in school, my girlfriend came over (from Czechoslovakia) and we started living together. It was all new and very exciting. I was playing tennis a lot but she was not in school and had a lot of time. She brought more stability to my life. I think I got a lot more peace and rest. (Wrisberg et al., 2000)

A college baseball player said that the fact that his girlfriend was also an athlete made it easier for her to provide him with the kind of support he needed.

— My girlfriend is an athlete too so she helps me put things in perspective. She really understands what I'm going through. (Wrisberg et al., 2000)

The fact that intimate relationships can also be a source of stress for athletes is illustrated by the comments of the following collegiate swimmer.

— My relationship with my girlfriend was such a roller coaster. She'd let me in close and then just push me away. It just about drove me crazy. (Wrisberg et al., 2000)

A female track and field athlete spoke of the stress she experienced when a prospective suitor refused to leave her alone.

— One guy I dated a few times started harassing me . . . wanting me to go out all the time,

sending me flowers and stuff like that. Finally, I had to call the cops to make him stop. It was kind of scary. (Wrisberg et al., 2000)

In summary, primary social functioning is one aspect of athletes' lives that has the potential to provide significant support and encouragement or to create considerable stress and deplete emotional energy. Athletes appreciate the support of significant others who help them achieve an optimal recovery-stress balance and maintain a healthy perspective on their lives. However, when many athletes speak of their families, they describe them as sources of stress rather than of enjoyment. It is particularly stressful for athletes when one or more of their family members is in crisis or when they feel that their sport participation represents a significant drain on their family's financial resources. Intimate relationships can either energize or stress athletes, depending on whether their significant other is a source of support or of trauma.

Secondary Social Functioning

In addition to relationships with family members and significant others, athletes encounter a variety of other types of people within the context of their sporting experiences. Such secondary social functioning represents another possible source of support or stress. Moreover, it is clear from the comments of athletes that they are abundantly aware of the expectations people they encounter in the sport context have of them. As one elite figure skater put it:

— Expectations are definitely a concern and they are not a superficial one. Will I measure up to other people's expectations? It is much easier when you don't have any expectations, because if you don't do very well, people just don't notice you; you can always do better next year. But if you do bad with expectations upon you, they condemn you, so that's a stress factor. (Gould, Jackson, & Finch, 1993a, p. 147)

The pressure of others' expectations can be compounded when athletes perceive that their prospects for success are threatened by the presence of more experienced or talented competitors. The following comment by a college swimmer illustrates how stressful such perceptions of inadequacy can be.

— I went to NCAA's and it was unbelievable the people I saw there. It was huge names in swimming and I felt so out of place . . . like I didn't

belong in the same pool with them. I had a really bad asthma attack and I think maybe part of that could have been the anxiety. I was completely psyched out. (Wrisberg et al., 2000)

Athletes who compete at the international level know that they must be politically astute if they hope to have any chance of succeeding. This type of awareness is reflected by the following comment of an elite figure skater who knew that she had

— to politic, because once you hit the national scene, even though you may be on the bottom of the pile somewhere, politics is where it's all at. So here you go—you have to be pleasant to all the right people. (Gould et al., 1993a, p. 141)

For many scholarship student-athletes, the expectations of athletic department officials are a common source of stress. A college soccer player commented about the high expectations she and her teammates felt as representatives of her university's athletic department.

— The athletic department standards are so high here. At the beginning of the season we came home from our first road trip and we were ashamed to tell people we lost. We felt like we let the whole department down. We were sitting in study hall and I don't know who it was came in and asked me, "Did you win yet?" I said, "No, we lost." She said, "Both games?" I said, "Yeah." And I felt just like "Ugh," you know. (Wrisberg et al., 2000)

An additional concern for university athletes is the pressure placed on them by professors who are unsympathetic to the demands of athletic participation. Such treatment prompted the following basketball player to disguise her athletic identity.

— I don't like being known as a basketball player. There are some professors who seem to like to punish people who are athletes. Like one I had wouldn't let me take a test (that was scheduled on the day of an important game) early or late. He told me I could make it up on the final but that puts more pressure on me to get a really high grade on the final to get an "A" in the class. That's too much pressure to go into a cumulative final with. (Wrisberg et al., 2000)

Without question, the most prominent members of an athlete's secondary social group are coaches and teammates. Coaches represent perhaps the most powerful secondary social influence on athletes' lives. Whereas some coaches provide helpful support for their athletes, others exert a negative influence (Johnson, 1998). A college springboard diver spoke of the positive experience she had with her coach and of the strong support she received from him.

> — *My coach definitely has been a major impact, helping me through all the tough times. He's always said that if I need him—whatever, however, whenever—to just call him and he will be there or try to do whatever he can. I trust him completely. (Wrisberg et al., 2000)*

Such was not the experience of the following college tennis player who spoke of a different type of experience he had with his coach.

> — *I think that coach failed to see the individual needs of players. Some people just couldn't practice for three hours in 90-degree heat. It got to them. Quite a few were sick off and on and half our team was injured. (Wrisberg et al., 2000)*

The worst case scenario is one in which athletes experience physical or mental abuse at the hands of their coaches. The following comment by a college volleyball player illustrates how one coach abused her power and became a serious source of stress for her athletes.

> — *All [coach] knew how to do was bitch at us. She made us feel like we were fat . . . real big. She called me names and told me how mentally disabled I was. She had something for everybody—I just happened to be the retarded one in her eyes. She liked to make cracks about our bodies. We were already pretty self-conscious about being big. So around her, we always felt so fat—just horrible and ugly. And our uniforms didn't help us one bit because they were real short . . . they came up to here, and they were pretty much a see-through, spandex material that would ride up even higher when we played. We just never felt very good about ourselves and she had a lot to do with that. (Wrisberg et al., 2000)*

Athletes are keenly aware of their coaches' moods and behavior, and as a result, they sometimes experience stress when they observe problems their coaches are having. One college softball player expressed the frustration she and her teammates experienced as a result of the poor communication they witnessed between the coaches on their team.

> — *There was miscommunication between the coaches, coaches were yelling at each other . . . it was really disorganized and it had a negative impact on me and the other players. (Wrisberg et al., 2000)*

Most sport participants agree that a genuinely unique relationship exists among the members of an athletic team. Teammates compete with each other, for each other, and against each other. Members of a team are challenged to sacrifice individual glory for the pursuit and achievement of a larger group goal. Most significantly, elite athletes spend an incredible amount of time with each other. They train together, suffer pain together, travel together, and experience success and failure together.

For many athletes, memories of intense shared experiences of sport participation remain with them for the rest of their lives. One retired athlete spoke of the bond he continued to feel with former teammates.

> — *Even now (that competitive days are over), we're still really close, we're still teammates. We would do about anything for each other. We went through the wringer together so many times in the past. That kind of experience builds a bond between people that is truly special. (Wrisberg et al., 2000)*

The words of the following college swimmer describe the positive feelings he had for his most recent group of teammates.

> — *Last year was one of the most amazing things I ever saw. Everybody just came together as such a team. There was so much support for everybody and it was really a lot of fun. (Wrisberg et al., 2000)*

The prolonged and intensive association athletes have with each other can serve to increase team cohesiveness. One college baseball player said that he felt that all the time he and his teammates spent together on road trips helped them build a strong team unity.

> — *I like the road trips. We (team members) eat together, we sleep at the same hotel, we wake up, we go to the same places. We experience the same things and that builds team unity. (Wrisberg et al., 2000)*

On the other hand, when members of a team have expectations of each other, it can create stress if some team members are not sufficiently committed to the goals of the others. A college baseball player expressed such a frustration with some of his teammates from the previous season.

—Last year some (team members) were slacking off and not doing the right thing. No one said anything but it upset a lot of us. (Wrisberg et al., 2000)

Similar stress is possible for athletes whose goal achievement depends on the performance of a partner. Scanlan, Stein, and Ravizza (1991) found that one source of stress for elite figure skaters was wanting, but not getting, a pairs partner to do what it takes to excel.

Perhaps because their association with team members is such an important part of athletes' lives, it is sometimes stressful when individuals are prevented from engaging in normal team activities or when they feel disconnected from their teammates. Such is often the experience of athletes who sustain serious injuries. The following comment by a college volleyball player reveals the feeling of disconnection from teammates she experienced after suffering an injury.

— I just had knee surgery two weeks ago. I've been pretty much out of it . . . five, six, seven hours a day. It keeps me away from practice, it keeps me away from my entire team. I don't eat lunch with them anymore. I spend all my time alone rehabbing my knee. (Wrisberg et al., 2000)

Unfortunately, some athletes resort to dysfunctional coping strategies when they feel disconnected from their teams. Such was the experience of the following college swimmer.

— One year I didn't perform well at all and I felt like I was missing something. I wasn't really part of the team. That's when I started drinking. I don't know if it's just my personality being kind of obsessive compulsive . . . once I started to drink, I couldn't stop. (Wrisberg et al., 2000)

Because athletes spend so much time together during training and competition, they are often more comfortable socializing with one another rather than with individuals who are not athletes or who are not a part of their team. As one college distance runner observed,

— When you're an athlete, you sort of stick to your little (athletic) community, you know. It's like a little clique you stick to. You don't seem to branch out much from that. (Wrisberg et al., 2000)

One college swimmer expressed the pleasure he derived from socializing with his teammates.

— I really enjoy things we do together away from the pool. Yesterday we went down to the rugby field and played mud football. We've also been to the rock quarries around here and that's a lot of fun . . . jumping off all the different levels of the cliff surface and things like that. (Wrisberg et al., 2000)

Not all athletes, however, prefer to spend their discretionary time with teammates. A college basketball player expressed this attitude when discussing the matter of choosing a roommate.

— I could never live with one of my teammates . . . just because you go through the same things all day long and then you come home—who are you going to—you know, you've got to have someone to vent towards. You can't vent towards your teammate. (Wrisberg et al., 2000)

A college golfer said he preferred to socialize with nonteam members because he liked the fact that they were interested in things other than golf. For this individual, active recovery included being around individuals who allowed him to temporarily escape the demands of his sport.

— I'm closer to guys that aren't on the team. Guys on the team are always talking golf and always worried about their golf game. It's important for me to get away from golf once in a while. (Wrisberg et al., 2000)

Regardless of whether their social activities include other athletes or nonathletes, individuals experience the most enjoyment when they are with people and in situations that allow them to relax and be themselves. One college springboard diver mentioned how much she enjoyed dinner invitations to the homes of teammates who resided near the university.

— Some of my teammates that lived locally would invite me over to their parents' home for some of their mom's home cooking. I really enjoyed that. (Wrisberg et al., 2000)

A college golfer said he had learned that to relax and recover, he needed to be around people who had a sense of humor and who accepted him unconditionally.

— I have to be around people who have a sense of humor. It's fun to go to their house, watch a movie, just hang out. Being with them is fun and they are not a drain on me. (Wrisberg et al., 2000)

Unfortunately, some athletes face social-cultural barriers that limit their options for active recovery activities. The experience of the following African-American female athlete is just one illustration.

— You've got to be careful about what parties you go to. Sometimes there are people who drink too much and there are fights. There are just not a lot of safe places for black athletes to go for fun. (Wrisberg et al., 2000)

In summary, secondary social functioning is a prominent aspect of athletes' lives and multidimensional in nature. Athletes encounter many types of individuals as part of their sporting experience and are abundantly aware of the expectations these individuals have of them. At times, athletes experience stress as a result of encounters with athletic officials, other competitors, university personnel, coaches, and teammates. Of these individuals, coaches and teammates exert the greatest influence on athletes' lives. In some cases, athletes experience support and speak of a special bond they have with coaches and teammates. In other cases, athletes must find ways to tolerate or even endure such relationships. Most athletes seem to prefer secondary social relationships with people who allow them to be themselves and who accept them unconditionally. Occasionally, it is difficult for some athletes to engage in social activities outside their immediate sporting environment because of their high-profile status or because of cultural biases. When athletes' secondary social groups include supportive individuals, they may have more opportunities to engage in the kinds of active recovery activities that promote the maintenance of an optimal recovery-stress balance.

Encouraging Recovery by Optimizing Athletes' Quality of Life

The following recommendations for sport practitioners and participants are offered based on the comments of the athletes quoted in this chapter. Generally speaking, athletes' QOL is optimized when the following criteria are met:

1. They are allowed and encouraged to achieve balance among the various components of their life experience.

2. They are allowed and encouraged to balance the physical demands of training with adequate rest, proper nutrition, and enjoyable active recovery activities.

3. They are allowed sufficient discretionary time to deal adequately with nonsport-related matters and to enjoy relationships and activities that contribute to their personal growth.

4. They experience the unconditional support and encouragement of the members of their primary social group (i.e., family members and significant others).

5. They experience the support and acceptance of coaches and teammates and maintain a realistic perspective regarding the expectations of other members of their secondary social group (e.g., athletic administrators, sport officials, other competitors, university professors, friends, acquaintances, etc.).

Summary

In this chapter, an attempt was made to characterize some of the sources of stress and recovery that athletes experience on a regular basis. To achieve this purpose, the results of several qualitative studies with high-performance athletes were examined, and quotes from athletes were selected and categorized within the context of Pflaum's (1973) four components of life quality (see figure 14.1, p. 257). Whereas the majority of quotes emanated from the lone qualitative study to date that has directly examined athletes' life quality (Wrisberg et al., 2000), an effort was made to characterize other athletes' experiences within the context of the results of previous qualitative research (see table 14.1, p. 256).

An important assumption of this chapter is that a given individual's recovery-stress balance is a strong indicator of that person's QOL at a given point in time. The responses of athletes reported in interview studies demonstrate how various sources of stress and recovery might fall within each of the QOL categories of biophysical functioning, personal growth and self-development, primary social functioning, and secondary social functioning (Pflaum, 1973).

The overriding conclusion of this chapter is that elite athletes experience stress and recovery from both competition and noncompetition sources. In addition, individual differences exist with respect to the specific aspects of athletes' lives that enhance or upset their recovery-stress balance. Obviously, the elements of athletes' experiences included in this chapter are limited to the experiences of the specific individuals who were interviewed. Nevertheless, it is reasonable to assume that these elements are representative of the experiences of the majority of high-performance athletes.

Acknowledgments

The authors thank Joe Whitney for helpful comments on an earlier draft of this chapter and Linda Whitney for technical assistance. Appreciation is extended to Gina Brooks for assistance with data collection and analysis.

References

Adang, E.M.M., Kootstra, G., Baeten, C.G.M.I., & Engel, G.L. (1997). Quality-of-life ratings in patients with chronic illnesses. *Journal of the American Medical Association, 277,* 1038.

American Institutes for Research. (1988a). *Report No. 1: Summary results from the 1987-88 national study of intercollegiate athletes.* Palo Alto, CA: Center for the Study of Athletics.

American Institutes for Research. (1988b). *Report No. 2: Methodology of the 1987-88 national study of intercollegiate athletes.* Palo Alto, CA: Center for the Study of Athletics.

Berg, B. L. (1995). *Qualitative research methods for the social sciences* (2nd ed.). Boston: Allyn and Bacon.

Dalkey, N.C., Lewis, R., & Snyder, D. (1972). *Studies in life quality.* Boston: Heath.

Dijkers, M. (1999). Measuring quality of life: Methodological issues. *American Journal of Physical Medicine and Rehabilitation, 78,* 286-300.

Fabian, E.S. (1990). Quality of life: A review of theory and practice implications for individuals with long-term mental illness. *Rehabilitation Psychology, 35,* 161-170.

Farquhar, M. (1995). Definition of quality of life: A taxonomy. *Journal of Advances in Nursing, 22,* 502-508.

Giorgi, A. (1970). *Psychology as a human science.* New York: Harper & Row.

Gould, D., Guinan, D., Greenleaf, C., Medbery, R., & Peterson, K. (1999). Factors affecting Olympic performance: Perceptions of athletes and coaches from more and less successful teams. *The Sport Psychologist, 13,* 371-394.

Gould, D., Jackson, S., & Finch, L. (1993a). Sources of stress in national champion figure skaters. *Journal of Sport and Exercise Psychology, 15,* 134-159.

Gould, D., Jackson, S., & Finch, L. (1993b). Life at the top: The experiences of U.S. National Champion figure skaters. *The Sport Psychologist, 7,* 354-374.

Gould, D., Tuffey, S., Udry, E., & Loehr, J. (1996). Burnout in competitive junior tennis players: II. Qualitative analysis. *The Sport Psychologist, 10,* 341-366.

Gould, D., Tuffey, S., Udry, E., & Loehr, J. (1997). Burnout in competitive junior tennis players: III. Individual differences in the burnout experience. *The Sport Psychologist, 11,* 257-276.

Henschen, K.P. (1998). Athletic staleness and burnout: Diagnosis, prevention, and treatment. In J.M. Williams (Ed.), *Applied sport psychology: Personal growth to peak performance* (pp. 393-408). Mountain View, CA: Mayfield.

Johnson, M.S. (1998). *The athlete's experience of being coached: An existential-phenomenological investigation.* Unpublished doctoral dissertation, University of Tennessee, Knoxville.

Klonoff, P.S., Costa, L.D., & Snow, W.G. (1986). Predictors and indicators of quality of life in patients with closed-head injury. *Journal of Clinical and Experimental Neuropsychology, 8,* 469-485.

Kreitler, S., Chaitchik, S., Rapoport, Y., Kreitler, H., & Algor, R. (1993). Life satisfaction and health in cancer patients, orthopedic patients, and healthy individuals. *Social Science Medicine, 36,* 547-556.

Lomas, J., Pickard, L., & Mohide, A. (1987). Patient versus clinician item generation for quality-of-life measures: The case of language disabled adults. *Medical Care, 25,* 764-769.

Mor, V., & Guadagnoli, E. (1988). Quality of life measurement: A psychometric tower of Babel. *Journal of Clinical Epidemiology, 41,* 1055-1058.

Morris, A.F., Lussier, L., Vaccaro, P., & Clarke, D.H. (1982). Life quality characteristics of national class women masters long distance runners. *Annals of Sports Medicine, 1,* 23-26.

O'Boyle, C.A., McGee, H., Hickey, A., O'Malley, K., & Joyce, C.R.B. (1992). Individual quality of life in patients undergoing hip replacement. *Lancet, 339,* 1088-1091.

Pflaum, J.H. (1973). *Development of a life quality inventory.* Unpublished doctoral dissertation, University of Maryland, College Park.

Scanlan, T.K., Stein, G.L., & Ravizza, K. (1989). An in-depth study of former elite figure skaters: II. Sources of enjoyment. *Journal of Sport and Exercise Psychology, 11,* 65-83.

Scanlan, T.K., Stein, G.L., & Ravizza, K. (1991). An in-depth study of former elite figure skaters: III. Sources of stress. *Journal of Sport and Exercise Psychology, 13,* 103-120.

Wrisberg, C.A. (1996). Quality of life for male and female athletes. *Quest, 48,* 392-408.

Wrisberg, C.A., Johnson, M.S., & Brooks, G.D. (2000). Assessing the quality of life of NCAA Division I collegiate athletes: A qualitative investigation. Unpublished data.

Beckmann, J. (2002). Interaction of volition and recovery. In M. Kellmann (Ed.), *Enhancing recovery: Preventing underperformance in athletes* (pp. 269-282). Champaign, IL: Human Kinetics.

15

Interaction of Volition and Recovery

Jürgen Beckmann

Although it is widely accepted that an exposure to stressors is not detrimental per se, prolonged exposure may cause memory deficits, decreases in performance, and health problems. A person's vulnerability to the effects of stress, however, depends to a large degree on how she reacts to the stressful situation and how she deals with stress and its effects. Individual characteristics play an important role in these processes. One person may interpret a situation as threatening and react with heightened physiological arousal (including a secretion of cortisol), negative affective reactions (worry), and feelings of uncontrollability and helplessness. Eventually this experience of negative stress, referred to as distress, leads to the negative effects described earlier (Selye, 1974). Another person may consider the same situation a challenge that she can master (cf. Lazarus & Folkman, 1984). Thus, the objectively equal situation evokes a completely different pattern of physiological and psychological reactions in this second person. Her generally positive reactions, referred to as eustress by Selye (1974), include heightened (specific) activation (secretion of catecholamines but no cortisol), feelings of self-efficacy, positive affect, and vigor.

The individual differences in the reaction to stressors can be based on different cognitive structures or experiences, or on different self-regulation skills. When speaking of self-regulation, Kuhl and Beckmann (1994a) referred to auxiliary (usually meta-) processes that aid individuals in generating or maintaining a state that is optimal for their transactions with the environment. Self-regulation involves the control of thinking, emotion, attention, and concentration. These auxiliary processes are required, and hence activated, whenever the situation involves adverse conditions (external or internal barriers or obstacles) that cannot be mastered by the basic emotion and motivation processes alone (cf. Ach, 1910; Atkinson & Birch, 1970).

Stressors constitute adverse conditions that demand the employment of self-regulatory skills that should help to reduce the stress load or define a stressful situation as a challenge to master. External adverse conditions producing stress include a strong opponent in a competition, a large and loud audience, and adverse weather conditions in outdoor sports. Internal stressors can turn athletes into their own worst enemies. They may "psych themselves out" in a competition because of negative thinking or intrusive thoughts that reduce their self-efficacy and concentration and interfere with recovery between trials (cf. Harris & Harris, 1984). Recovery can suffer from adverse external conditions (e.g., a noisy environment when trying to rest between trials, an uncomfortable bed, etc.) as well as from adverse internal conditions (e.g., worrying about being dismissed from the team after a bad performance, conflicts, etc.). Self-regulation skills can help athletes cope with these adverse conditions and thereby further recovery.

This chapter will address individual athletes' unique reactions to stressors and the repertoire of self-regulation skills that can help them cope. In addition, the more overarching personality disposition of action versus state orientation, which determines the acquisition and efficient implementation of self-regulation skills, will be addressed. A two-factor volitional model of the recovery process will be presented. Factors and processes that lead to full recovery on the one extreme or overtraining and underperformance on the other extreme will be discussed.

Volition and Self-Regulation

Wanting to do something is one thing; actually doing it successfully is another. Normally, we have more than one goal at a time with several action tendencies competing for access to the (limited) executive system (cf. Atkinson & Birch, 1970). Whereas the selection of action alternatives is labeled "motivation" in a narrow sense, a commitment to one action alternative and its implementation and completion are referred to as acts of will, or volition (cf. Heckhausen, 1991).

In short, volition refers to processes that support the initiation, perseverance, and deactivation of intentions. Initiation addresses which of the competing action tendencies are to be implemented through action and when they are to be initiated. Perseverance deals with carrying out an activity until the goal is reached rather than jumping to another action alternative before the task is completed. Deactivation refers to the process of decreasing the strength of an action tendency or, more specifically, reducing the activation of the underlying intention after some kind of end state (result) has been reached. All of these processes help individuals to stay in control over what they intend to do. Therefore, the problems volition deals with are also referred to as issues of action control (Kuhl, 1984).

In their everyday training routine as well as during competitions, athletes may face all of these problems of volition. At times athletes will find it hard to pull themselves together to, for example, go to the gym for another unit of strength training (initiation problem). During the exhausting strength training they might choose to perform only 6 repetitions instead of the scheduled 12 in the third series (perseverance problem). Most important in the context of this chapter on volition and recovery is the deactivation problem. When athletes do not manage to deactivate the

underlying intentions of activities already performed, which is most likely the case after a slump has occurred, their subsequent performance is negatively affected. The tennis player who has just lost an important point must escape from this failure to fully concentrate on the next point. After losing the final match at Wimbledon, the tennis player must come to terms with that experience and deactivate the underlying intention in order to recover and regain motivation and self-confidence for upcoming tournaments. The failure to deactivate will thus lead to proximal underperformance (in the case of concentrating on the next point) or distal underperformance (in the case of regaining motivation for future matches). Whereas the first is mainly mediated through a lack of concentration, the second is primarily mediated by disturbed recovery.

Deactivation is of special interest in this chapter. If an intention is not deactivated after an outcome has been obtained, its activation will remain at a high level. Thoughts related to that activity are likely to intrude into consciousness, thereby interfering with concentration on a new activity (Beckmann, 1994b, 1998). The intrusions can disturb proactive as well as passive recovery (for a definition of proactive and passive recovery, see Kellmann, this volume, chapter 1). Sleep is an important form of passive recovery. Thoughts about failing to reach a goal during the day may result in sleep disruption. If a change of activity is planned as a form of proactive recovery, the intrusions may impair this new activity and thus ruin recovery.

Consider a manager who enjoys golfing as a form of recovery. During her busy working day, which includes many meetings, problems to be solved, and decisions to be made, she is looking forward to playing a round of golf in the evening. Because she was delayed at the office, she must rush to the golf course to make her tee time. Not all problems have been solved or all decisions made, so while driving she continues to negotiate on her mobile phone. As she approaches the first tee, she is still engaged in business conversations. After her first shot, she realizes that she is unable to concentrate and enjoy her round of golf. Consequently, she does not find recovery in her golfing.

Obviously, the manager did not succeed in distancing herself from the problems at work and took them onto the golf course. As a consequence she was unable to fully orient herself to the new activity that was intended to lead to recovery. Thus, distancing and new orientation seem to be essential prerequisites of recovery (cf. Allmer, 1996). Deactivation, distancing, and orientation are major functions of volition achieved through self-regulation.

Individuals have a set of volitional strategies at their disposal that execute these self-regulatory functions. These volitional strategies are acquired during socialization. How many of them are acquired, whether they are actually employed, and how efficiently they are executed depends to a large degree on the action control dispositions of action and state orientation, which will be addressed later in this chapter. According to Davis, Botterill, and MacNeill (this volume, chapter 9, p. 173): "The ability to control thinking, attention, and concentration is an important element of optimal recovery." Thus, self-regulation should be an important element in the recovery process.

Volitional Components

Volition has various components with different levels of sophistication and differing demands for cognitive and energetic resources. The more sophisticated components are usually based on (meta-) knowledge (i.e., knowledge of which emotional processes support and which impair performance, knowledge of how decreasing motivation can be stabilized on a level sufficient to maintain the action until the goal is reached, etc.). Research on action control has shown that efficient employment of such processes supports high levels of performance and goal achievement (Beckmann, 1994a).

Less sophisticated volitional components have a different functionality in the support of action control. These lower-level volitional components are less effective than the first and may produce negative side effects in the long run, but they require fewer resources (Beckmann, 1987). In general, two categories of the volitional components can be distinguished: self-control and self-regulation (cf. Kuhl & Beckmann, 1994b).

Self-Control

Self-control describes a mode of volition in which an individual acts according to an internal model of an action requested or desired by another person without necessarily integrating this model into his own system of beliefs, needs, and values (Deci & Ryan, 1991; Kuhl & Beckmann, 1994b). Self-control includes "self-denial" (i.e., self-discipline against one's own needs).

Alienation (i.e., the inability to behave according to one's own needs) is a behavioral consequence of the mode of self-control. Because it involves the loss of personal autonomy, it is also accompanied by procrastination, susceptibility to mental intrusions, rumination, and sometimes passive avoidance (Kuhl & Beckmann, 1994b). It becomes obvious that the self-control mode of volition promotes the increase and perseveration of stress and interferes with adequate recovery. Although it may be effective in the completion of an activity for which incentives are no longer present (e.g., completing strength training when it has lost its appeal), it may become detrimental in the long run, when a person begins to experience a loss of autonomy. The loss of autonomy can take the form of an aggravating cycle. This loss-of-autonomy cycle starts with chronic exposure to external control, which initiates four stages of an escalating loss-of-autonomy cycle: (1) chronic external control stabilizes a tendency toward self-control (suppression of personal needs), which (2) accumulates conflicts (e.g., between suppressed personal needs and compliance to external control); (3) uncontrollable intrusive thoughts can result from this conflict; (4) these intrusions impair self-regulatory efficiency. To compensate for these volitional impairments, the individual resorts to more self-control further promoting a loss of autonomy (Kuhl & Beckmann, 1994b).

In short, continued suppression of the self leads to an accumulation of conflicts between what a person would actually like to do and what she feels obliged to do and actually does. This leads to intrusive thoughts about wishes that could not be enacted. These intrusions impair sophisticated volitional strategies. In such a situation, maintaining some degree of action control can only be countered by more self-control—that is, further suppression of the self.

Self-Regulation

In contrast to self-control, self-regulation can be regarded as an integrated, self-determined, autonomous, or nonalienated mode of volition. In self-regulation, the personality subsystems of motivations, emotions, and intentions are organized in a congruent way. An intention is not maintained through an inhibition of the other systems, if, for example, the motivation is gone and the emotions do not fit as is the case in self-control. Instead, motivations and emotions are brought in line, for example, through finding positive incentives for a continuation of strength training. The intention may also be abandoned if there is no way to bring the other systems in line. Volitional components of self-regulation are self-determination, positive self-motivation, emotional control, self-relaxation, initiative, and volitional self-efficacy. These components should help an individual realize the best thing to do at a certain time, whether it is time to take a break, and the best personal strategy for recovery.

Individual Differences: Action and State Orientation

Individual differences have been a major focus in the analysis of the will. Lay psychologists see individuals as differing in terms of strength of will, or willpower. These concepts also played a role in the traditional scientific psychology of the will from the turn of the 20th century to the 1930s (see Kuhl & Beckmann, 1985, for an overview). There are individual differences regarding the volitional components, which might be associated with the term *strength of will*. Some of these differences are based on better or more (meta-) knowledge of one's reactions, for example, knowing that one becomes more focused and energized in competition when one gets angry (mood management). Action and state orientation are more fundamental individual differences that determine the general approach to dealing with adverse conditions or, in other words, determining the basic action control modes.

State Orientation

A continued preoccupation with a past, present, or future state characterizes the state-oriented action control mode. This means that a person with a disposition to state orientation is likely to ruminate on a past failure, an uncompleted intention, what to do in a given situation, and the chances and potential consequences of an upcoming event. In this case attentional capacity is split between concentration on the task at hand and uncontrollable and dysfunctional mental intrusions about these states. A study by Beckmann and Hazlett (1989) showed that state-oriented cross-country skiers were much more occupied during the race with their potential finishing place and what consequences would follow from this finishing place than cross-country skiers who were action-oriented. If attention control or keeping to a competition plan is essential, state

orientation negatively affects athletic performance (Beckmann & Kazen, 1994). Furthermore, it is probably related to long-term underperformance, as it interferes with recovery. State orientation is usually associated with the self-control mode of decision making and the loss-of-autonomy cycle.

Action Orientation

Action orientation, in contrast to state orientation, is described as the ability to facilitate the enactment of context-adequate intentions. Stronger context sensitivity exists in persons with an action orientation as opposed to a state orientation. This means that intentions would not be maintained if the context signaled that continuation would be a waste of energy, or the actor could no longer find incentives to continue, as is the case in self-control. Thus, action orientation is associated with self-regulation. The personality subsystems are self-organized in a way that promotes the maintenance of the current intention. If goal attainment appears impossible, the intention will be deactivated. Action orientation, therefore, supports processes promoting the actual realization of an intention but also volitional components that further detachment from an unrealistic intention or one that has been brought to a (successful or unsuccessful) conclusion. Consequently, it can be assumed that action orientation is a personality disposition promoting recovery and preventing underperformance.

A Process Model of Recovery

As stated earlier, an important precondition of recovery is the detachment from a past activity (i.e., a complete deactivation of its underlying intention, a distancing from its content, and an orientation toward a new activity), which, in the context of the present discussion, is aimed at recovery. The question is, how do individuals manage to achieve a thorough detachment so that they can fully enter into a recovery-oriented activity undisturbed from intrusive thoughts related to that past activity?

Detachment from the past activity followed by an engagement in a new activity can be regarded as a volitional process. The Rubicon model of action phases (Heckhausen, 1987) specifies a postactional phase that describes this volitional process. This model will be used as a starting point for the development of a more comprehensive model of the recovery process and its effects on performance.

The Rubicon model, as depicted in figure 15.1, differentiates among four phases during the course of an action. The predecisional motivation phase ends when individuals commit themselves to a specific action alternative and thus cross the intention Rubicon. This phase is followed by two volitional phases: the preactional volition phase and the actional volition phase. In contrast to the predecisional motivation phase, which is characterized by objective and impartial information processing, the volitional phases are characterized by a realization orientation. Information processing is now biased in favor of the chosen action alternative. Once some kind of an outcome has been obtained, the actional volition phase ends and the postactional motivation phase begins. Information processing becomes reality oriented again. The goal of the postactional phase is to deactivate the executed intention and switch attention forward to a new activity (Heckhausen, 1991).

The postactional phase postulated in the Rubicon model is the crucial phase in the recovery process. It serves mainly two functions. First, it helps the individual disengage from the past activity and deactivate the respective goal. Second, after the individual has achieved deactivation, the postactional phase helps her orient herself toward a new activity. The new activity could be some kind of recovery. In the example of the manager trying to recover from work while golfing, the attempt to find recovery failed. All the unsolved problems of the day, and all the decisions she had to make continued to fill her mind while she tried to play golf. Consequently, she was unable to concentrate on her golfing, played terribly, and eventually got upset with herself. Instead of finding recovery in golfing, the round of golf became an additional stress experience. Thus, a necessary condition for recovery is deactivation from the past activity.

Several studies have shown that deactivation is an active process. A past activity does not become deactivated by simply turning to something else or distracting oneself. A series of studies by Beckmann (1998) showed that blocking a retrospective evaluation left the activity in a state of heightened activation, which made recurrent thoughts of the past activity likely. In another study, Beckmann (1994b) found that after failing on ego-involving tasks (i.e., tasks that are relevant to an important aspect of a person's self-concept), individuals differed in their retrospective evaluations of those experiences. Some individuals went through a systematic evaluation sequence of their performance (i.e., a task-oriented analysis). They first summarized the result of the whole task: *I did not succeed on a single task of the test.* They then analyzed what went wrong on a performance-related level: *What did I forget to take into account?* Usually, they came up with what the flaw might have been. The result of their task analysis told them what to do on a possible future encounter with the same task. These individuals succeeded in effectively turning off the past activity. Individuals who instead focused on the consequences the failure had for themselves tended to get captured in self-evaluation loops that blocked deactivation. Typically, these self-evaluation loops started with a statement of the failure *(I did not even solve a single problem).* This led to internal stable attributions blaming the failure on a lack of ability, which became an endless loop leaving them without clues what to do in a possible future encounter with the same task. Consequently, the past task could not be turned off.

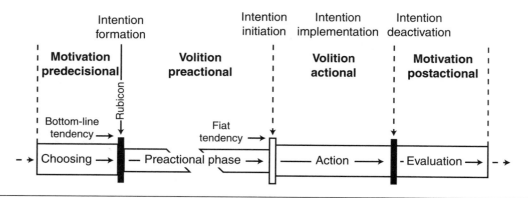

Figure 15.1 The Rubicon model of action phases.

After Heckhausen, 1986.

This generated a potential for intrusive thoughts that interfered with future activities (e.g., proactive recovery).

The personality disposition of action versus state orientation and the related volitional components play an important role in these postactional processes. State-oriented individuals are unable to disengage from a past activity and remain preoccupied with that activity. Empirical findings support the assumption that state-oriented individuals are especially likely to end up in self-evaluation loops (see Beckmann, 1994b).

However, it should be noted that it is impossible in most cases to simply switch from one activity to the next without effort. The golf-playing manager's recovery intention was probably ruined by this faulty assumption. A premature change of activity, as well as an ineffective postactional evaluation, will not lead to a deactivation of the past activity. Instead, the past activity will likely persist as a constant source of stress or will produce intrusive thoughts (see Beckmann, 1994b).

Certain volitional components mediate the deactivation process. Components that promote and inhibit detachment, as well as an engagement in proactive recovery, can be described in a two-factor model of the recovery process. One of these factors affects the disengagement from the past activity and thus determines whether the stress load from a past activity will persevere. Therefore, this factor is referred to as the perseveration factor. Other volitional components promote recovery. These components are subsumed under the orientation factor.

As figure 15.2 shows, factor 2, the perseveration factor, instigates the persistence of the stress load. A high level of self-discipline may render it impossible for a person, for example, to accept that he was unable to complete the full training program that either he or his coach intended him to complete. As a consequence the person will not be able to let go and relax (passive recovery) afterward. Also, when he tries to do something else for a change, such as read a book (proactive recovery), he may find that he cannot concentrate on reading because thoughts about the uncompleted training keep intruding.

Factor 1, the orientation factor, shows the opposite effect. Factor 1 subsumes the self-regulation components of volition. Efficient self-regulation will help the person fully focus attention on something new, for example, some kind of proactive recovery. At the same time, it will help the person detach from the past activity, thereby decreasing the stress load. This will promote passive recovery. Self-regulaton will also facilitate proactive recovery, resulting in a reduction of intrusive thoughts, for example.

Deactivation is a necessary condition for efficient recovery. If no deactivation is achieved, passive or proactive recovery is likely to be disturbed. But deactivation is not a sufficient condition for recovery. Recovery is a highly individualistic process. Thus, individuals must find the form of recovery that best suits their situation and personal preferences, and then implement an optimal recovery strategy (cf. Kellmann, this volume, chapter 1). The volitional components of factor 1, the orientation factor, are focused on a promotion of this process.

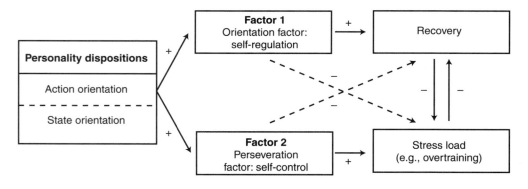

Figure 15.2 A two-factor model of the recovery process.

Empirical Findings on Volition and Recovery

According to the theoretical consideration stated previously, volitional components should be associated with the perseveration of the stress load and passive and proactive recovery. Also, the personality disposition of action versus state orientation should moderate stress reactions and recovery.

These assumptions were tested in several studies (Beckmann & Kellmann, 2002). In these studies the participants usually completed the Volitional Components Questionnaire (VCQ; Kuhl & Fuhrmann, 1998), the Action Control Scale (ACS; Kuhl, 1994), and the Recovery-Stress Question-

naire for Athletes (RESTQ-Sport; Kellmann & Kallus, 2000). In a study of 58 members of the 1998 German Junior National Rowing Team clear-cut distinctions between six volitional components affecting stress load and six volitional components supporting recovery emerged. As table 15.1 shows, the volitional components that are significantly related to recovery are *Self-Determination, Positive Self-Motivation, Emotion Control, Self-Relaxation, Initiative,* and *Volitional Self-Efficacy.* This means that persons who feel they decide for themselves, find positive incentives for what they have to do, generate mood states that promote the execution of an action, know how to relax in states of stress, easily get started on an activity, and have generally high confidence in their abilities are more likely to achieve high states of recovery.

Table 15.1 Relationship of the VCQ Components to Stress and Recovery

| | Recovery-stress state patterns | | | | | | | |
VCQ scales	Pattern I MW SD $n = 14$		Pattern II MW SD $n = 18$		Pattern III MW SD $n = 17$		Pattern IV MW SD $n = 9$		P(R) df (1,54)	P(S) df (1,54)	P(RxS) df (1,54)
1 Self-Determination	1.70	.49	1.51	.49	2.11	.49	2.07	.39	.000	.383	.566
2 Positive Self-Motivation	1.64	.33	1.42	.52	1.98	.39	1.76	.34	.005	.058	.999
3 Emotion Control	1.63	.34	1.43	.55	1.84	.62	1.82	.42	.038	.461	.519
4 Self-Relaxation	1.57	.36	1.18	.33	1.98	.61	1.53	.60	.005	.002	.850
5 Initiative	1.63	.37	1.40	.42	1.89	.39	1.80	.48	.004	.154	.549
6 Volitional Self-Efficacy	1.79	.40	1.69	.54	2.14	.46	2.02	.64	.014	.432	.936
7 Procrastination	0.79	.48	1.08	.49	0.79	.52	1.02	.52	.847	.059	.832
8 Susceptibility to Intrusions	0.59	.46	1.19	.44	0.59	.60	1.07	.67	.682	.000	.669
9 Alienation	1.03	.29	1.30	.38	0.84	.39	1.02	.29	.017	.020	.662
10 Rumination	1.06	.43	1.42	.53	0.95	.51	1.24	.54	.308	.020	.789
11 Passive Avoidance	0.77	.47	1.24	.60	0.53	.46	1.09	.50	.162	.001	.759
12 Self-Discipline	1.30	.27	1.68	.41	1.37	.43	1.62	.47	.966	.005	.581

$n = 58$

Recovery-stress state patterns: (I) low stress, low recovery; (II) high stress, low recovery; (III) low stress, high recovery; (IV) high stress, high recovery

Main effect recovery: ($F[12,43] = 1.85$; $p = 0.07$)

Main effect stress: ($F[12,43] = 2.31$; $p < 0.05$)

Interaction: ns

Another six volitional components are related to stress. These components are *Procrastination, Susceptibility to Intrusions, Alienation, Rumination, Passive Avoidance,* and *Self-Discipline.* Persons who tend to fail on the actual execution of implemental intentions; experience a high degree of intrusive thoughts that impair concentration; have an impaired access to their actual (implicit) self, their own needs, and wishes; chronically ruminate and experience negative affect; show passive avoidance characterized by feeling paralyzed in stressful situations; and show a high degree of self-discipline experience a higher degree of stress than persons who have low scores on these volitional components.

The relationship of high self-discipline and high stress load may appear surprising at first, but as stated before, high self-discipline implies the exertion of high self-control in the sense that per-

sons continue to execute an activity for which they have no positive incentives. Thus, personal preferences and the execution of this activity (often an externally imposed duty) are in conflict. It was found that the volitional components subsumed under the orientation factor in the two-factor model are in fact positively related to recovery, whereas those volitional components subsumed under the perseveration factor are related to a high stress load.

Table 15.2 presents the findings regarding recovery that were replicated in a study of 93 athletes with separate levels of expertise in different sports. A similar pattern was found regarding the relationship of the previously described volitional components and stress load. Only *Procrastination, Susceptibility to Intrusions,* and *Self-Discipline* did not reach the conventional level of statistical significance.

Table 15.2 Relationship of the VCQ Components to Stress and Recovery

VCQ scales	Pattern I MW n = 12	Pattern I SD	Pattern II MW n = 25	Pattern II SD	Pattern III MW n = 29	Pattern III SD	Pattern IV MW n = 10	Pattern IV SD	P(R) df (1,72)	P(S) df (1,72)	P(RxS) df (1,72)
1 Self-Determination	1.55	.46	1.69	.57	2.07	.49	1.96	.51	.004	.912	.350
2 Positive Self-Motivation	1.28	.64	1.33	.43	1.95	.40	1.80	.37	.000	.663	.411
3 Emotion Control	1.05	.53	1.22	.50	1.88	.45	1.78	.56	.000	.802	.288
4 Self-Relaxation	1.33	.45	1.23	.52	1.81	.57	1.52	.38	.005	.142	.480
5 Initiative	1.50	.46	1.42	.44	1.90	.59	1.76	.51	.006	.403	.797
6 Volitional Self-Efficacy	1.68	.46	1.78	.54	2.41	.39	2.24	.40	.000	.750	.267
7 Procrastination	0.62	.37	1.22	.60	0.90	.59	1.30	.37	.184	.001	.465
8 Susceptibility to Intrusions	1.12	.57	1.42	.65	0.90	.61	1.08	.47	.074	.120	.707
9 Alienation	1.08	.45	1.20	.50	0.86	.41	1.14	.59	.239	.100	.498
10 Rumination	1.03	.78	1.38	.61	0.81	.57	0.98	.27	.045	.096	.561
11 Passive Avoidance	0.83	.61	1.06	.56	0.57	.50	0.76	.46	.044	.135	.897
12 Self-Discipline	1.33	.48	1.65	.38	1.28	.57	1.50	.47	.426	.035	.695

n = 93; of the 93 participants in this study, only 76 fully completed the RESTQ as well as the VCQ.
Recovery-stress state patterns: (I) low stress, low recovery; (II) high stress, low recovery; (III) low stress, high recovery; (IV) high stress, high recovery
Main effect recovery: (F[12,61] = 5.53; p < 0.001)
Main effect stress: (F[12,61] = 2.13; p < 0.05)
Interaction: ns

The personality disposition of action and state orientation is closely related to the volitional components. Whereas the volitional components related to recovery are usually found in action-oriented individuals, the volitional components related to stress are usually found in state-oriented individuals (Kuhl & Beckmann, 1994a). The results of a study of 221 participants engaged in various sports show a relationship between (failure-related) action versus state orientation and the RESTQ-Sport, which reflects the relationship between action/state orientation and the volitional components.

As figure 15.3 shows, state-oriented and action-oriented participants differ significantly on a con-

siderable number of the RESTQ-Sport stress scales as well as recovery scales. On the one hand, scores for *General Stress, Emotional Stress, Social Stress, Lack of Energy,* and *Physical Complaints* were significantly higher for state-oriented than for action-oriented participants. On the other hand, the state-oriented participants had significantly lower scores on *General Well-Being* and on *Physical Recovery* than the action-oriented participants (Beckmann & Kellmann, 2002).

So far, the results support several aspects of the two-factor model of the recovery process. The data of yet another study with 58 members of the year 2000 German Junior National Rowing Team more directly addressed the specified processes

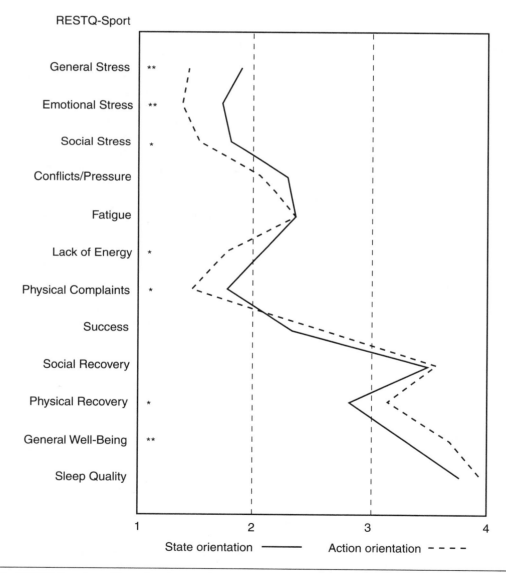

Figure 15.3 RESTQ-Sport profiles of action- and state-oriented athletes. Asterisks indicate significant differences ($* = p < 0.05$; $** = p < 0.01$).

by submitting the data to a path analysis. This path analysis included action versus state orientation as an independent variable, the perseveration and orientation factors as mediator variables, and recovery as a dependent variable. At the point of the highest training load in minutes per day (see Kellmann, Altenburg, Lormes, & Steinacker, 2001) during the preparation camp for the Junior World Championships significant correlations were found in the directions predicted by the two-factor model. There was a significant negative correlation between failure-related action/state orientation and RESTQ-Sport *General Stress* (the mean of all stress-related scales of the RESTQ-Sport, $r = -.32$, $p < 0.02$), and a significant positive correlation between action/state orientation and *Recovery* (the mean of all recovery-related scales of the RESTQ-Sport, $r = .30$, $p < 0.025$). This means that, as expected, recovery is related to action orientation, whereas "general stress" is related to state orientation. There were significant correlations between the VCQ perseveration factor and *General Stress* ($r = .36$, $p < 0.01$) as well as *Recovery* ($r = -.32$, $p < 0.02$). The VCQ orientation factor also correlated significantly with these RESTQ factors but in reverse directions: *General Stress*, $r = -.28$, $p < 0.05$; *Recovery*, $r = .50$, $p < 0.001$.

Entering all of these variables into one equation generates the pattern depicted in figure 15.4. As shown, the correlations between failure-related action/state orientation and the RESTQ-Sport (*General Stress*, $r = -.32$; *Recovery*, $r = .30$) are significantly reduced by entering the VCQ factors into the equation (*General Stress*, $r = -.16$; *Recovery*, $r = .20$). This means that the disposition factors do not exert a strong, direct influence on stress load and recovery. The crucial

mediators are obviously the volitional component factors. The effect of these mediators on the relationship between action/state orientation and the RESTQ-Sport factor is partialed out in figure 15.4. These factors are affected by the individual difference dimension of action versus state orientation.

The Dynamics of Overtraining and Staleness

Some further assumptions may be ventured based on the previously described process model of recovery and the empirical findings supporting this model. Although these assumptions are hypothetical, they can be derived from the previously mentioned model. Overtraining and staleness can be addressed from a dynamic systems perspective. Nonlinear dynamics especially appear to appropriately describe the processes underlying overtraining and staleness.

Davis et al. (this volume, chapter 9, p. 161) describe the relationship of self-regulation and recovery as a reciprocal process: ". . . poor self-regulation and low mood may sometimes *result in* poor athletic performance and prolong inadequate recovery; at other times, these factors may directly *result from* inadequate recovery." In accordance with Kuhl and Beckmann's (1994b) loss-of-autonomy cycle outlined earlier, the relationship may be described as a dynamic, feed-forward circle.

A disposition toward state orientation may be a starting point. This disposition provokes recovery deficits via the paths of volitional components. The tiredness and lack of motivation caused by recovery deficits can be countered by self-discipline. But prolonged execution of self-

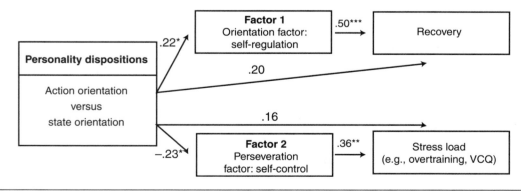

Figure 15.4 A structural-equation analysis of the two-factor model of recovery (see Beckmann & Kellmann, 2002). Note that the correlation computed between the volitional perseveration factor and action versus state orientation employed the failure-related subscale of the Action Control Scale resulting in the negative correlation depleted in the figure (* = $p < 0.10$; ** = $p < 0.05$; *** = $p < 0.01$).

discipline with the resulting negative emotions promotes or intensifies state-oriented reactions. The data given earlier show that state orientation amplifies stress reactions and blocks effective recovery mediated through the specified two factors of orientation and perseveration. Consequently, when an individual continues for a long period of time to execute large amounts of high-intensity training either by exerting high self-discipline or self-control or being other directed (e.g., through the coach), the stress load will increase disproportionally. If these self-reinforcing processes continue, the whole system may reach a point of collapse. For some period of time, although the load is already too high, the individual will perform quite normally; that is, she will show no signs of overtraining. At a certain point, however, "a straw may break the camel's back."

Thus, stress and recovery can be considered elements that interact in a complex, often nonlinear way to produce patterns of optimal performance, overtraining, or staleness. The nature of the feedback among the elements can promote complex dynamics and the emergence of a new order of the system, optimal performance preconditions, or overtraining.

In recent years such a dynamic systems perspective "has emerged as an integrative metatheory for many otherwise distinct domains of science." It "redirects the focus of science to the evolution and spontaneous self-organization of natural phenomena" (Vallacher & Nowak, 1994, p. xv). This perspective allows us to describe the sudden and dramatic changes in individual states and reactions that seem to apply well to the field of recovery, overtraining, and staleness. Researchers have often found that two athletes in the same training group, with the same training and recovery schedule, will experience opposite states at one point during preparation for the season—one enters the state of overtraining, whereas the other feels optimally prepared and energetic. Also, with the same amount of rest after a season, the latter athlete will recover fully, whereas the other will remain in a state of overtraining.

This may be described by the cusp-catastrophe model illustrated in figure 15.5. The original model goes back to the theorizing of the French mathematician Rene Thom (1975). Thom's central theorem was that, with certain qualifications, all naturally occurring discontinuities could be classified as being of the "same type" as (i.e., topologically equivalent to) one of seven fundamental catastrophes. The most commonly applied of these seven

fundamental catastrophes is the cusp catastrophe, which has been applied frequently in the behavioral sciences. Hardy and Fazey (1987), for example, used it to develop an intriguing account of the relationship between anxiety and performance (see also Hardy, 1990). It appears to be a very useful model to account for the relationship between stress/recovery and underperformance (overtraining).

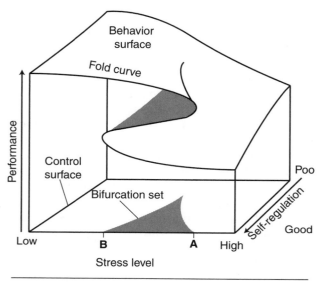

Figure 15.5 A cusp-catastrophe conceptualization of performance and the recovery process.

Adapted, by permission, from R. Thom, 1975, *Structural stability and morphogenesis* (New York: Benjamin-Addison Wesley).

The cusp-catastrophe model is three dimensional. The discussion of the processes involved in the recovery process in this chapter involved more factors. As a first approximation the cusp-catastrophe model will be discussed merging the VCQ perseveration and VCQ orientation factor into one self-regulation factor. Within the three-dimensional model, the horizontal plane is called the control surface and is defined by the two control dimensions, in this case, stress (training load and other stressors) and self-regulation. These are the independent variables. The vertical dimension is the behavior dimension (e.g., the state of the organism or an athlete's form, performance, or underperformance in the case of overtraining), and the top with the fold curve is the behavior surface. Assuming that the behavior surface is translucent, if one were to shine a light directly above the figure, a shadow would be cast on the control surface directly below and conforming to the shape of the fold curve (in two dimensions). The cusp-shaped area the shadow defines is called the bifurcation set. In this case the behavioral prediction is bimodality.

To make predictions from this model, one seeks out a point on the control surface, for example, the training load established for a particular athlete plus the diagnosed self-regulation skills of this athlete. The level of the behavior surface directly above this point is the predicted behavior. Note that the model gives two behavior surfaces in the case of good self-regulation skills, due to the fold above the bifurcation set. In this case, the behavioral prediction is bimodality, which will be specified now.

Consider the case of an athlete with high self-regulation skills. As stress (training load and other stressors) is increased, this athlete will reduce the stress and find recovery. Thus, he is able to stabilize himself and not exhaust his resources. Suppose, as the athlete goes into the competition season, stress further increases (although training load is reduced, he experiences stress from competition, traveling, trouble with personal relationships, etc.). Still, these may result in only small decrements in the athlete's form and performance. But when stress reaches a high enough level, just a small increase in stress will exceed the threshold and result in a large and sudden decrement in form/performance and thus a sudden change to a state of overtraining (i.e., a catastrophic change in the state and behavior of the individual). The model predicts that just beyond point A there is a catastrophic drop from the upper to the lower surface. The model also tells us that it will be difficult to return to the upper surface. Once on the lower surface, one has to reduce the stress load far more than it was before the drop (at point A) occurred, as far as point B, where there will be another catastrophic jump from the lower to the upper surface. The higher the stress load, the longer it will take to get back to the upper level through reduction of stress (no training).

For individuals low in self-regulation skills the change in state/behavior will not be as large and sudden. It is represented by the rear side of the figure. The (hypothetical) athlete without self-regulation skills is unable to deal with increases in stress load and shows decrements in behavior proportional to the increasing stress.

Thus, the higher the self-regulation skills of athletes, the higher the training load they can master. Overreaching is possible, but the individual, and the coach, should know that if the high load is continued for a longer period of time, the dynamics described by the cusp-catastrophe model will set in and inevitably lead to a sudden breakdown that requires a disproportionally long recovery time. As in a cusp catastrophe (see figure 15.5), it is hard to get out of this state. It now takes disproportional amounts of recovery to set the system back to equilibrium.

What Can Be Done

Action versus state orientation is assumed to affect the stress experience, its persistence, and the recovery process. In general, a person's personality disposition seems to enhance or interfere with recovery. Recent research on twins showed that action/state orientation has a genetic component (Geppert & Halisch, 2001). Nevertheless, a person's orientation is not completely resistant to change. Hartung and Schulte (1994) showed that through behavior therapy, state-oriented individuals can become more action oriented. Also, the personality disposition becomes effective only through the respective action control state. But the occurrence of this state can be prevented, or the negative effects of the state can be mitigated.

Intervention programs can directly address the factors in the two-factor model discussed earlier. The perseveration factor can be disabled through relaxation techniques. Relaxation programs help to block out intrusive thoughts, negative emotionality, and alienation in action-oriented individuals, and thus help to reduce the stress load (Kuhl, 2001). In the long run the negative effects of this factor may be shut off by breaking the loss-of-autonomy cycle, which involves changes in personality. Self-determination should be promoted. Athletes should learn to focus on what they feel and want, and then decide on that basis. Participation is a key term in modern leadership promoting motivation and performance. Anecdotal evidence reported by several top-level coaches, including the author, also shows that top athletes usually have a very good sense of their optimal training and stress loads. Promoting self-determination is usually the best way to find the optimal training load for them.

The orientation factor is supported by several standard interventions employed by sport psychologists. To a great extent mental training in sport teaches athletes volitional strategies that help them to stay focused, mobilize energy, and relax and recover when appropriate.

Recommendations

In general, this chapter attempts to further the understanding of stress effects and the recovery process. Personality factors are taken into account in this approach. Some concrete recommendations can be given to the practitioner for how to deal with this process to prevent overtraining and underperformance.

- First of all, it must be realized that stress experience and recovery is a highly individualistic process. Thus the acceptable stress load (e.g., training load) and type and extent of recovery must be tailor-made for a specific individual.

- Personality factors play an important role in this process. To influence this process it is helpful to know if an individual is action- or state-oriented.

- Perseveration of stress load can be disabled through relaxation techniques. Relaxation prevents intrusions, negative emotionality, and alienation especially in state-oriented individuals.

- After a stressful event (e.g., a failure experience) distraction is not the right thing to do. Distraction will not turn off the stress load. To achieve recovery individuals have to go through a systematic evaluation of the stressful experience. This evaluation should lead to a conclusion that helps the individual know how to deal with this situation in the future and do better.

- The higher the self-regulation skills of individuals, the higher the training load they can master. Thus, psychological skills training can help to master higher training loads (i.e., avoiding overtraining).

- Whereas state-oriented individuals benefit from explicit directions on self-regulation strategies, the same directions can probably interfere with the action-oriented individual's self-regulation strategies (which are usually effective) and may lead to reactance (Antoni & Beckmann, 1990).

- Self-determination should be promoted. Individuals should learn to get better access to what they feel and want.

References

Ach, N. (1910). *Über den Willensakt und das Temperament* [On the act of will and temper]. Leipzig, Germany: Quelle & Meyer.

Allmer, H. (1996). *Erholung und Gesundheit* [Recovery and health]. Göttingen, Germany: Hogrefe.

Antoni, C.H., & Beckmann, J. (1990). An action control conceptualization of goal setting and feedback effects. In U. Kleinbeck, H. Quast, H. Thierry, & H. Häcker (Eds.), *Work motivation* (pp. 41-52). Hillsdale, NJ: Erlbaum.

Atkinson, J.W., & Birch, D.A. (1970). *A dynamic theory of action*. New York: Wiley.

Beckmann, J. (1987). Metaprocesses and the regulation of behavior. In F. Halisch & J. Kuhl (Eds.), *Motivation, intention and volition* (pp. 371-386). Berlin, New York: Springer.

Beckmann, J. (1994a). Volitional correlates of action and state orientation. In J. Kuhl & J. Beckmann (Eds.), *Volition and personality: Action and state orientation* (pp. 155-166). Seattle: Hogrefe & Huber.

Beckmann, J. (1994b). Rumination and the deactivation of an intention. *Motivation and Emotion, 18,* 317-334.

Beckmann, J. (1998). Intrusive thoughts, rumination, and incomplete intentions. In M. Kofta, G. Weary, & G. Sedek (Eds.), *Personal control in action. Cognitive and motivational mechanisms* (pp. 259-278). New York: Plenum.

Beckmann, J., & Hazlett, S. (1989). *Facilitating and inhibiting thoughts during competition: A study with cross-country skiers and ski jumpers.* Unpublished manuscript. Max-Planck-Institute for Psychological Research, Munich.

Beckmann, J., & Kazen, M. (1994). Action and state orientation and the performance of top athletes. In J. Kuhl & J. Beckmann (Eds.), *Volition and personality: Action and state orientation* (pp. 439-451). Seattle: Hogrefe & Huber.

Beckmann, J., & Kellmann, M. (2002). *Self-regulation and recovery.* Manuscript: University of Potsdam.

Deci, E.L., & Ryan, R.M. (1991). A motivational approach to self: Integration in personality. In R.E. Dienstbier (Ed.), *Nebraska Symposium on Motivation, 1990* (pp. 237-288). Lincoln, NE: University of Nebraska Press.

Geppert, U., & Halisch, F. (2001). Genetic vs. environmental determinants of traits, motives, self-referential cognitions, and volitional control in old age: First results from the Munich Twin Study (GOLD). In A. Efklides, J. Kuhl, & R. Sorrentino (Eds.), *Trends and prospects in motivation research* (pp. 359-387). Dordrecht, Netherlands: Kluwer.

Hardy, L. (1990). A catastrophe model of performance in sport. In J.G. Jones & L. Hardy (Eds.), *Stress and performance in sport* (pp. 81-106). Chichester, U.K.: Wiley.

Hardy, L., & Fazey, J. (1987). *The inverted-U hypothesis: A catastrophe for sport psychology?* Paper presented at the Annual Conference of the North American Society for the Psychology of Sport and Physical Activity, Vancouver.

Harris, D.V., & Harris, B.L. (1984). *The athlete's guide to sport psychology. Mental skills for physical people.* New York: Leisure Press.

Hartung, J., & Schulte, D. (1994). Action and state orientation during therapy of phobic disorders. In J. Kuhl & J. Beckmann (Eds.), *Volition and personality: Action and state orientation* (pp. 217-229). Seattle: Hogrefe & Huber.

Heckhausen, H. (1986). Wiederaufbereitung des Wollens: Eine Einführung [Reprocessing the will: An introduction]. In H. Heckhausen, J. Beckmann, P.M. Gollwitzer, F. Halisch, P. Lütkenhaus, & M. Schütt, *Wiederaufbereitung des Wollens* (pp. 1-9). München, Germany: Max-Planck-Institute for Psychological Research Paper 19/1986.

Heckhausen, H. (1987). Perspektiven einer Psychologie des Wollens [Perspectives of a psychology of the will]. In H. Heckhausen, P.M. Gollwitzer, & F.E. Weinert (Eds.), *Jenseits des Rubikon. Der Wille in den Humanwissenschaften* (pp. 121-142). Berlin: Springer.

Heckhausen, H. (1991). *Motivation and action.* New York: Springer.

Kellmann, M., Altenburg, D., Lormes, W., & Steinacker, J.M. (2001). Assessing stress and recovery during preparation for the world championships in rowing. *The Sport Psychologist, 15,* 151-167.

Kellmann, M., & Kallus, K.W. (2000). *Der Erholungs-Belastungs-Fragebogen für Sportler; Handanweisung.* [The Recovery-Stress-Questionnaire for Athletes: Manual]. Frankfurt, Germany: Swets Test Services.

Kuhl, J. (1984). Motivational aspects of achievement motivation and learned helplessness: Toward a comprehensive theory of action control. In B.A. Maher & W.B. Maher (Eds.), *Progress in experimental personality research* (Vol. 13, pp. 99-171). New York: Academic Press.

Kuhl, J. (1994). Action versus state orientation: Psychometric properties of the Action Control Scale (ACS-90). In J. Kuhl & J. Beckmann (Eds.), *Volition and personality: Action and state orientation* (pp. 47-59). Seattle: Hogrefe & Huber.

Kuhl, J. (2001). *Motivation und Persönlichkeit: Interaktionen psychischer Systeme* [Motivation and personality. Interactions of psychic systems]. Göttingen, Germany: Hogrefe.

Kuhl, J., & Beckmann, J. (Eds.). (1985). *Action control: From cognition to behavior.* New York: Springer.

Kuhl, J., & Beckmann, J. (Eds.). (1994a). *Volition and personality.* Seattle: Hogrefe & Huber.

Kuhl, J., & Beckmann, J. (1994b). Alienation: Ignoring one's preferences. In J. Kuhl & J. Beckmann (Eds.), *Volition and personality: Action and state orientation* (pp. 375-390). Seattle: Hogrefe & Huber.

Kuhl, J., & Fuhrmann, A. (1998). Decomposing self-regulation and self-control: The volitional components inventory. In J. Heckhausen & C. Dweck (Eds.), *Life span perspectives on motivation and control* (pp. 15-49). Hillsdale, NJ: Erlbaum

Lazarus, R.S., & Folkman, S. (1984). *Stress, appraisal, and coping.* New York: Springer.

Selye, H. (1974). *Stress without distress.* Philadelphia: Lippincott.

Thom, R. (1975). *Structural stability and morphogenesis.* New York: Benjamin-Addison Wesley.

Vallacher, R.R., & Nowak, A. (Eds.). (1994). *Dynamical systems in social psychology.* San Diego: Academic Press.

Kallus, K.W. (2002). Impact of recovery in different areas of application. In M. Kellmann (Ed.), *Enhancing recovery: Preventing underperformance in athletes* (pp. 283-300). Champaign, IL: Human Kinetics.

16

Impact of Recovery in Different Areas of Application

K. Wolfgang Kallus

The Recovery-Stress Questionnaire (RESTQ) turned out to be a useful tool in sport psychology, helping to monitor training, predict performance, and so on. This chapter addresses the question of whether or not a person's RESTQ score reflects the person's psychosomatic recovery-stress states validly as implied from a biopsychological perspective. Recent research on the recovery-stress state in various professions shows that the scores of the RESTQ reflect a "biopsychosocial" state that persists for a fair amount of time. The RESTQ may therefore be useful in areas other than sport. Although the instrument has exhibited a broad range of validity, we are clearly in need of a better understanding of and more research on recovery after stress as research on stress-recovery sequences is less than sparse outside the area of physical training.

Recovery-Stress Approach

The basic idea of a recovery-stress approach is that long-term negative effects of stressors occur if the organism is unable to "unwind" (Frankenhaeuser, 1978), to restore resources and regain homeostatic and biorhythmic balance—in other words, to recover. The positive effects of recovery are at least threefold. First, stress effects are compensated; these may include changed hormonal status, changed metabolism, changed immune functioning, exhausted resources, cellular damage, changed thresholds in neurochemi-

cal functioning and neurochemical imbalance, as well as dysregulations in mood, action regulation, and social functioning. Second, the organism regains its normal reactivity, which allows it to cope adequately with subsequent taxing situations. Finally, recovery allows the organism to consolidate adaptive processes, thereby "learning" from stress and optimizing resources.

Fitness and a high degree of competence and functioning will result from stress combined with optimal recovery. Increasing empirical evidence shows that recovery processes are impaired in subjects with high risks of psychophysiological stress disorders (cf. Rau & Richter, 1995). Stress and recovery are considered basic biopsychological states that have a strong biological basis and are continuously modulated by physiological adaptation, psychological processes, the social context, and environmental conditions. A transactional perspective is helpful in understanding and analyzing recovery-stress states (cf. Lazarus & Launier, 1978); such a perspective views the individual as actively acting in an environment, which requires actions, reactions, and adaptive coping with the actual conditions.

The recovery perspective changes the view from the current mainstream perspective on stress, stress mediators, and stress moderators in the following ways:

- Time window: According to a recovery-stress approach, reactions due to stressful conditions should be monitored until a state of homeostatic balance has been reestablished or new stressors occur, which could cause further disturbance of the individual.

• Systems: Stress research focuses on the ergotrophic sympathetic vegetative system and the HPA (hypothalamic-pituitary-adrenal) axis and its impact on immune functioning and central nervous system, emotional, motivational, cognitive, and behavioral changes accompanied by the general mobilization of resources to cope with stress. The recovery-stress approach, by contrast, directs attention to those processes that compensate for the expenditure of resources, control excessive activation, and lead to the reestablishment of a homeostatic equilibrium and normal reactivity.

• Symptoms/indicators: Stress research focuses on negative psychological and physiological symptoms and how to reduce stress, while the recovery-stress state includes positive mood, well-being, life satisfaction, performance increments, the reestablishment and optimization of resources, and biological rhythms.

Thus, the concept of the individual's recovery-stress state affords a better understanding of the adverse and beneficial effects of stress than does a mere analysis of stress reactions and coping, because recovery processes are explicitly taken into account.

The recovery-stress perspective allows us to look at mediators and moderators of stress reactions in a new way. For example, individuals are encouraged to seek social support, which offers social recovery. In the case of decision and action latitude (Karasek, 1979), individuals under stress are more encouraged to create their own schedules and plan their own recovery activities and breaks.

Recovery focuses on the (limited) resources of the individual. Resources can be divided into permanent resources and consumptive resources according to Schönpflug (1983). The resources concept allows us to define recovery as the reestablishment and optimization of resources after they have been taxed by stress due to challenges or threats to the individual.

Defining recovery can be difficult. We wonder, for example, whether recovery processes from qualitatively different stress reactions are comparable or qualitatively different. While a brief rest during strenuous work, recovery from a stressful emotional state, recovery from a test or sport competition, and recovery from surgery may all share a general definition of recovery, they may differ in specific features.

Recovery processes occur on all levels of subsystems of the organism. They range from cellular mechanisms, which reestablish the functional state of neurons, to recovery in social aggregates such as teams. This chapter looks at recovery from the macroscopic level of the individual. The recovery-stress state depends on stress and recovery processes, which take place more or less regularly in the course of a few days or nights. The recovery-stress state is considered to be stable up to 72 hours. On the other hand, changes during a whole week or an extremely stressful day of business or training can well be expected. Not considered in this chapter are recovery processes on a microscopic level (e.g., cellular mechanisms) and long-term recovery processes such as recuperation or rehabilitation, which take more than one or two weeks.

The basic approach of this chapter is outlined in figure 16.1.

Stressors are rarely imposed on a passive person (radiation is one example); rather, people generally evaluate situations and act planfully. Even simple physical stimulations such as noise will actively be appraised by the person (cf. Glass & Singer, 1972; Lazarus & Launier, 1978). When an individual's resources are taxed by a task and the situational context of that task, and the individual then achieves proper recovery, the individual is said to be in a fitness loop. The individual's recovery-stress state is optimized continuously, and stress offers positive consequences. Social support, relaxation skills, and off-time activities, which allow the individual to move away from stress (diversion), support regeneration. The fitness loop is accompanied by increased well-being and other positive attributes, such as a sense of coherence (Antonovsky, 1987) and self-efficacy (Bandura, 1997).

Underrecovery, which sets the person in a "burnout loop," is accompanied by negative symptoms. When recovery is insufficient, omitted, or disturbed, the individual can become exhausted or burned out. Negative coping and poststress rumination enhance the chance of underrecovery, which causes an imbalance between stress and recovery. This imbalance will cause negative consequences of stress, such as performance decrements, physical symptoms, impaired immune system functioning, fatigue, motivational decrements, and dropping out, just to mention a few.

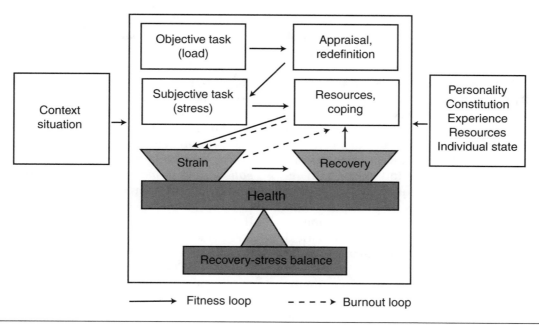

Figure 16.1   Recovery-stress process.

Adapted, by permission, from K.W. Kallus and T. Uhlig, 2001, Erholungsforschung: Neue Perspektiven zum Verständnis von Streβ [Recovery research: New perspectives for the understanding of stress]. In *Psychologie 2000* edited by R.K. Silbereisen and M. Reitzle (Lengerich: Pabst Science), 372.

Worth considering is whether increased stress (demanding increased recovery) will reach a threshold beyond which it is impossible for the organism to recover adequately. Kellmann and Kallus' scissors model of the interrelation of stress states and recovery demands (see this volume, chapter 1) addresses the question of whether there is really a fixed threshold that will lead to stress symptoms even if the individual tries to keep stress and recovery in a fair balance. Negative long-term consequences, including tissue damage, might be expected when a "high-load balance" is lost.

On the other hand, excessive rest (dolce vita) might cause problems due to inactivity. This is well known in the muscular system, which shows atrophy when not regularly used. Figure 16.1 reflects the rule that stress is necessary for maintaining fitness. This is well in accordance with notions from Selye (1993) and others who stated that stress should not be avoided under all circumstances.

The recovery-stress state, like stress, is a biopsychological construct that should be studied and assessed using a multilevel, multimethod approach. Until now, no suitable indicators for recovery have been described that are sensitive and specific. Many sensitive indicators are accompanied by positive emotional states, a sense of coherence, and general well-being. We know that a positive recovery-stress state is associated with

high performance potential (Kellmann & Kallus, 1999) and adaptive reactions to challenges. In the long run, dynamic indicators (e.g., reactivity measures, cf. Janke & Kallus, 1995; Uhlig, 1999) will be necessary to obtain a multidimensional picture, which has to take several dimensions into account simultaneously to qualify the recovery-stress state.

Options for checking for an optimal recovery-stress state should include reactivity tests. Reactivity tests, such as the stress-arithmetic test of v. Eiff, Czernik, and Zanders (1969), look at the changes and dynamics of psychophysiological measures under controlled conditions. The v. Eiff test takes cardiovascular measures before, during, and after the subjects perform arithmetic problems while they are disturbed by noise. Tests like this one allow a direct assessment of stress reactivity and subsequent recovery. For this reason reactivity tests should be used in the future.

One way to assess the recovery-stress state is to use the Recovery-Stress Questionnaire (RESTQ, Kallus, 1995; Kellmann & Kallus, 2001). The RESTQ addresses different levels of stress and recovery activities and states (physical indicators, emotional symptoms, behavioral and performance-related symptoms, and social activities) during the past three days/nights. A multilevel conception has been used to develop the different scales. It should be pointed out that the method (self-report) and the level of assessed variables (physical, emotional, behavioral, social) need not necessarily be in a one-to-one ratio. Of course, a direct measurement of all levels will help to better understand the underlying processes and check the validity of the self-report measures.

Reliability of the RESTQ has already been discussed by Kellmann (this volume, chapter 3). The RESTQ allows derivation of a profile of stress and recovery scores, which reflect the overall recovery-stress state of the individual with respect to the stress and recovery activities and episodes in different areas within the past three days or even longer. The profile can be summarized into three basic scores for brief statistical comparisons: general stress, performance-related stress (tiredness), and recovery.

The idea of creating a symmetrical picture for stress and recovery turned out to be too simplistic. Correlation analysis of the scales (Kallus, 1995; Kellmann & Kallus, 2000) showed that stress and recovery cannot be treated as two sides of the same coin.

Table 16.1 summarizes the scales of the RESTQ and shows the factorial structure based on a sample of 420 subjects who attended a sports conference. Principal component analysis with Kaiser's extraction criterion (eigenvalue 1) resulted in three factors. Table 16.1 gives the loadings above .25, which resulted from varimax rotation. Stress and recovery scales are relatively independent and do not emerge as two ends of a bipolar factor. Furthermore, stress can be divided into two subfactors: general/emotional stress and performance-related/work-related stress (such as *Fatigue* and *Somatic Complaints*). Especially in work settings the three-factor interpretation seems to be quite useful. Sometimes a two-factor solution turned out to be the best option as the two stress factors (factors 1 and 2) show high side-loading on each other.

The RESTQ has been used in different areas of application. The large amount of convergence and positive results leads to the conclusion that the recovery-stress state is of high relevance from a biological, psychological, and performance-related point of view. Recovery scores especially often show an impressive incremental validity in the prediction and moderation of responses in highly demanding situations. The different areas of re-

Table 16.1   Three-Factor Solution (*a* > .25) of the RESTQ-72* (*n* = 420)

RESTQ scales	Factor 1	Factor 2	Factor 3	h²
1 General Stress	.54	.67	−.28	.83
2 Emotional Stress	.31	.85	-	.85
3 Social Stress	-	.90	-	.84
4 Conflicts	.63	.49	-	.68
5 Fatigue	.80	-	-	.70
6 Lack of Energy	.56	.58	-	.68
7 Physical Complaints	.74	-	−.31	.68
8 Success	-	-	.79	.72
9 Social Recovery	-	-	.71	.53
10 Physical Recovery	−.43	-	.74	.78
11 General Well-Being	−.43	−.28	.75	.83
12 Sleep Quality	−.64	-	.49	.67
Eigenvalue	5.89	1.89	1.00	
Variance in %	49.1	15.8	8.3	

* RESTQ-72 is the basic version of the RESTQ and measures subscales 1-12 of the RESTQ-Sport with six items per subscale.
Adapted, by permission, from K.W. Kallus, 1995, *Der Erholungs-Belastungs-Fragebogen (EBF)* [The Recovery-Stress Questionnaire] (Frankfurt, Germany: Swets & Zeitlinger), 29.

search with the RESTQ, outlined here, will be discussed in the following sections of this chapter.

- Biopsychological stress research: Primarily concerned with changes in psychological and physiological variables, this area shows that the recovery-stress state is an important predictor for the individual's stress reactivity.

- Work psychology: An applied setting in which performance under high demands and recovery processes are of high importance. Interestingly, classical work on work, tiredness, and rest schedules (Graf, 1961; Kraepelin, 1903) is currently neglected in many areas.

- Health and clinical psychology: The role of recovery in surgical patients is an example of a clinical application.

Before starting with the different areas of recovery research, we will address one of the frequently asked questions: Is recovery a new disguise for coping with stress? The interrelation between recovery and coping is less simple than expected. Effective coping with stress in many instances is implicitly considered as adequate recovery from stress. At the same time dysfunctional coping, such as rumination, is likely to impair recovery (see also Beckmann, this volume, chapter 15). Thus, there are close conceptual links between recovery and coping. The intercorrelations of the German version of the RESTQ (Kallus, 1995) and the Stress Coping Inventory (Janke et al., 1985) are rather low, as there is less than 10% common variance for most of the scales. In the 12 by 19 matrix the highest correlations were obtained (r .40) for *Rumination* and *Resignation* with *General Stress*.

The only area of moderate correlations has to do with more or less dysfunctional poststress coping modes. All in all, the weak correlations show that the processes have to be analyzed in detail to shed light on the similarities and differences between recovery and coping. For the time being, we can state that the recovery-stress state is only moderately related to coping strategies.

Recovery-Stress State and Biopsychological Stress Research

Research has increasingly shown that a person's state, as assessed by the RESTQ, is well reflected in changes in biological state indicators (Kallus &

Uhlig, 2001; Uhlig, 1999). This is an important result of biopsychological recovery-stress research, which uses a multilevel approach to assess the state of the individual. Performance measures and behavioral indicators, self-reported emotional and motivational indicators, and physiological and biological state markers are used to infer the recovery-stress state of the individual. The dynamic properties of the state are far better understood if reactivity measurement (assessment under stimulating conditions) is included. In many instances laboratory stressors, such as mental arithmetic or bicycle ergometer work, are used to provoke a reaction. Changes in reactivity can be observed in many instances of changed individual state (e.g. tiredness, depression, overtraining; cf. Janke & Kallus, 1995).

Different emotional reactions for subjects who score low and high in overall recovery in the RESTQ can be shown under experimental laboratory conditions (simulated public speaking and mental arithmetic; see figure 16.2).

Forty subjects were studied under stress conditions (public speaking) in phase 1 of the experiment, while 26 were randomly assigned to the control condition. After public speaking, subjects were given a recovery period. Finally, all subjects were subjected to a second laboratory stressor (mental arithmetic with noise). Measures were taken at baseline, after the announcement of the task (task), directly before the speech (prespeech), after finishing the speech (postspeech), after the announcement of a break (recovery start), by the end of the 10-minute recovery period (recovery stop), and before and after the mental arithmetic task of v. Eiff (v. Eiff et al., 1969). To show the impact of the recovery-stress state, researchers divided the subjects into low- and high-recovery groups (median split) according to the preexperimental RESTQ score for total recovery.

Preexperimentally badly recovered subjects (lines with squares) show a clear-cut aftereffect of public speaking, which results in increased lack of energy. This unfavorable state is not compensated by the break. Instead, it is prolonged into the second laboratory stressor. This result supports the hypothesis that low recovery impairs the adaptation to subsequent stressful conditions. Resources were exhausted by the first stressor for those subjects with low preexperimental recovery. After exhaustion the break is not sufficient enough to meet the second stressor in the same way as in the preexperimentally well-recovered subjects.

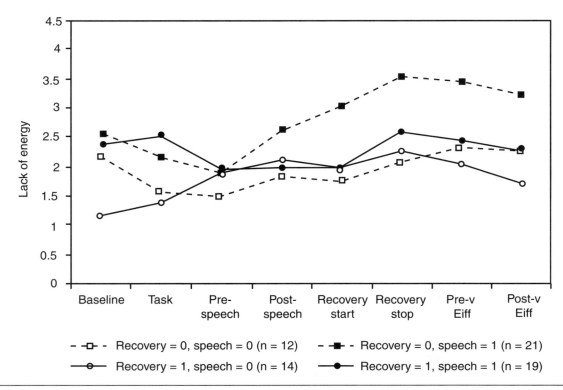

Figure 16.2 Lack of energy (exhaustion: 0 = not at all, 6 = very strong) in an experimental stress experiment for groups with low (below-median) and high (above-median) preexperimental recovery (recov. = 0: RESTQ-Recovery below median; recov. = 1: RESTQ-Recovery above median; speech = 0: no simulated public speaking; speech = 1: simulated public speaking). Lack of energy was assessed by an adjective checklist based on Janke and Debus (1978).

Adapted, by permission, from K.W. Kallus and T. Uhlig, 2001, Erholungsforschung: Neue Perspektiven zum Verständnis von Streß [Recovery research: New perspectives for the understanding of stress]. In *Psychologie 2000* edited by R.K. Silbereisen and M. Reitzle (Lengerich: Pabst Science), 374.

Uhlig (1999) published an overview across empirical investigations on recovery-stress state, as assessed by the RESTQ, and biological parameters. His field studies showed that the recovery-stress state in healthy subjects is related to several reactivity indicators. These comprise self-report data, cardiovascular measures (heart rate, blood pressure), catecholamines (blood samples of epinephrine and norepinephrine), indicators of the HPA axis (adrenocorticotrophic hormone [ACTH], cortisol), growth hormone, and renin. Blood samples were analyzed for hormone levels. Fine-grained analysis of hormone release (pulsatility) could not be included in the applied settings. (For a detailed discussion of various hormones in psychological stress experiments, see Stanford & Salmon, 1993.)

In these studies subjects were divided into different groups according to the RESTQ scores: those with high stress and low recovery scores and those with high recovery and comparably low stress scores. This typology overcomes the prob-

lem that frequency-based stress and recovery scores in the Recovery-Stress Questionnaire comprise two independent factors. The typology of high stress/low recovered versus high recovered/low stress is supported by configuration frequency analyses of two large samples (Uhlig, 1999). Inferring on the functional state, the above-median stress scores and the lower-tercile recovery scores seem to indicate a psychological state accompanied by drastic changes in reactivity compared with those subjects who score below median in the stress scores of the RESTQ and at the same time show medium to high recovery scores.

In a study with bicycle ergometry, Uhlig, Seifert, Kallus, and Schmucker (1998) studied the reactivity of participants in a fitness program. Blood samples were taken for baseline measures (before first ergometrics), after first ergometrics, during a break, after a second ergometry, and after a final rest period (after break). Levels of renin were determined to compare the results with those from clinical samples. Renin is the key hormone of renal blood pressure regulation. It directly reflects changes in sympathetic stimulation. Renin is part of the renin-angiotensin-aldosterone system, which increases blood pressure if activated due to loss of salt, loss of blood volume, low (renal) blood pressure, or sympathetic stimulation. The overall status of the subjects was assessed by a questionnaire, and subjects with irregularities in physical or psychological functions were excluded. During the test all subjects followed the same protocol (standard physical work capacity [pwc] 170 ergometry, no additional fluid intake, etc.). Despite its functional importance, renin is rarely used in psychophysiological reactivity tests with healthy subjects.

Subjects with a low recovery and a high stress score (group low recovery) showed elevated values of renin in the recovery period and throughout a subsequent ergometer trial, including the second recovery period (see figure 16.3). This showed that an unfavorable recovery-stress state increases the probability of dysfunctional physiological reactions in demanding situations. Uhlig (1999) reported further studies, which support the view that the two types (high stress/low recovery and low stress/high recovery) also show different catecholaminergic reactions under moderate physical and psychological stress conditions.

The functional approach has already been stressed by Frankenhaeuser (1978). The better the recovery score and the less the stress scores, the better the adaptivity of the physiological reac-

tions to challenges. Later in this chapter results with clinical samples will briefly be addressed, which will strengthen the view that the recovery-stress state can be considered a biopsychologically founded state.

Recent empirical evidence shows that the recovery-stress state as assessed by the RESTQ corresponds also with reactivity indicators of the stress state, which parallel sport-medical blood parameters such as lactate, pH-value, and so forth. Porta et al. (1993) proposed provoked changes in serological parameters to assess the stress state. Porta's poststress provocation test (see also Bacher et al., 1999) is based on the rationale that moderate physical activity will result in adaptive responses, which differ for persons in different stress states. At the same time physical activity will bring those catecholamines of the blood into circulation, which accumulate at the walls of the larger vessels during and after stress conditions. Peripheral blood samples taken from the fingertip before and after moderate physical exercise reveal metabolic and catecholaminergic stress indicators (Porta et al., 1993). Many problems related to the assessment of catecholamines can be overcome by using Porta et al.'s (1993) reactivity approach.

Two studies have used the RESTQ to assess the self-reported recovery-stress state and at the same time the serological stress indicators used by Porta. The first study by Porta and Kallus (2000) was conducted with 35 subjects who attended a fitness studio for training. Correlations up to $r = .5$

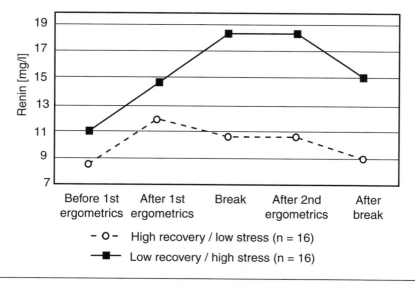

Figure 16.3 Recovery-stress state and renin reactivity for two groups of participants in a health-related promotion program. Groups were built using the overall stress and recovery scores of the RESTQ.

Drawn, by permission, from T. Uhlig, 1999, *Erholung als biopsychologisches Konstrukt.* [Recovery as a biopsychological construct]. Dissertation, Julius Maximilians University, Würzburg, Germany, 106.

were obtained between RESTQ scores and the biological stress state indicators. The largest correlation was obtained for RESTQ *Physical Complaints,* which correlated with the pH scores after exercise ($r = -.52$). Similar spearman correlations were obtained for lactate levels, which trigger blood pH. These results indicate that elevated stress levels (especially if reflected in *Physical Complaints*) might be accompanied by a reduced capacity to buffer lactate-induced acidosis in the blood, which might be of high importance for trainers and athletes.

Porta, Fleck, and Hueber (2000) obtained similar results by studying 21 parachute jumpers before and after the parachute jump. Blood pH correlated positively with recovery scores in this instance. The spearman correlation was as high as $r = .59$ before jumping and $r = .51$ after jumping. Correlations with recovery-stress scores were significant despite the small sample size in this study. These results fit neatly into the picture that the recovery-stress balance is a good predictor not only of performance in sports but also of poststress adaptation.

Subjects who show an unfavorable recovery-stress balance prior to examinations have a higher risk of poststress physical complaints. This was documented in the RESTQ manual by Kallus (1995) and was also reported by Deinzer and Schuller (1998). Changes in RESTQ scores after vacation are to be expected and were shown by Strauss-Blasche, Ekmekcioglu, and Marktl (2000) and Kellmann, Johnson, and Wrisberg (1998). All in all, there is accumulating evidence that the recovery-stress state reveals important biopsychological characteristics of the individual, which is of special importance in predicting what will happen if the individual is taxed by challenging situations. One very challenging situation for the organism is the occurrence of medical interventions. These will be considered in the final section of this chapter.

Recovery-Stress State and Job-Related Work

Stress at work is a function of workload and moderators such as action latitude, social support, and work motivation. Workload depends on the amount of work to be done, the tools available, the quality of the work, and the distribution in time. Since the historic studies of Kraepelin (1903) and Graf (1922), it has been known that distributed short breaks are far more effective than single long breaks as far as performance measures are concerned. Recent studies on the "spillover" of work into the off-time show that recovery from work stress takes substantial amounts of time and determines the off-time state to a large degree (cf. Frankenhaueser, 1993). Rau and Richter (1995) showed that daytime stress affects the time it takes to unwind in the night, especially for subjects with high control ambitions.

Stress moderators as well as the stress-rest distribution in time are conceptually linked to the recovery-stress state. The recovery-stress state is an important moderator of performance in athletes. Is the recovery-stress state related to performance in work settings as well? This is especially relevant for professionals with high levels of responsibility, such as pilots, air traffic controllers, brokers, physicians, nurses, and managers. Besides performance, another aspect of the recovery-stress state in work settings is health, as a long-term imbalance of stress and recovery will increase the risk of disorders.

A study of 77 air traffic controllers from 12 different air traffic control centers in Europe showed that a considerable amount of variability exists in the recovery-stress state of active controllers. Extreme values, as obtained repeatedly (see figure 16.4) certainly bear the risk of suboptimal performance, which is normally ensured by the team in air traffic control.

Schwarhofer and Kallus (2000) assessed the recovery-stress state during two shift cycles in 12 railway traffic controllers. This study examined changes in recovery-stress state due to shift work; the RESTQ was filled out four times—at the beginning and end of two consecutive shift cycles. Each shift cycle consisted of two day and two night shifts with 24 hours of recovery between each. The two shift cycles were separated by a three-day (72 hours) off period.

Results showed that recovery-stress states changed as expected from the beginning to the end of the shift cycles. The average change for both shift cycles is given in figure 16.5. Note that recovery scores are not affected in the same way as stress scores.

Shift cycles of day-night-day-night with a shift period of 12 hours and a recovery period of 24 hours were shown to lead to an accumulation of stress. Further analyses showed that this effect was compensated in the 72 hours of off-time between the two shift cycles.

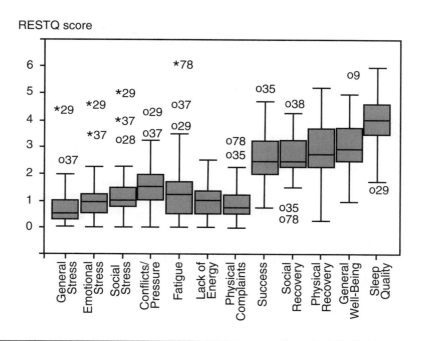

Figure 16.4 Box-whiskers plots of recovery-stress profiles of 77 air traffic controllers (o = outliers; * = extremes).

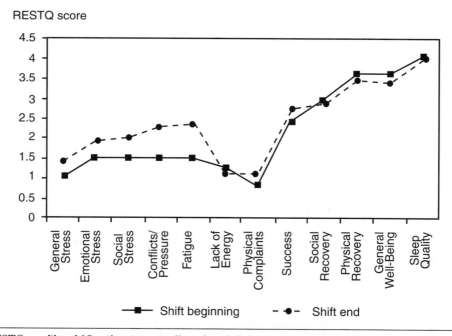

Figure 16.5 RESTQ profile of 12 railway controllers for shift beginning and shift end.

Monitoring the recovery-stress state might well be worthwhile in high-responsibility white-collar jobs. Our first results indicated that the recovery-stress state, as assessed by the RESTQ, shows considerable variation between and within subjects in work settings (Kallus & Uhlig, 2001). As such, recovery-stress states can probably be use-

ful for predicting performance and ensuring safety and health at work.

By examining recovery-stress states, we can look at stress moderators from a process-oriented point of view, which can help us to understand how they impact stress in a variety of work settings. Consider, for example, the stress buffer of decision latitude (Karasek, 1979; Karasek & Theorell, 1990), in which individuals are permitted to choose their goals and how to achieve them. This buffer can be explained within a recovery-stress framework (Meijman & Mulder, 1998). Individuals with adequate decision latitude can distribute their work and recovery periods optimally according to their own resources. Thus, resources can be used optimally to achieve work goals. On the other hand, reduced decision latitude (low stress buffers) can lead to under-recovery. With respect to coping with occupational stress, social support can be viewed as an additional resource for the individual, serving to reduce her workload, help her cope with stress, and foster recovery. Social support shows a considerable overlap with social recovery as far as item content is concerned. All in all we can conclude that factors identified as stress buffers in work-related stress research are accompanied by lower stress scores and higher recovery scores in the RESTQ.

Data from a larger study in Austria (Pelzl, 1999) support this empirically. The recovery-stress state was assessed in 415 participants from different occupational groups (computer workers, nurses, and blue-collar workers). A version of the RESTQ, which covers seven instead of three days as a reference period, was used to assess the recovery-stress state. Since the manual permits changes in RESTQ time windows, seven days of reference were selected to cover a whole working week (Kallus, 1995). RESTQ scores were aggregated, which resulted in a first score for general stress (mean of scales *General Stress, Emotional Stress,* and *Social Stress*), a second score for performance stress (mean of *Conflicts/Pressure, Fatigue, Lack of Energy,* and *Physical Complaints*), and a third score for recovery (mean of *Success, Social Recovery, Physical Recovery, General Well-Being,* and *Sleep Quality*).

Of the 415 subjects, 396 completed a second questionnaire called AVEM (work-related patterns of behavior and psychic states) developed by Schaarschmidt and Fischer (1997), which assesses work-related behavior and appraisal patterns. Scales of the AVEM can be summarized into three factors:

- Factor 1, *Engagement,* is characterized by high engagement and ambition.
- Factor 2, *Ability to Switch Off,* assesses the ability to "switch off" after work and relax.
- Factor 3, *Satisfaction,* is characterized by social support, success, and life satisfaction.

The bivariate spearman correlations show negative correlations with stress and positive correlations with recovery for all factors (even *Engagement*) of work-related behavior and appraisal patterns (see table 16.2).

The AVEM scale of *Social Support/Satisfaction* showed the highest correlation to RESTQ *Recovery.* Note that even *Engagement* showed a negative correlation with stress and a positive correlation with recovery. This is rather astonishing at first glance, as high engagement and ambition are considered contributing factors to the type A behavior pattern identified in cardiovascular risk research by Friedman and Rosenman (1974); type A behavior is positively related to stress. *Engagement* without the negative attributes of type A behavior (hostility, high perfectionism, low *Ability to Switch Off,* and low *Satisfaction*) showed a negative relation to stress and a positive relation to recovery. Thus, this result adds interesting arguments to the type A behavior debate from a recovery-stress perspective. It shows that an ability to switch off (or in other words, recover) is an important intervention-related characteristic that probably circumvents the negative consequences of high job engagement.

Table 16.2 Spearman Correlations Between RESTQ Factors and Factors of Work-Related Behavior and Appraisal Patterns (AVEM)

			AVEM Engagement	AVEM Ability to Switch Off	AVEM Satisfaction
Spearman-Rho	RESTQ General Stress	Corr.	−.29	−.49	−.42
	RESTQ Performance Stress	Corr.	−.26	−.49	−.33
	RESTQ Recovery	Corr.	.36	.45	.51

All correlations are significant ($p < 0.001$) because of the large sample size ($n = 396$).

Another result that validates the RESTQ in work psychology was obtained by a short Questionnaire for Work Analysis (Kurzfragebogen zur Arbeitsanalyse [KFZA] Prümper, Hartmannsgruber, & Frese, 1995; see table 16.3). The single-scale scores of the KFZA were also grouped to higher-order scales.

- Scale 1, *Work Quality,* is based on action latitude, variability of work, and completeness of work.
- Scale 2, *Social Quality of Work,* is composed of social support, cooperation, information/participation, and organizational support.
- Scale 3, *Workload,* is the mean of qualitative workload, quantitative workload, work interruptions, and environmental stressors.

Results from this study showed a pattern of correlations that were consistent with expectations. *Social Work Quality* shows the highest correlation to *Recovery,* and *Work Quality* is also positively related to *Recovery.*

Before interpreting the absolute values of the previously reported correlations, we must bear in mind that RESTQ scores are state dependent and not specifically related to work, which means that the correlations reported should be considered as lower bounds of the true relationships. A work-specific version of the RESTQ is currently under construction (Kallus, in preparation).

A comparison of two subsamples of 141 female office workers and 143 female nurses resulted in unexpected differences showing high stress scores and low recovery scores for the office tasks with

Table 16.3   Spearman Correlations of RESTQ and a Questionnaire of Subjective Task Analysis (KFZA)

KFZA		RESTQ General Stress	RESTQ Performance Stress	RESTQ Recovery
Score 1	Work Quality	−.16	−.15	.28
Score 2	Social Quality of Work	−.37	−.30	.36
Score 3	Workload	.46	.47	−.34

All correlations are significant ($p < 0.003$; $n = 396$).

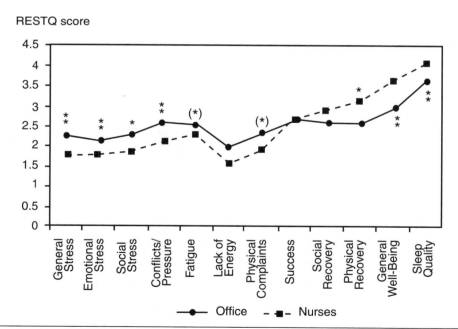

Figure 16.6   Recovery-stress profile of nurses and office employees. Results of pairwise t-tests: (*) = 0.1 < p 0.05; * = 0.05 < p 0.01; ** = $p < 0.01$.

Drawn from Pelzl, 1999.

a large amount of computer work (see figure 16.6). This is accompanied by more emotional exhaustion and less work satisfaction reported by the subjects with a high amount of computer work. This highlights the fact that people with high-tech jobs have a high risk for stress-related disorders and need special attention.

The unexpected high stress levels of office personnel were also reflected in the subjective task analysis results of KFZA (Scale *Workload*). A possible explanation can be derived from the higher score in *Social Quality of Work* of nurses. This quality might act as a stress buffer, reducing overall stress. Problems in recovery-stress balance clearly do not occur only in classical populations at risk for burnout, such as nurses. Office work, call-center work, and others might turn out to be the future's new high-stress jobs.

Different work conditions are also reflected in the recovery-stress state. In a study by Kallus and Wagner (1996) a sample of 57 nurses from different wards was studied. Wards were classified according to high versus low staff turnover and manning. Manning refers to the number of people working in a work setting in relation to the number of people that are necessary to "run" the work setting. Figure 16.7 shows that wards with high fluctuation showed significantly higher scores in *Emotional Stress* and *Social Stress*. Other differences showed p-values above 0.1 in the pairwise

U-tests, which were used for statistical comparison. Performance-related scales *(Conflicts/Pressure, Fatigue, Lack of Energy,* and *Physical Complaints)* did not support the result from the general stress scales *(General Stress, Emotional Stress,* and *Social Stress)*.

Other results from the Recovery-Stress Questionnaire in this study showed that the recovery-stress state is also related to features of the tasks on a microscopic level; for example, the number of objects needed to conduct the task or the necessity to switch rooms often as well as communication patterns were related to RESTQ scores.

The recovery-stress state might contribute to the understanding of the role of rest and recovery in occupational settings. Future application areas range from creating optimal work schedules to providing for sufficient unwinding after work (Frankenhaeuser, 1978) in order to reduce the risk of work-related cardiovascular and other psychosomatic diseases (Frankenhaeuser et al., 1989; Rau, 1998).

Recovery-Stress State in Clinical and Health Psychology

A huge number of prevention programs in health psychology as well as psychological intervention programs in clinical psychology focus on stress

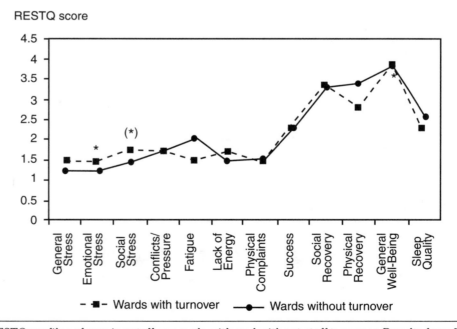

Figure 16.7 RESTQ profiles of nursing staff on wards with and without staff turnover. Results from U-tests: (*) = 0.1 < p 0.05; * = 0.05 < p 0.01.

From Kallus and Wagner, 1996.

and coping. Improvement in the recovery-stress state is an important benchmark for those prevention and intervention programs. Consequently, the assessment of changes in stress management programs was one of the early validation criteria of the RESTQ.

Participants in a stress-reduction program showed overall changes in stress and recovery scores in a pre-post design, which was validated against a waiting list control group (Kallus, 1995). A similar effect could be replicated for a health-related activity program. Over 700 participants completed the Recovery-Stress Questionnaire before and after participating in health-promoting physical activity programs. The programs were conducted in weekly courses over three months and were held by trainers with special health-related qualifications. Results were evaluated using a group of students who also attended sports activities on a weekly basis as a control group. Change scores for both groups are shown in figure 16.8.

Sport students show only marginal changes, with slight increases in work-related stress scales—probably due to increasing workloads as the term went on. Participants in the health-promotion program showed a very pronounced decline in all stress scales and an increase in recovery, which was very pronounced in *Physical Recovery*. Changes for participants turned out to be highly significant due to the large sample size.

Results again showed that expected changes in the recovery-stress state due to stress-reducing conditions are quite validly assessed by the Recovery-Stress Questionnaire.

From a practical point of view an interesting question to ask is, Must one remove stress and then enhance recovery, or can enhanced recovery result in an organism that is better able to cope with stressful situations? Data from the previously mentioned study on health sports (cf. figure 16.8) allows us to look at the processes a bit more closely because the recovery-stress state was assessed repeatedly by a short version of the Recovery-Stress Questionnaire during the courses (beginning, week 2, week 5, week 8, week 10). Over a third of the subjects were available for repeated-measures analysis. The RESTQ with 24 items was used to reflect changes in the recovery-stress state.

General Stress and *Performance Stress* scores are depicted in figures 16.9a and 16.9b, respectively. The results indicate that after the first sessions of the health-promotion program a substantial decline in *General Stress* scores is already achieved (see figure 16.9a, program start to 5th course). *Recovery* (see figure 16.9c) shows an increase, which is most pronounced in the first weeks. Both effects stabilize during the course of the program. Interestingly, *Performance Stress* shows a slower change (see figure 16.9b). While these results do not determine "what comes first," they do show that different areas show different

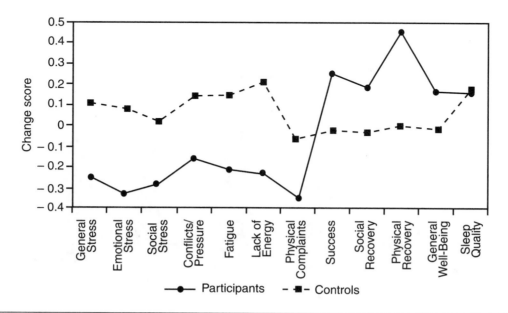

Figure 16.8 Change scores (begining of program, end of program) of the RESTQ for participants in a health-promotion program and a control group of students who exercised regularly.

Data from Kallus and Uhlig, 1997.

General Stress

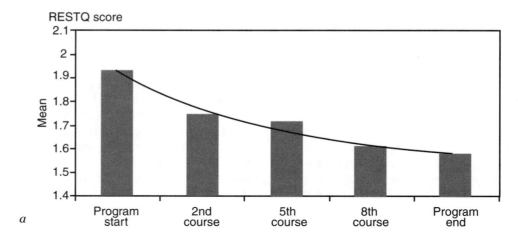

a

Performance Stress

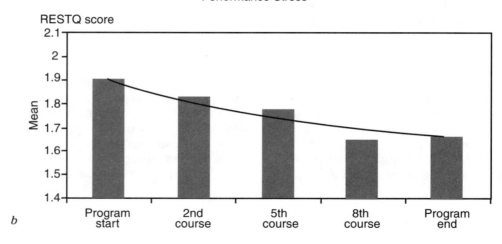

b

Recovery

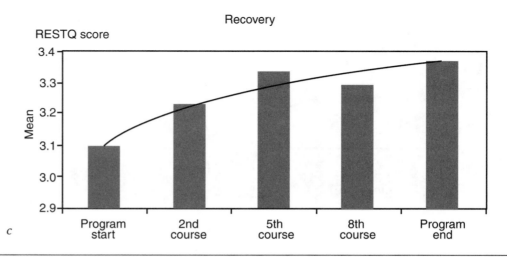

c

Figure 16.9 Changes of recovery-stress state in the course of a health-promoting fitness program. *General Stress (a); Performance Stress (b); Recovery (c).*

dynamics. Results raise the hypothesis that increases in recovery are obtained most quickly.

Deinzer, Kleineidam, Stiller-Winkler, Idel, and Bach (2000) also addressed the dynamics of changes in the recovery-stress state data. These data show that while the recovery-stress state changes before and after examinations, the HPA axis seems to be much less sensitive to changes. This also supports the idea that recovery behaviors, such as sleeping, relaxing, and reducing stressful activities, must be increased before the overall biological state of the organism can recover.

Finally, we will review some evidence of the clinical impact of the recovery-stress state. Uhlig (1999) reported data from heart surgery patients (*n* = 66). After dividing the patients into two groups—positive and negative recovery-stress states (as described earlier in this chapter), he looked for changes in the course of preparation for surgery. Different reactivity was found for these two groups of patients. Measures of renin were taken when patients entered the surgical procedure and again just before the heart/lung machine took over cardiovascular functioning. Highly stressed and badly recovered patients showed a dysfunctional elevation of renin during surgery, which was not observed in those who were in a positive recovery-stress state (see figure 16.10). An unfavorable recovery-stress state also contributed to more problems during surgery and more problems with postsurgical recovery.

The recovery-stress state as assessed by the RESTQ allows us to predict how persons will adapt to extremely stressful conditions, such as surgical intervention, and how processes such as recovery from surgery will develop. The increasing evidence on the biological bases of the recovery-stress state explains why RESTQ scores predict performance and have turned out to be valuable in training monitoring, as these scores are related to the ability to cope with extremely taxing situations. From this point of view the recovery-stress concept will also be helpful in optimizing performance in repeated competitions or in competitions that have to be carried out in spite of minor injuries. Even monitoring recovery from injuries might be considered as an area of application of the recovery-stress approach.

Conclusions

Recent research on the validity of the RESTQ shows that the scores reflect the state of a person not only on a self-report level but also on a biopsychological level, which is reflected in vegetative reactivity, hormonal stress indicators, and serological indicators of physical fitness. Areas of application cover biopsychological stress research, sport psychology, work and health psychology, and clinical psychology.

The first lesson learned in RESTQ research was that recovery and stress are not simply two parts of the same process. Some processes, such as performance-related recovery (breaks and rest periods) and sleep, have no direct stress-related counterpart. This led to the model of a recovery-stress balance (cf. figure 16.1, p. 285),

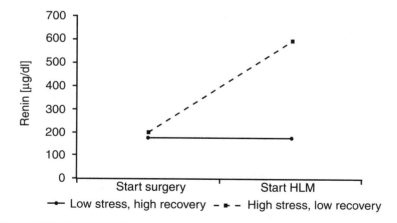

Figure 16.10   Recovery-stress state and renin reactivity of surgical patients. Groups were built based on presurgical RESTQ data for social stress and overall recovery. Blood samples were taken at the start of the surgery and when anesthesia began to work and the heart/lung machine was switched on (start HLM).

Reprinted, by permission, from T. Uhlig, 1999, *Erholung als biopsychologisches Konstrukt* [Recovery as a biopsychological construct]. Dissertation, Julius Maximilians University, Würzburg, Germany, 133.

which is a resource-oriented interpretation of the recovery-stress state (for resource-oriented models, see also Hobfoll, 1988). In addition, we learned that recovery and coping with stress overlap only to a small extent.

The recovery-stress state is linked to mood as assessed by adjective checklists or the Profile of Mood States (McNair, Lorr, & Droppleman, 1992). High correlations with vigor show that the impact of recovery should probably be considered along with the impact of positive mood states (Kellmann & Kallus, 2001). Clearly, positive mood seems to be an important feature of recovery activities. This is also reflected in the recovery items of the RESTQ, which include a positive evaluation throughout. Classical stress moderators such as controllability, decision latitude, and social support also correlate considerably highly with recovery scores. Further research is needed for a closer look at the process components to clarify the mechanisms of stress moderation and recovery. Some stress moderators do not only affect the stress process but seem to allow the individual to make optimal use of recovery, probably in a synergistic sense (Meijman & Mulder 1998).

The diagnostic value of the recovery-stress state has been well demonstrated in the preparation for high-performance events. Now the impact of recovery-stress states on work-related health and performance, health psychology, and recovery after surgery is being studied. First results on the role of the recovery-stress state in these new areas are very encouraging.

The empirical results support our initial argument that we are in need of a systematic study of recovery processes in all areas that address the costs and benefits of stress. At this point we do not know too much about how people manage to keep stress and recovery in a fair balance—especially under extreme conditions.

References

Antonovsky, A. (1987). *Unraveling the mystery of health. How people manage stress and stay well.* San Francisco: Jossey-Bass.

Bacher, H., Mischinger, H.J., Cerwenka, H., Werkgartner, G., El-Shabrawi, A., Supancic, A., & Porta, S. (1999). Liver ischemia, catecholamines and preoperative condition influencing postoperative tachycardia in liver surgery. *Life Sciences 66*(1), 11-18.

Bandura, A. (1997). *Self-efficacy: The exercise of control.* New York: Freeman.

Deinzer, R., Kleineidam, C., Stiller-Winkler, R., Idel, H., & Bach, D. (2000). Prolonged reduction of salivary immunoglobulin A (sIgA) after a major academic exam. *International Journal of Psychophysiology, 37*(3), 219-232.

Deinzer, R., & Schuller, N. (1998). Dynamics of stress-related decrease of salivary immunoglobulin A (sIgA): Relationship to symptoms of the common cold and studying behavior. *Behavioral Medicine 23*(4), 161-169.

Eiff, A.W. von, Czernik, A., & Zanders, H. (1969). Zur medikamentösen Beeinflussung der Sympathikus-hyperaktivität: Parasympathomimeticum und Beta-Rezeptoren-Blocker im Kurzdauernden, pharmakologischen Experiment am Menschen [Pharmacological effects of the sympathetic nervous system: A parasympathicomimeticum and a beta-receptor-blocker in acute, pharmacological trials with humans]. *Klinische Wochenschrift, 47,* 701-708.

Frankenhaeuser, M. (1978). Psychoneuroendocrine approaches to the study of emotion as related to stress and coping. In H.E. Howe (Ed.), *Nebraska Symposium on Motivation* (pp. 123-161). Lincoln: University of Nebraska.

Frankenhaeuser, M. (1993). Current issues in psychobiological stress research. In M. Vartiainen (Ed.), *European Views in Psychology—Keynote Lectures* (pp. 1-11). Tampere, Finland: Third European Congress of Psychology.

Frankenhaeuser, M., Lundberg, U., Fredrikson, M., Melin, B., Tuomisto, M., Myrsten, A.L., Hedman, M., Bergman-Losman, B., & Wallin, L. (1989). Stress on and off the job as related to sex and occupational status in white-collar workers. *Journal of Organizational Behavior, 10,* 321-346.

Friedman, M., & Rosenman, R.H. (1974). *Type A behaviour and your heart.* New York: Knopf.

Glass, D.C., & Singer, J.E. (1972). *Urban stress.* New York: Academic Press.

Graf, O. (1922). Über lohnende Arbeitspause bei geistiger Arbeit [About worthwhile breaks in mental work]. In Kraepelin, E.K. (Ed.), *Psychologische Arbeiten Band 7* (pp. 548-611). Berlin: Verlag von Julius Springer.

Graf, O. (1961). Arbeitszeit und Arbeitspausen. In A. Mayer & B. Herwig (Eds.), *Betriebspsychologie* (pp. 95-117). Handbuch der Psychologie, Band 9. Göttingen, Germany: Hogrefe.

Hobfoll, S.E. (1988). *The ecology of stress.* Washington, DC: Hemisphere.

Janke, W., & Debus, G. (1978). *Die Eigneschaftswörterlist (EWL)* [The Adjective Checklist (EWL)]. Göttingen, Germany: Hogrefe.

Janke, W., Erdmann, G., & Kallus, K.W. (1985). *Der Streßverarbeitungsfragebogen (SVF)* [The Stress Coping Inventory]. Göttingen, Germany: Hogrefe.

Janke, W., & Kallus, K.W. (1995). Reaktivität [Reactivity]. In M. Amelang (Ed.), *Enzyklopädie der*

Psychologie. Verhaltens- und Leistungsunterschiede. Differentielle Psychologie und Persönlichkeitsforschung (Part 2, pp. 1-89). Göttingen, Germany: Hogrefe.

Kallus, K.W. (1995). *Der Erholungs-Belastungs-Fragebogen (EBF)* [The Recovery-Stress Questionnaire]. Frankfurt, Germany: Swets & Zeitlinger.

Kallus, K.W. (in preparation). *Der arbeitsspezifische Erholungs-Belastungs-Fragebogen (EBF-67/7)* [The work-specific Recovery-Stress Questionnaire (RESTQ-Work)]. Manuscript, University of Graz, Austria.

Kallus, K.W., and Uhlig, T. (1997). *Projekt 'fit und gesund'* [The fitness program "fit and healthy"]. Würzburg, Germany: IFB (project report).

Kallus, K.W., & Uhlig, T. (2001). Erholungsforschung: Neue perspektiven zum verständnis von stress [Recovery research: New perspectives for the understanding of stress]. In R.K. Silbereisen & M.Reitzle (Eds.), *Psychologie 2000* (pp. 364-379). Lengerich: Papst Science.

Kallus, K.W., & Wagner, S. (1996). *Stress and Behaviour settings.* Manuscript, University of Würzburg, Germany.

Karasek, R.A. (1979). Job demands, job decision latitude and mental strain: Implications for job redesign. *Administrative Science Quarterly, 24,* 285-308.

Karasek, R.A., & Theorell, T. (1990). *Healthy work. Stress, productivity, and the reconstruction of working life.* New York: Basic Books.

Kellmann, M., Johnson, M.S., & Wrisberg, C.A. (1998). Auswirkungen der Erholungs-Beanspruchungs-Bilanz auf die Wettkampfleistung von amerikanischen Schwimmerinnen [The effects that the recovery-stress state has on the performance of American female swimmers]. In D. Teipel, R. Kemper, & D. Heinemann (Eds.), *Sportpsychologische Diagnostik, Prognostik und Intervention* (pp. 123-126). Cologne, Germany: bps.

Kellmann, M., & Kallus, K.W. (1999). Mood, recovery-stress state, and regeneration. In M. Lehmann, C. Foster, U. Gastmann, H. Keizer, & J.M. Steinacker (Eds.), *Overload, fatigue, performance incompetence, and regeneration in sport* (pp. 101-117). New York: Plenum.

Kellmann, M., & Kallus, K.W. (2000). *Der Erholungs-Belastungs-Fragebogen für Sportler; Handanweisung* [The Recovery-Stress Questionnaire for Athletes; Manual]. Frankfurt, Germany: Swets Test Services.

Kellmann, M., & Kallus, K.W. (2001). *Recovery-Stress Questionnaire for Athletes: User manual.* Champaign, IL: Human Kinetics.

Kraepelin, E. (1903). Über Ermüdungsmessungen. [About fatigue measures]. *Archiv für die Gesamte Psychologie, 1,* 9-30.

Lazarus, R.S., & Launier, R. (1978). Stress-related transactions between person and environment. In L.A. Pervin & M. Lewis (Eds.), *Perspectives in interactional psychology* (pp. 287-327). New York: Plenum.

McNair, D.M., Lorr, M., & Droppleman, L.F. (1992). *Profile of Mood States manual.* San Diego: Educational and Industrial Testing Service.

Meijman, T.F., & Mulder, G. (1998). Psychological aspects of workload. In P.J.D. Drenth, H. Thierry,& C.J. de Wolff (Eds.). *Handbook of work and organizational psychology. Vol. 2: Work psychology* (2nd ed., pp. 5-33). Hove, UK: Psychology Press/Erlbaum.

Pelzl, K. (1999). *Psychische Belastungen am Arbeitsplatz [Psychic stress at work].* Thesis, Karl-Franzens University, Graz, Austria.

Porta, S., Emsenhuber, W., Petek, W., Purstner, P., Vogel, W.H., Schwaberger, G., Salwitsch, P., & Korstako, W. (1993). Detection and evaluation of persisting stress-induced hormonal disturbances by a post stress provocation test in humans. *Life Sciences, 53,* 1583-1589.

Porta, S., Fleck, G., & Hueber, B. (2000). *Stress and bungee.* Unpublished manuscript, University of Vienna.

Porta, S., & Kallus, K.W. (2000, May). Acid based metabolism and stress [Abstract]. Acid-Base Metabolism Congress, Freising, Germany.

Prümper, J., Hartmannsgruber, K., & Frese, M. (1995). KFZA. Kurzfragebogen zur Arbeitsanalyse. [KFZA, Short Questionnaire for Work Analysis]. *Zeitschrift für Arbeits-und Organisationspsychologie, 39,* 125-131.

Rau, R. (1998). Ambulantes psychophysiologisches Monitoring zur Bewertung von Arbeit und Erholung. [Ambulant psychophysiological monitoring for assessing work and recovery]. *Zeitschrift für Arbeits-und Organisationspsychologie, 42*(4), 185-196.

Rau, R., & Richter, P. (1995). *24-Stunden-Monitoring zur Prüfung der Reaktivität psychophysiologischer Parameter in Belastungs- und Erholungsphasen* [24-hour monitoring to examine the reactivity of psychophysiological parameter in stress and recovery episodes]. Forschungsbericht der Bundesanstalt für Arbeitsmedizin. Bremerhaven, Germany: Wirtschaftsverlag.

Schaarschmidt, U., & Fischer, A. (1997). AVEM—ein diagnostisches Instrument zur Differenzierung von Typen gesundheitsrelevanten Verhaltens und Erlebens gegenüber der Arbeit [AVEM—A diagnostic instrument to differentiate between types of health-related behavior and work experiences]. *Zeitschrift für Differentielle und Diagnostische Psychologie 18,* 151-163.

Schönpflug, W. (1983). Coping efficiency and situational demands. In R. Hockey (Ed.), *Stress and fatigue in human performance* (pp. 299-326). Chichester, UK: Wiley.

Schwarhofer, M., & Kallus, K.W. (2000). *Stress and recovery in railway-traffic controllers.* Department of Psychology, Karl-Franzens University, Graz, Austria.

Selye, H. (1993). History of the stress concept. In L. Goldberger & S. Breznitz (Eds.), *Handbook of stress* (pp. 7-18). New York: The Free Press.

Stanford, S.C., & Salmon, P. (1993). *Stress. From synapse to syndrome.* London, CA: Academic Press.

Strauss-Blasche, G., Ekmekcioglu, C., & Marktl, W. (2000). Does vacation enable recuperation? Changes in well-being associated with time away from work. *Occupational Medicine 50*(3), 167-172.

Uhlig, T. (1999). *Erholung als biopsychologisches Konstrukt* [Recovery as a biopsychological construct]. Dissertation, Julius Maximilians University, Würzburg, Germany.

Uhlig, T., Seifert, C., Kallus, K.W., & Schmucker, P. (1998). Befinden und sympathoadrenege Reaktivität in Abhängigkeit von der subjektiven Erholungs-Beanspruchungs-Bilanz [Well-being and sympathico-adrenergic reactivity as determined by the subjective recovery-stress balance]. In W. Hacker (Ed.), *41 Kongreß der Deutschen Gesellschaft für Psychologie.* [Abstracts]. Disc/Konpro. University of Technology, Dresden, Germany.

Kellmann, M. (2002). Current status and directions of recovery research. In M. Kellmann (Ed.), *Enhancing recovery: Preventing underperformance in athletes* (pp. 301-311). Champaign, IL: Human Kinetics.

17

Current Status and Directions of Recovery Research

Michael Kellmann

The applied case studies discussed in this book emphasize that recovery is an important factor in athletic and nonathletic life and that optimal recovery may prevent underperformance. As shown, an interdisciplinary approach is very valuable for the integration of psychological and physiological knowledge as well as for the use of applied intervention and prevention strategies. Despite the fact that the contributors of this book are from different disciplines and countries, they touch on the same fundamental issues of recovery. Kellmann (this volume, chapter 1) points out that whereas underrecovery and overtraining have the same impact (a decline in performance), underrecovery can be identified as the precursor/cause of overtraining. Based on this assumption, this book deals with the connections among underrecovery, overtraining, and underperformance.

A connecting link throughout the book is the availability and replenishment of resources. According to Schönpflug (1983, 1987) and others, reactions to stress depend on permanent and consumptive resources, which offer a person some resistance to stress. Consumptive resources refer to regeneration and recovery, while permanent resources refer to the person's own skills and abilities. Consumptive resources (e.g., effort, tension, willpower, and energy with limited reserves and clear proportional reduction) activate and support permanent resources, which are long-term available internal performance requirements

such as talent, competence, and capacity. Limited consumptive capacities, or a failure to replenish the consumptive resources one has, negatively affects the regeneration of the permanent resources immediately. This consequently increases the risk of a total exhaustion of resources. Therefore, athletes should be encouraged to create, care for, use wisely, repair after use, and replace both resources when lost (Schönpflug, 1987). Overtraining may be the consequence if athletes do not adequately replenish consumptive and permanent resources.

Relevance of Recovery and Overtraining in Sports

As a result of several studies of high-performance athletes, Gould and Dieffenbach (this volume, chapter 2) point out the relevance of overtraining in high-performance sports and its importance as a performance-influencing factor. In a study by Gould et al. (1998) 84 of 298 U.S. Atlanta Olympic athletes (28%) reported that they had overtrained for the Games and that this overtraining had had a negative impact on performance. Similarly, in open-ended responses 35 of the athletes said that they identified overtraining/not getting enough rest as the number one coaching decision that hurt their performance. Among the 1998 U.S. Nagano Winter Olympians 10% of the respondents felt that overtraining had

301

had a negative impact on their performance (Gould, Greenleaf, Dieffenbach, Chung, & Peterson, 1999). Gould and Dieffenbach warn against assuming that this results from inappropriate physical training alone. Other factors such as psychological stress, inadequate rest, type of recovery activity, travel, personality, and sociological issues must be examined in multifaceted models.

Holistic Perspective on Recovery

The results reported by Gould and Dieffenbach (this volume, chapter 2) support the definition by Lehmann and colleagues (e.g., Lehmann et al., 1997; Lehmann, Foster, Gastmann, Keizer, & Steinacker, 1999), who state that overtraining is due to an imbalance between stress and recovery (including all training, competition, and additional nontraining stress factors). Too much stress combined with too little regeneration is the cause for overtraining. Social, educational, occupational, economical, nutritional, and travel factors; time stress; and the monotony of training act to increase the risk of an overtraining syndrome. Smith and Norris (this volume, chapter 5) refer to Noakes (1991), who suggested that training holism encompasses two ideas: (1) training must be balanced and varied, and (2) nontraining time has a major influence on training itself. It is important therefore that all factors outside the realm of the training session, including diet, sleep, other physical effort, and work stress, be evaluated as to their possible negative influence on total fatigue (Noakes, 1991). Coaches should be aware that athletes have to coordinate training with educational or professional responsibilities, friendships, and personal matters.

Balance of life and quality of life are key issues, implying that recovery is a dynamic process (Wrisberg & Johnson, this volume, chapter 14). As in Antonovsky's (1979, 1987) breakdown continuum, a person can also be located on a current recovery-stress state. The recovery-stress state can be changed positively either by stress reduction or, more important, by self-initiated recovery activities, which are outlined in the model describing the interrelations of stress states and recovery demands (see Kellmann, this volume, chapter 1; Paskevich, this volume, chapter 13). Both resource approaches can be described on various levels, and they credit passive, active, and proactive recovery activities. Kenttä and

Hassmén (this volume, chapter 4) developed their conceptual model to understand when optimal training and underperformance occurs. From these authors we can conclude that applying a holistic perspective (i.e., considering the individual's whole life) to training and recovery will change the planning, monitoring, and evaluation conditions.

Following the previous arguments, a holistic perspective on recovery should be assessed continually as a multilevel process. This is also suggested by the biopsychological stress model (Janke & Wolffgramm, 1995), which implies that recovery and stress should be addressed using a multilevel approach, that is, by dealing with physiological, emotional, cognitive, behavioral, performance, and social aspects of the problem both separately and together. This model suggests that instruments used to assess stress or recovery should be able to achieve this on various levels (see Kellmann, this volume, chapter 3). Ideally the assessment of recovery should occur in conjunction with clinical parameters, medical/physiological data (Steinacker & Lehmann, this volume, chapter 6), and training logs in order to properly address emotional management and encourage a holistic perception of recovery.

Emotion, Debriefing, and Volition

Botterill and Wilson (this volume, chapter 8) highlight the importance of emotions and emotional management in the recovery process. Fitness involves at least three major components—(1) physical, (2) mental, and (3) emotional—that are dynamically related. Each component involves both a set of capacities and a state. Athletes work hard to develop their physical capacities, but if their state is not good because of lack of rest, poor nutrition, poor hydration, or inadequate recovery, their capacities will be "masked" or lost. In addition to developing physical capacities, elite performers develop impressive mental skills or capacities to facilitate training, performance, and recovery. If an elite athlete is feeling mentally "overloaded" or exhausted because of "overanalysis" or mental fatigue, these important capacities (focusing, goal setting, visualizing, relaxing, relating, communicating, energizing) will be eroded or dramatically limited.

Emotion is an issue before, during, and after competition. Even more important, emotions can influence performance if they are not dealt with properly. Hogg (this volume, chapter 10) focuses on the debriefing of athletes after competition as an important process designed to facilitate necessary change and guide the athlete to the next level of performance. If debriefing after low or even high performances does not occur properly, the recovery process may be disturbed and performance may decline. Hogg identifies various activities that athletes and coaches can perform to reduce that risk. In this context, Beckmann (this volume, chapter 15) points out the importance of detachment from the past activity followed by engagement in a new activity. This can be regarded as a volitional process. Beckmann asserts that the postactional phase in Heckhausen's (1987) phase model of action is crucial for the recovery process. It serves mainly two functions: First, it helps the athlete disengage from the past activity and deactivate the respective goal, and second, it serves to orient the athlete toward a new activity after achieving deactivation. Allmer (1996) described the phases of the complete process necessary for recovery as dissociation (distancing oneself physically and mentally from the event), regeneration (recovery), and reorientation (preparing for the new activity). In all discussed models the stepwise completion of all phases is necessary to appropriately process previous events and prepare for subsequent performance.

Specificity of Training

The concept of specificity of training indicates that training programs should be custom made to best meet athlete's unique, individual needs (Foss & Keteyian, 1998). "Thus a particular training schedule may improve the performance of one individual, be insufficient for another, and be damaging for a third" (Raglin, 1993, p. 842). Individualized training recognizes that athletes have differing backgrounds and levels of tolerance. Younger athletes in particular show earlier signs of overtraining but do not relate those to the training process. Goss (1994) reported that older swimmers possessed fewer mood disturbances than younger swimmers. Monitoring is important for everybody but especially for younger athletes such as juniors. Consequently, training monitoring should be started early in the career so it can be integrated into the daily routine.

Monitoring Athletes and Avoiding Training Errors

As Kellmann (this volume, chapter 3) discussed, training logs can also be used to monitor warning signs of overtraining, especially if they are completed in conjunction with the Profile of Mood States (McNair, Lorr, & Droppleman, 1971, 1992), Borg's Rating of Perceived Exertion (Borg, 1975, 1998), the method of Total Quality Recovery (Kenttä & Hassmén, 1998), the Recovery-Stress Questionnaire for Athletes (Kellmann & Kallus, 2000, 2001), the Recovery-Cue (Kellmann, Botterill, & Wilson, 1999), or the Individual Zones of Optimal Functioning model (Hanin, 1997, 2000). In addition to using psychometric instruments, Davis, Botterill, and MacNeill (this volume, chapter 9) suggest assessing underrecovery by asking specific questions dealing with poor self-regulation, negative affect, learned helplessness, low self-efficacy, anxiety, and fear.

Physiological, behavioral, and performance monitoring, such as heart rate; blood test; Rusko orthostatic heart rate test (Rusko, Härkönen, & Pakarinen, 1994; see Smith & Norris, this volume, chapter 5); face check (looking in the athlete's eyes); reactions before, during, and after workouts; and the athlete's movements, can also help to prevent overtraining. For all measurements, baseline assessments are recommended to judge whether the athlete's recovery state is stable or unstable, and if a specific pattern occurred. In addition, Kellmann and Kallus (2001) pointed out that as a rule, internal consistency increases with the familiarity of the subjects to a questionnaire (the "Socrates effect;" Jagodzinski, Kühnel, & Schmidt, 1987). Only when coaches and athletes monitor on a regular basis does the time and effort pay off. While monitoring does consume time, the effect of enhanced self-awareness is worth it.

Adequate rest or recovery training must be learned, planned, and implemented within a training program. Athletes should be encouraged to train easily enough on easy days so that they can train hard enough on hard days (Seiler, 1997). Sometimes athletes have to learn what easy training feels like. Even if the coach schedules an easy speed run or swim, it often turns into a higher speed because athletes feel uncomfortable going easy. Not only the planning but also the evaluation of training should be part of the training routine. Often a training plan exists, but a training log in which the actual training is reported is less often completed precisely. Only an analysis of training can prevent future training errors and enhance performance.

Individualizing Recovery

In addition to having individual recovery strategies, athletes should also have more than one recovery strategy available. Sometimes the first choice cannot be used or does not work because of external or internal circumstances. As pointed out in chapter 1 of this volume, a person's number one recovery strategy of going for a run may work perfectly in a familiar environment, but in the first few days after traveling overseas and crossing several time zones, the same recovery activity may stress the organismic systems. As a result the person is more likely to be stressed than recovered. A second, third, or fourth backup recovery strategy should be available and applied, depending on current personal and situational factors. Hanin (this volume, chapter 11) points out that each individual has specific recovery strategies that match her personal situation and preferences. He underlines that an intraindividual approach is useful in finding the best recovery strategies for a person.

Floodgate Function of a Break

Recovery processes in competitive sports support the restoration of individual activity conditions and well-being after training and competition demands (Allmer, 1996). The optimal use of the available recovery time is imperative for success in sports. Top performances can only be reached by athletes who can recover quickly during competition and optimally navigate the transition from stress to recovery to further stress (Renzland & Eberspächer, 1988).

In this connection, Eberspächer (1995) introduced the concept of the floodgate function of a competition break. This model proposes that the optimal break between two periods of stress (e.g., between races in rowing) covers three phases. The *evaluation phase* enables the athlete to process the results from the first heat and to cope with psychological and physiological stress. During this phase

regeneration occurs and energy reservoirs are replenished. The *transitional phase* takes the most time and serves as recovery. This phase can include many different activities, including eating, drinking, dozing, sleeping, playing cards, meeting friends, or other mostly unplanned activities. Because not all will bring the desired recovery effect, however, each person should develop his own strategy and consciously think how to make the most effective use of a break. Optimal recovery has to take individual peculiarities into account. While some feel great after a nap, others are absolutely wiped out. There is no general valid formula. The final phase of a break, the *preparing phase,* starts with the physiological warming up for, and the mental focusing on, the next race. During this phase the athlete restores the preparedness of mind and body for the next performance.

Toolbox for Planning Rest Days

Since recovery is specific to each individual, it is important for a coach to develop a toolbox for planning rest days during regular training, in training camps, and during competition, respectively. A toolbox also helps to individualize recovery. Obviously, individualizing recovery will be easier for coaches dealing with few athletes and more complex for coaches of large teams. However, coaches of large teams usually need not offer a high number of disparate recovery activities as long as they keep in mind that not every activity has the same recovering effect for each athlete.

Athletes can perform recovery activities either individually or with a group. Sometimes athletes should be left by themselves to do whatever they want to, and other times it could be profitable to give some direction. Most important to remember is that recovery is a proactive, self-initiated process for replenishing psychological and physiological resources. From this perspective athletes are responsible for initiating their own activities, such as going to a movie, visiting close friends, or going for a run. While numerous possibilities for recovery are available in regular life, options are limited during training camps.

Table 17.1 lists activity options for rest days during training camps. For most activities, important thoughts to consider are also listed.

Table 17.1 Activity Options for Rest Days in Training Camps

Indoor activities	Important thoughts/considerations
Massage/sauna	Are you used to massages/saunas?
Relaxation programs/techniques	These help to block intrusions.
Listening to music	This can be done indoors, outdoors, or while walking.
Visiting museums	Don't walk around too long.
TV	This is positive only if you control the remote.
Team dinner/lunch/brunch/breakfast	Eat away from the location of daily training; you need a change!
Dancing	Plan to get enough sleep—you need to be fit for training or competition.
Going out/meeting friends	Spend time with people not involved in your sport, other sport people, or family. Take care that you get enough sleep!
Stretching program	
Indoor games (e.g., board games, word games, card games)	
Reading a book	
Group evening with guitar	
Going to the movies, theater, opera	
Sleeping in	

Outdoor activities	Important thoughts/considerations
20- to 30-minute regeneration activity: Running, swimming, biking, inline skating, etc.	Choose an activity you are used to. New sports can cause muscle pain or make you more tired.
Inline skating/bike tour	Use proper equipment.
Going for a walk/hiking	Consider the level of difficulty, distance, and weather.
Walking or bike tour with picnic	Consider the profile, distance, and weather.
A trip to a lake including picnic and swimming or an easy run	Consider weather conditions.
Sightseeing	This can be done by bus, by boat, or on foot,
Shopping	Don't walk around so long that you have tired legs the next day.
Amusement park/miniature golf	
Festival of any kind: public, art, music, and so on	

Activities include 20-30 minutes of running, swimming, biking, or inline skating. It is recommended to choose activities that the athletes are used to. New sports can cause muscle pain or enhance tiredness. In the example of taking a sauna, coaches should remember that some athletes feel uncomfortable in a sauna and perceive it as a stressor. Consequently, they would not feel recovered after a sauna. Athletes and coaches can add activities to the list and specify which recovery activities are appropriate for themselves or their team during the season and off-season.

Frequency of Performing

Norris and Smith (this volume, chapter 7) focus on the planning, periodization, and sequencing of training and competition. As they point out, major components of planning, periodization, and sequencing are the frequency of competitions and the decision as to when performance should peak. The length of time (weeks, months, or even years) available to achieve the relevant and identified objectives, together with the competition calendar, sets the overall structure and tone for the periodized plan (Norris & Smith, this volume, chapter 7). This works better in some sports than in others. However, there are different implications for low, medium, and high density of performing, which will be outlined in the following sections.

Low Density of Performing

Rowing, cycling, modern pentathlon, track and field, speed skating, and other sports have up to three major competitions (e.g., National Championships, World and European Championships, and the Olympics). Of course, athletes compete more often during the regular season (e.g., in World Cups), but the periodization is planned around the major events (see Norris & Smith, this volume, chapter 7). Since the season usually lasts four to five months, periods of hard and light training can be scheduled easily. Sometimes the trials to qualify for world championships or the Olympics are more important than the events themselves. In that case the critical question is whether there is enough time between the trials and the final competition to go through the complete periodization process or only part of it (this problem is discussed extensively in chapter 7). In the United States only one big event for qualification exists, for example, in track and field. In comparison, German athletes have to achieve

qualification results (e.g., times) defined by the Deutscher Leichathletik-Verband (German Track and Field Association) twice within a certain period of time during the season. If qualification times are not successfully reached by the time of the target competition, athletes focus on lower-rated events. The short-notice modification of the original training schedule, however, does not necessarily lead to the desired result in the lower-rated events.

Medium Density of Performing

Medium-density performance sports are categorized as sports that have almost a full-year competition schedule. Examples of these sports are tennis, soccer, basketball, and so on. In the German First Division Soccer League, a regular season consists of 34 games, plus National Cup and additional international championship games if the team qualifies. The examples of Hertha BSC and of the Colorado Avalanche were given in chapter 1. Hertha BSC played more games than any of the other German professional soccer teams in the first half of the 1999/2000 season—29 games within 18 weeks, an average of one game every 4.3 days, including travel time. According to the official game schedule, the Colorado Avalanche, like any other NHL team, played an average of one game every 2.3 days during the regular season. When athletes play two or three games a week, physical and mental recovery is often incomplete. Consequently, time between games (competitions) is used differently than in low-density performance sports. Here, the main focus is on regenerative training and not on aiming for high training load or high-intensity training. High-intensity training is usually only possible before the season starts or during the winter break (e.g., in the German Soccer League).

Focusing on the seasonal schedule in soccer, for example, the question arises, When do successful players have a complete recovery period? German National Soccer Team athletes mostly play for clubs that participate in the European Soccer Cup, the German First Division Soccer League (34 games a season), and the National Cup. Such athletes have little time for complete recovery as other time is filled with training camps in preparation for the season or after the winter break. For example, the 2000/2001 winter break was about six weeks long, and the majority of players had a 10-day (nonpractice) break between Christmas and New Year's Day. After the break a training camp for the second part of the season took place at the end of January. Coaches are aware of the problem of incomplete recovery and often rotate players so that occasionally an athlete does not play even if he is fit. Consequently, teams require more players. This raises the costs and increases the economic pressure to be successful in order to finance the players. Sometimes this is the beginning of a vicious circle.

High Density of Performing

High-density performance sports compete more often than medium-density performance sports. The athletes of the Cirque du Soleil have approximately 400 shows a year (mostly two shows a day), plus daily training to maintain performance and further the development of new acrobatic elements. The goal of the training methodology is threefold: to (1) prevent overtraining, (2) maintain a level of physical conditioning that enables the artist to perform at a high level throughout a long and demanding schedule, and (3) maintain a level of motivation for training. Here, maintaining performance rather than achieving peak performance is the key element. In other words, the best "overall long-term performance" is rated when 95% of the maximum performance can be achieved in every show. Spectators usually cannot judge the missing difference of 5%, but notice when the task is performed only at the 60% level. Therefore, the goal is a decrease of variability in performance. Mathematically described, the goal is to have a mean performance of 95% of the personal best with almost zero standard deviations. Therefore, the professional supporting staff strive to optimize the surroundings and conditions in the work environment of their athletes.

Maintaining Performance and Recovery

Maintaining performance is also an issue in our regular work environment. Interestingly, vacation time in Germany is described as a "recovery holiday." Its purpose is to refresh and rejuvenate people. But is that goal always reached? Vacation time in Germany ranges from five to six weeks a year, which is higher than in other countries. The trend, however, is to divide this time into three, four, or five vacations. Rarely does someone take three weeks off at one time. However, this time period is most often necessary to deeply replenish one's resources. Two weeks are usually not sufficient (within that time, the recovery process just begins). A one-week trip often includes travel

time, resulting in a loss of profit from the vacation. Of course, a weekend at the beach or in the mountains can provide recovery and replenish resources, but in most cases, just to a certain level. While it is important to plan these activities several times a year, they should not be a substitute for a long-term vacation.

Lehmann et al. (1999) defined short-term overtraining as lasting less than three weeks, and long-term overtraining as lasting at least three weeks or more. According to the arguments in chapter 1, overtraining is due to underrecovery, and therefore, the new terms should actually be *short-term underrecovery* and *long-term underrecovery*. Approaching the problem of overtraining from a perspective that complements this book, Budgett et al. (2000) redefined the overtraining syndrome as unexplained underperformance syndrome. "Underperformance syndrome is a persistent unexplained performance deficit (recognized by coach and athlete) despite two weeks of relative rest" (p. 67).

Whether the recommended time frame for complete recovery is two or three weeks, recovery depends on personal situations and needs. If self-awareness and understanding are developed, and the individual learns at what time a certain activity is needed, a huge step toward adequate recovery is taken. A trial phase is suggested to discover which recovery strategy fits best in different situations. This applies not only to sports, but also to other related areas. Kallus (this volume, chapter 16) discusses the impact of recovery in different professions. Naturally we hope that people working in professions that have responsibility for other people achieve a balanced recovery-stress state. Pilots, surgeons, flight controllers, and bus drivers, for example, should be made aware of recovery and be mindful of replenishing their resources.

Future Perspectives of Recovery Research

The need for a conscious integration of recovery phases during the competition and training cycle is one of the common themes of this book. To achieve optimal performance, it is essential to recognize the reasons for overloading as early as possible for effective elimination. The coach is a key factor when it comes to underrecovery. The coach is responsible not only for the specificity of training, but also for the type of training. In addition, coaches must learn to deal with stress themselves. Coaches' own capacities to cope with stress affect their athletes, who often look to them as role models. Furthermore, coaches who deal poorly with stress find that their behavior during competitions is affected, as is their ability to analyze that behavior.

The Coach

Kellmann (1997) and Kallus, Kellmann, Eberspächer, and Hermann (1996) reported results of a study with 195 semiprofessional and professional coaches who completed the Stress-Coping Inventory (Janke, Erdmann, & Kallus, 1985), the Recovery-Stress Questionnaire for Coaches (RESTQ-Coach; e.g., Kallus & Kellmann, 1995, 2000), and an adjective checklist dealing with their behavior during rest periods (Kellmann & Kallus, 1994). Based on selected post-hoc comparisons, this survey revealed deficits in coping strategies in younger coaches as well as differences in coping strategies between coaches of team sports and coaches of individual sports. Coaches of individual sports use more cognitive reevaluation and active, positive coping strategies in dealing with stress. In addition, they search for self-affirmation and pity themselves more than coaches from team sports. The focus on coaches' status show different ways of coping. Semiprofessional coaches use more positive self-instruction, active coping, and relaxation than their professional colleagues. In summary, full-time coaches are more burned out and highly stressed, experience less recovery, and are less fit than semiprofessional coaches.

Feedback workshops with the coaches supported the assumption that the findings reflected changes in lifestyle. Apparently, professional coaches have lost their hobby: they can no longer compensate their occupational stress by coaching during leisure time. Furthermore, they have less continuous contact with their athletes and spend more time traveling. Coaches' recovery-stress states and coping strategies are important in terms of retention. The risk of burnout is higher for professional than for semiprofessional coaches. Professional coaches also show deficits in coping strategies as measured by the Stress-Coping Inventory and therefore may possibly react less effectively in critical situations. Group differences in the recovery-stress state are not influenced by variables such as age. Kallus and Kellmann (2000) concluded that:

Stress + Recovery Deficit + Deficient Coping → High Risk of Burnout

Furthermore, the results revealed that coaches' behavior during rest periods in competition (e.g., halftimes, time-outs) is closely related to the experienced psychological stress. Analyses indicated that coaches who were highly stressed rated themselves as significantly less active and less authoritarian during rest periods than their lower-stressed colleagues.

Kellmann (1997) also surveyed 76 professional coaches using the Rest-Period Questionnaire for Coaches (Kellmann & Kallus, 1995), the RESTQ-Coach, and a biographic measure. Subjects were classified post hoc using different criteria (e.g., age, sport, performance expectations, extent of psychological stress). Coaches who were highly stressed described their behavior during rest periods in competition as more directive and angrier compared to the lower-stressed group. Age revealed an important mediator for behavior, because older coaches showed more positive behavior during rest periods in competition than their younger colleagues. These results matched the findings of an earlier study showing that coaches' behavior during rest periods was closely related to experienced psychological stress (see Kellmann & Kallus, 1994).

Interdisciplinary Work

Athletes' optimal performance requires a close cooperation among coaches, athletes, sport physicians, and sport psychologists to utilize the available medical, psychological, and performance data on an interdisciplinary basis (Botterill & Wilson, this volume, chapter 8; Froehlich, 1993; Harre, 1982; Kellmann & Altenburg, 2000; Kenttä & Hassmén, 1998; Norris & Smith, this volume, chapter 7). Such an interdisciplinary approach also provides better research opportunities to find reliable markers for overtraining. Putting an optimal interdisciplinary approach successfully into practice depends on the participation of the people involved. Perhaps it is worth mentioning that respect for colleagues is a necessary interdisciplinary function. This starts with open communication, adherence to agreements, quick reaction to feedback, and an openness to learn from one another. Various publications present results from different perspectives (e.g., Berger et al., 1999; Kellmann, Altenburg, Lormes, & Steinacker, 2001; O'Connor, Morgan, & Raglin, 1991; Steinacker et al., 1999, 2000).

Figure 17.1 reveals the approach of the German Junior National Rowing Team. The athlete is the center of interest; she has to perform at a top level

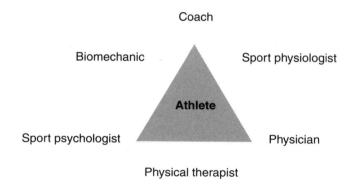

Figure 17.1 Interdisciplinary counseling approach of the German Junior National Rowing Team.

at the World Championships. The coach receives the information dealing with different areas provided by the staff and makes decisions based on this broad database. In addition, daily team meetings ensure that all staff members have the same level of information. Every year since the 1995 training camp for the World Championships, athletes on the team have been monitored using the Recovery-Stress Questionnaire for Athletes (e.g., Kellmann, Kallus, Günther, Lormes, & Steinacker, 1997; Kellmann & Kallus, 1999). During the six-week training camp (and before the championships), the athletes complete the Recovery-Stress Questionnaire for Athletes (see Kellmann, this volume, chapter 3; Kellmann, Patrick, Botterill, & Wilson, this volume, chapter 12). Parallel to the questionnaire measurements, a sport medical assessment (i.e., lactate, creatine kinase) takes place. One goal is to identify those athletes whose recovery-stress states deviate from those expected based on individual or group profiles. As athletes complete questionnaires, the coaches and physicians involved receive fast feedback and are therefore able to provide immediate interventions. Today, recovery-stress state assessments are as much a part of the preparation routine before the World Championships as lactate testing.

Summary

This book posits that optimal recovery is a key factor of performance. It is suggested that a constant lack of recovery or disturbed recovery may turn into overtraining. Being slightly under-recovered over a longer period of time may result in underperformance, not only in athletics but also in nonathletes. The multilevel concept also emphasizes that physical training is just one part of an athlete's life. Worries or problems outside of the training environment (e.g., fights, parents' divorce) affect athletes and often disturb their recovery time. Therefore, coaches and athletes need to know about the importance of the integration of recovery during practice and in everyday life.

While practice is clearly important in improving performance, the focus should be on the quality rather than on the quantity of training. Most athletes should be discouraged from doing additional workouts simply because they feel particularly good during training. When athletes understand that a weekend off training is part of the training schedule—meaning that they should not train on their own or go for a heavy bike ride—they take a huge step toward adequate recovery.

Recovery research is a young field especially when compared to stress research. However, stress and recovery affect each other, and a lot of underlying recovery mechanisms still need to be examined. For example, how long does it take before underrecovery in children has a major effect on involvement in sports and school performance? In this context it is relevant to find the right balance between practice and recovery when children start to become involved in athletics. Often athletes who as children and junior athletes achieved top performance sometimes stagnate as senior athletes. Frequently they report a loss of fun and feelings of being physically and mentally drained. Counseling with these athletes reveals that training errors during their younger years didn't influence their performance until much later.

Measurement tools for assessing acute recovery levels also need further development, as do underrecovery coping strategies. In addition, managers of sport organizations and club owners should understand the importance of recovery. As in other business fields, understanding at the top levels of management is necessary if coaches and athletes are to be able to achieve the aimed recovery. While this book provides the current status of recovery research, it is the underlying hope of all contributors that in the future more publications will deal with enhancing recovery to prevent underperformance in sport.

References

Allmer, H. (1996). *Erholung und Gesundheit: Grundlagen, Ergebnisse und Maßnahmen* [Recovery and health: Basics, results and interventions]. Göttingen, Germany: Hogrefe.

Antonovsky, A. (1979). *Health, stress, and coping.* San Francisco: Jossey-Bass.

Antonovsky, A. (1987). *Unraveling the mystery of health.* San Francisco: Jossey-Bass.

Berger, B.G., Motl, R.W., Butki, B.D., Martin, D.T., Wilkinson, J.G., & Owen, D.R. (1999). Mood and cycling performance in response to three weeks of high-intensity, short-duration overtraining, and a two-week taper. *The Sport Psychologist, 13,* 444-457.

Borg, G. (1975). Perceived exertion as an indicator of somatic stress. *Scandinavian Journal of Rehabilitational Medicine, 2,* 92-98.

Borg, G. (1998). *Borg's Perceived Exertion and Pain Rating Scales.* Champaign, IL: Human Kinetics.

Budgett, R., Newsholme, E., Lehmann, M., Sharp, C., Jones, D., Petro, T., Collins, D., Nerurkar, R., & White, P. (2000). Redefining the overtraining syndrome as the unexplained underperformance syndrome. *British Journal of Sport Medicine, 34,* 67-68.

Eberspächer, H. (1995). *Mentales Training* [Mental training]. Munich, Germany: Sportinform.

Foss, M.L., & Keteyian, S.J. (1998). *Fox's physiological basis for exercise and sport* (6th ed.). Boston: WCB/McGraw-Hill.

Froehlich, J. (1993). Overtraining syndrome. In J. Heil (Ed.), *Psychology of sport injury* (pp. 59-70). Champaign, IL: Human Kinetics.

Goss, J. (1994). Hardiness and mood disturbances in swimmers while overtraining. *Journal of Sport & Exercise Psychology, 16,* 135-149.

Gould, D., Greenleaf, C., Dieffenbach, K., Chung, Y., & Peterson, K. (1999). *Positive and negative factors influencing U.S. Olympic athletes and coaches: Nagano Games assessment.* U.S. Olympic Committee Sport Science and Technology Final Grant Report. Colorado Springs, Colorado.

Gould, D., Guinan, D., Greenleaf, D., Medbery, R., Strickland, M., Lauer, L., Chung, Y., & Peterson, K. (1998). *Positive and negative factors influencing U.S. Olympic athletes and coaches: Atlanta Games assessment.* Final grant report submitted to the U.S. Olympic Committee Sport Science and Technology Division, Colorado Springs, Colorado.

Hanin, Y.L. (1997). Emotions and athletic performance: Individual Zones of Optimal Functioning model. In R. Seiler (Ed.), *European Yearbook of Sports Psychology* (Vol. 1, pp. 29-72). St. Augustin, Germany: Academia.

Hanin, Y.L. (2000). Individual Zones of Optimal Functioning (IZOF) model: Emotion-performance relationships in sport. In Y.L. Hanin (Ed.), *Emotions in sport* (pp. 65-89). Champaign, IL: Human Kinetics.

Harre, D. (1982). *Principles of sports training: Introduction to the theory and methods of training* (English version; 1st ed.). Berlin: Sportverlag.

Heckhausen, H. (1987). Perspektiven einer Psychologie des Wollens [Perspectives of a psychology of the will]. In H. Heckhausen, P.M. Gollwitzer, & F.E. Weinert (Eds.), *Jenseits des Rubikon. Der Wille in den Humanwissenschaften* (pp. 121-142). Berlin: Springer.

Jagodzinski, W., Kühnel, S.M., & Schmidt, P. (1987). Is there a "Socratic Effect" in nonexperimental panel studies? *Sociological Methods & Research, 15,* 259-302.

Janke, W., Erdmann, G., & Kallus, K.W. (1985). *Streßverarbeitungsfragebogen* [Stress-Coping Inventory]. Göttingen, Germany: Hogrefe.

Janke, W., & Wolffgramm, J. (1995). Biopsychologie von Streß und emotionalen Reaktionen: Ansätze interdisziplinärer Kooperation von Psychologie, Biologie und Medizin [Biopsychology of stress and emotional reactions: Starting points of an interdisciplinary cooperation of psychology, biology, and medicine]. In G. Debus, G. Erdmann, & K.W. Kallus (Eds.), *Biopsychologie von Streß und emotionalen Reaktionen* (pp. 293-349). Göttingen, Germany: Hogrefe.

Kallus, K.W., & Kellmann, M. (1995). The Recovery-Stress Questionnaire for Coaches. In R. Vanfraechem-Raway & Y. Vanden Auweele (Eds.), *Proceedings of the 9th European Congress on Sport Psychology in Brussels* (Vol. 1, pp. 26-33). Brussels: FEPSAC/Belgian Federation of Sport Psychology.

Kallus, K.W., & Kellmann, M. (2000). Burnout in athletes and coaches. In Y.L. Hanin (Ed.), *Emotions in sport* (pp. 209-230). Champaign, IL: Human Kinetics.

Kallus, K.W., Kellmann, M., Eberspächer, H., & Hermann, H.-D. (1996). Beanspruchung, Erholung und Streßbewältigung von Trainern im Leistungssport [Stress, recovery, and coping with stress of coaches in elite sports]. *Psychologie und Sport, 3,* 114-126.

Kellmann, M. (1997). *Die Wettkampfpause als integraler Bestandteil der Leistungsoptimierung im Sport: Eine empirische psychologische Analyse* [The rest period as an integral part of optimizing performance in sports: An empirical psychological analysis]. Hamburg, Germany: Dr. Kovac.

Kellmann, M., & Altenburg, D. (2000). Betreuung der Junioren-Nationalmannschaft des Deutschen Ruderverbandes [Consultation of the German Junior National Rowing Team]. In H. Allmer, W. Hartmann, & D. Kayser (Eds.), *Sportpsychologie in Bewegung—Forschung für die Praxis* (pp. 67-80). Cologne, Germany: Sport und Buch Strauss.

Kellmann, M., Altenburg, D., Lormes, W., & Steinacker, J.M. (2001). Assessing stress and recovery during preparation for the World Championships in rowing. *The Sport Psychologist, 15,* 151-167.

Kellmann, M., Botterill, C., & Wilson, C. (1999). *Recovery-Cue.* Unpublished recovery assessment instrument. Calgary, AB: National Sport Centre.

Kellmann, M., & Kallus, K.W. (1994). Interrelation between stress and coaches' behavior during rest periods. *Perceptual and Motor Skills, 79,* 207-210.

Kellmann, M., & Kallus, K.W. (1995). The Rest-Period Questionnaire for Coaches: Assessing the behavior of coaches during rest periods. In R. Vanfraechem-Raway & Y. Vanden Auweele (Eds.), *Proceedings of the 9th European Congress on Sport Psychology in Brussels* (Part 1, pp. 43-50). Brussels: FEPSAC/Belgian Federation of Sport Psychology.

Kellmann, M., & Kallus, K.W. (1999). Mood, recovery-stress state, and regeneration. In M. Lehmann, C. Foster, U. Gastmann, H. Keizer, & J.M. Steinacker (Eds.), *Overload, fatigue, performance incompetence, and regeneration in sport* (pp. 101-117). New York: Plenum.

Kellmann, M., & Kallus, K.W. (2000). *Der Erholungs-Belastungs-Fragebogen für Sportler; Handanweisung* [The Recovery-Stress Questionnaire for Athletes; manual]. Frankfurt, Germany: Swets Test Services.

Kellmann, M., & Kallus, K.W. (2001). *Recovery-Stress Questionnaire for Athletes: User manual.* Champaign, IL: Human Kinetics.

Kellmann, M., Kallus, K.W., Günther, K.-D., Lormes, W., & Steinacker, J.M. (1997). Psychologische Betreuung der Junioren-Nationalmannschaft des Deutschen Ruderverbandes [Psychological consultation of the German Junior National Rowing Team]. *Psychologie und Sport, 4,* 123-134.

Kenttä, G., & Hassmén, P. (1998). Overtraining and recovery. *Sports Medicine, 26,* 1-16.

Lehmann, M., Foster, C., Gastmann, U., Keizer, H.A., & Steinacker, J.M. (1999). Definition, types, symptoms, findings, underlying mechanisms, and frequency of overtraining and overtraining syndrome. In M. Lehmann, C. Foster, U. Gastmann, H. Keizer, & J.M. Steinacker (Eds.), *Overload, fatigue, performance incompetence, and regeneration in sport* (pp. 1-6). New York: Plenum.

Lehmann, M., Lormes, W., Opitz-Gress, A., Steinacker, J.M., Netzer, N., Foster, C., & Gastmann, U. (1997). Training and overtraining: An overview and ex-

perimental results in endurance sports. *Journal of Sports Medicine and Physical Fitness, 37,* 7-17.

McNair, D., Lorr, M., & Droppleman, L.F. (1971). *Profile of Mood States manual.* San Diego: Educational and Industrial Testing Service.

McNair, D., Lorr, M., & Droppleman, L.F. (1992). *Profile of Mood States manual.* San Diego: Educational and Industrial Testing Service.

Noakes, T.D. (1991). *Lore of running* (3rd ed.). Champaign, IL: Human Kinetics.

O'Connor, P.J., Morgan, W.P., & Raglin, J.S. (1991). Psychobiologic effects of 3 d of increased training in female and male swimmers. *Medicine and Science in Sports and Exercise, 23,* 1055-1061.

Raglin, J.S. (1993). Overtraining and staleness: Psychometric monitoring of endurance athletes. In R.B. Singer, M. Murphey, & L.K. Tennant (Eds.), *Handbook of research on sport psychology* (pp. 840-850). New York: Macmillan.

Renzland, J., & Eberspächer, H. (1988). *Regeneration im Sport* [Regeneration in sports]. Cologne, Germany: bps.

Rusko, H.K., Härkönen, M., & Pakarinen, A. (1994). Overtraining effects on hormonal and autonomic regulation in young cross-country skiers. *Medicine and Science in Sports and Exercise, 26*(5), S64.

Schönpflug, W. (1983). Coping efficiency and situational demands. In R. Hockey (Ed.), *Stress and fatigue in human performance* (pp. 299-326). Chichester, U.K.: Wiley.

Schönpflug, W. (1987). Beanspruchung und Belastung bei der Arbeit—Konzepte und Theorien. Arbeitspsychologie [Strain and stress during work—Concepts and theories]. In U. Kleinbeck & J. Rutenfranz (Eds.), *Enzyklopädie der Psychologie* (Part III/1, pp. 131-184). Göttingen, Germany: Hogrefe.

Seiler, S. (1997). *Endurance training theory—Norwegian style* [Internet]. Available: http://home.hia.no/~stephens/xctheory.htm (20 June 2001).

Steinacker, J.M., Kellmann, M., Böhm, B.O., Liu, Y., Opitz-Gress, A., Kallus, K.W., Lehmann, M., Altenburg, D., & Lormes, W. (1999). Clinical findings and parameters of stress and regeneration in rowers before World Championships. In M. Lehmann, C. Foster, U. Gastmann, H. Keizer, & J.M. Steinacker (Eds.), *Overload, fatigue, performance incompetence, and regeneration in sport* (pp. 71-80). New York: Plenum.

Steinacker, J.M., Lormes, W., Kellmann, M., Liu, Y., Reißnecker, S., Opitz-Gress, A., Baller, B., Günther, K., Petersen, K.G., Kallus, K.W., Lehmann, M., & Altenburg, D. (2000). Training of junior rowers before World Championships. Effects on performance, mood state and selected hormonal and metabolic responses. *Journal of Sports Medicine and Physical Fitness, 40,* 327-335.

Index

Note: The italicized *f* and *t* following page numbers refer to figures and tables, respectively.

Recovery-Stress Questionnaire for Coaches (RESTQ-Coach) 308
recovery-stress states
    biopsychological approach to x, 5-6, 11, 14-15, 283-284
        nonsport applications of 287, 290-297
        research advantages of 283-287, 285f, 286t
        research results of 287-290, 288f, 289f, 297-298
    emotional markers of 207-208
    nontraining factors of 5-6, 66
    optimal balance of 208-209, 253, 261, 263, 266
        checking for 285-286, 286t
    performance connection in 4-5, 285
    as research approach
        on biopsychological stress 287-290, 288f, 289f
        in clinical and health psychology 287, 294-297, 295f, 296f, 297f
        directions for 283, 297-298, 302
        in job-related work 287, 290-294, 291f, 292t, 293f, 293t, 294f
        process advantages of 283-287, 285f, 286t
        summary results of 297-298
    training-stimulus and 10-11, 81
    training volume and 27-28
        mood states profile in 41-42
recovery time(s), for endurance training 83, 84t, 92
red blood cells, in training tolerance 90, 90t
regeneration
    clinically relevant parameters of 106-113
    neglect of 134-135
    recovery vs. 10, 18, 129, 284
    research directions for 302
    training strategies for 95, 127f
rehabilitation
    coping variables of 242
        social support impact on 245-247
    in overtraining case study 71-74, 73f
relationships, interpersonal. See social entries
relaxation
    of muscles. See muscle relaxation
    for recovery 4, 7, 18, 148, 280
    recovery points for 65-66, 70
    as stress management 242-243, 297
    as underrecovery intervention 171-172, 171t
    as volition factor 154, 275, 275t, 276t, 280
reliability, statistical, of Recovery-Stress Questionnaire for Athletes 43, 45-46, 46f
renin, in recovery-stress state 288-289, 289f, 297
reorientation, for goal achievement 303
repetition, as periodization principle 124-125
repression, emotional management of 149
research. See recovery research
resources, for optimal individualized recovery 212-213, 284, 285f, 301
respect, in team dynamics 150
responsibility
    in debriefing 184, 196
    shared, for training optimization 75, 225
    through sport involvement 150, 156
rest
    barriers to 210-212, 211t, 212t
    as burnout factor 25-26, 31, 33
    excessive 285
    as overtraining treatment 18-19
    in periodization 130
    recovery points for 65, 70

    self-awareness of 154
rest days, activity options for. See recovery activity(ies)
resting heart rate
    morning, in training tolerance 89-90
    in stress response 163-164, 164f
restlessness, with overtraining 15, 16t
Rest-Period Questionnaire for Coaches 10, 308
RESTQ-Coach. See Recovery-Stress Questionnaire for Coaches (RESTQ-Coach)
RESTQ-Sport. See Recovery-Stress Questionnaire for Athletes (RESTQ-Sport)
rewards, as burnout factor 30-32, 31f
roommates, quality of life and 260, 265
RPE. See Rating of Perceived Exertion (RPE)
RPs. See recovery points (RPs), in Total Quality Recovery
Rubicon model, of volitional action phases 273, 273f
rumination
    in recovery-stress process 284
    as volition factor 271, 275t, 276, 276t
running speed, endurance of 82, 82f
Rusko Heart Rate Test, as training indicator 137-138, 137f

S

sadness, emotional management of 149
salivary immunoglobulin-A, in training tolerance 93-94, 111
salutogenesis 12
Sampras, Pete 70
satisfaction rating
    in debriefing 190, 191f, 192, 192f, 198
    in job-related stress 292, 292t
Sauer, George 150
saunas, as recovery strategy 7-8, 306
schema, in negative affect 165
scissors model, of stress and recovery 11-12, 11f
secondary social functioning, in quality of life 255-257, 257f, 263-266
secondary stress 241
Seiler, S. 141
self-acceptance, in quality of life 255, 257, 257f, 259-261
self-analysis. See self-reflection
self-assessment. See self-evaluation
self-awareness
    in complete monitoring system 60, 61f, 63-64
    in debriefing 184-185, 193-195
    research directions for 303-304
    through sport involvement 150-151
    in training monitoring 151-154, 220, 225
self-blame 241
self-condition scale, for underrecovery assessment 38
self-confidence
    building interventions for 171t, 173-174
    in debriefing 193-195
self-consciousness, unhealthy, as debriefing issue 193
self-control. See also self-regulation
    as volition mode 271, 274f
self-criticism, in debriefing 184, 188, 193
self-determination
    debriefing impact on 9, 182
    as volition factor 275, 275t, 276t
        intervention programs based on 9, 280-281
self-development, in quality of life 255, 257, 257f, 259-261
self-discipline, as volition factor 271, 275t, 276, 276t
    in overtraining dynamics 278-279, 279f
self-efficacy
    in debriefing 193-195

supercompensation principle, of recovery 58-59, 61
in endurance training 85
suppleness, as training component 127, 127f
surgery
recovery-stress states with 297-298
social support impact on 245
surprise, emotional management of 149
sustenance, as training component 127-128, 127f
swimming
low self-regulation case study of 175-176
periodization case study of 135-136, 136f
training case study of 151-152, 224, 225f
switch off ability, in job-related stress 292, 292t
sympathetic overtraining 15, 16t, 95
as biphasic response 104-105, 104f
downregulation of 110-111, 110f
mood states and 112, 163
symptoms, in recovery-stress process 284
systems, in recovery-stress process 284

T

tactics, for global performance 96-97, 97f, 130-131, 130f
taper phase, of recovery 6, 26
mood states and 42
myopathy and 108
Recovery-Cue monitoring of 223, 224f
task analysis, for recovery-stress state 285f, 293-294, 293t
task behaviors, burnout and 30, 31f
Task 12 Program Design (Planning and Periodization)
138-139
teams and teamwork
emotional management for 150, 204, 205f, 206
quality of life and 263-266
testosterone, training tolerance and 94
testosterone/cortisol ratio, in training tolerance 94-95
test-retest reliability, of Recovery-Stress Questionnaire
for Athletes 43, 46
themes, in quality of life 254-255, 257
theory-driven interventions, for underrecovery 161-162
theory of planned behavior
health practices and 237-239, 237f
sports applications of 239
thinking control, as underrecovery intervention 171t, 173
threat, perceived 241
time, in endurance training
performance and 82, 82f, 85, 85f
theoretical modeling of 85-86, 86f, 87f
time dimension, of Individual Zones of Optimal
Functioning 206
time window, in recovery-stress process 283-284
time zones. *See also* travel
recovery strategies and 7
total fitness model 144-145, 145f
Total Quality Recovery (TQR)
action assessment guidelines 63-64
Action scale of 62-63, 62f
utilizing scores of 66-67
action scoring with 64-66
points earned by 63-66
use of information from 66-67
implementation of 63
initial purpose of 61-62
optimizing strategies for 74-75
overview of 63, 63f
Perceived scale of 62, 62f
utilizing scores of 66-67

Rating of Perceived Exertion scale *vs.* 61, 62f
subdimensions of 62-63
in underrecovery assessment 38
total recovery time 6
track and field, training case study of 223, 224f
traffic controllers, recovery-stress state of 290, 291f
trainable load, in endurance training 84
training
components of 127-130, 127f
emotional management for 149-150
energizing techniques for 149
global approach to 95-96, 97f, 130-131, 130f
goal of 69, 81, 87
holistic perspective on 95-96, 97f, 194, 202, 302
monitoring of. *See* monitoring system; monitoring tools
optimal strategies for 19, 33-34, 52. *See also* Individual
Zones of Optimal Functioning (IZOF)
criteria for 58-59, 121
evolutionary trends of 57-58, 103, 285
global 130-131, 130f
holistic 95-96, 97f
self-awareness of 151-154
as performance factor 14, 16
nontraining stressors interaction with 14-15, 69, 75
periodization planning of. *See* periodization, of training
research directions for 303
specificity of 303
training addiction 146-147
training camps
group monitoring tools for 47, 51, 63
psychological 112, 113f
health risks in 106
mood disturbances and 162
periodization case study of 136-138, 137f
training cycles. *See also* periodization, of training
applications of 103, 124, 138
competition-specific 306-307
Recovery-Cue monitoring of
after cycles 223
weekly during 219-223, 229
training demands, modern 145-146
training diary, for training tolerance 89
training duration
in complete monitoring system 59f, 60
in endurance training 88
mood profiles and 41-42
perceived exertion with 61, 61f
training effort, calculation of 87
training errors
research directions for 303-304
in sequencing 134-135
underperformance with 130
as underrecovery factor 4, 37-38, 65
training fatigue
as continuous goal 81, 83
decay time of 86, 87f
quantification of 87-88, 128
recovery times for 83, 84t
training history, in endurance training 84-85, 85f
training impulse (TRIMP), in endurance training 87
training intensity
in complete monitoring system 59-60, 59f, 128
in endurance training 84-85, 85f, 96
tolerance of 88, 92, 93f
mood states and 41-42
perceived exertion with 38-39, 41, 60-61, 61f

as training error 134
training load
    biphasic response to 104-105, 104*f*
    as burnout factor 28-29
    in complete monitoring system 59-60, 59*f*
    components of 103
    in endurance training 81, 83
        classification of 84-85
        quantification of 87-88
        sequencing strategies for 95, 130*f*
            errors of 134-135
        tracking methods for 87-88
    individualization of 5, 60, 95, 97
    mood state and 112, 113*f*
    overtraining and 15-16, 18, 28
        dynamic systems perspective of 279-280, 279*f*
        in elite athletes 27-28
        immune system impact of 110-112, 111*f*, 112*f*
        in young athletes 28
    in periodization monitoring 132, 133*f*, 134
    as recovery factor 4, 10-11
        clinically relevant parameters of 106-112
        intervention programs based on 280-281
        threshold maximization of 285
    in today's programs 145-146
    two-factor model of response to
        in competition preparedness 128-129, 129*f*
        intervention programs based on 280-281
        recovery sequence with 85-86, 87*f*
        volitional perspectives of 274, 274*f*, 278, 278*f*
training log
    analysis importance of 303-304
    for athletes, in underrecovery assessment 39, 40*t*
    for staff 52
    for training tolerance 97, 106
training reaction, in complete monitoring system 59-60,
        59*f*
training sequencing
    case studies of 135-138
    strategies for 95, 121-122, 130*f*. *See also*
            periodization, of training
        errors of 134-135
        summary of 138-139
    value of 121-122, 306
training stimulus
    in complete monitoring system 59, 59*f*
        perception of 59-60, 59*f*
        response to 59-60, 59*f*
    recovery-stress state and 10-11, 81
training strain, in endurance training 87
training stress, configuration of total physical 69
training threshold
    illnesses related to 88
    objective measurement of 38-39, 41
        in endurance training 88
training tolerance. *See also* monitoring system;
            monitoring tools
    fatigue *vs.* fitness in 84*t*, 85-86, 85*f*, 86*f*, 87*f*
    holistic approach to 95-96, 97*f*
    key components of 96-97
    load quantification in 87-88, 128
    nontraining stressors in 88-89, 95-96, 97*f*
    performance and endurance in 81-83, 82*f*, 83*f*
    practical methods for monitoring 88-96, 93*f*
    preventing overtraining syndrome with 88-89, 89*t*
    sequencing strategies. *See* training sequencing

training volume
    as burnout factor 27-28, 30
    in endurance training 84-85, 85*f*, 96
        tolerance of 88, 92, 93*f*, 128
    perceived exertion with 39, 41
    recovery-stress states and 27-28
        mood states profile in 41-42
trait anxiety, burnout and 30, 31*f*
transactional model, of stress 241
transition phase
    in break strategies 304
    Recovery-Cue monitoring of 223-224
travel
    as burnout factor 26, 31, 33, 34
    quality of life and 260-261, 264
    recovery strategies and 7, 132
triathlon training, case study of 221-222, 221*f*
TRIMP. *See* training impulse (TRIMP), in endurance training
trust, in debriefing 188-189, 195
tumor necrosis factor, in biphasic response to overload
        105, 111
TV watching, as recovery strategy 9, 148
two-factor model
    of preparedness for competition 128-129, 129*f*
    of recovery process
        intervention programs based on 280-281
        structural-equation analysis of 278, 278*f*
        training load sequence in 85-86, 87*f*
        volitional perspective in 274, 274*f*

U

unconditional acceptance, quality of life and 265-266
underdemanding situations, recovery and 6, 9
underperformance
    factors of 81, 88, 103
        global 96, 97*f*, 130*f*
    health relationship with x, 233-234
    in Individual Zones of Optimal Functioning 201
    prevention strategies for 33-34, 213-214
    research directions for 302, 307
underrecovery (UR)
    clinical mechanisms and findings of 103-114, 104*f*
    determinants of x, 4-5, 10, 37, 161
    empirical intervention model for 161-162, 176
    fatigue as 4, 41-42, 161
        assessment of 41, 45-46, 46*f*, 169*f*, 170
        case examples of 174-176
        interventions for 168-174, 169*f*
        mood disturbance with 162-163, 165-168, 168*t*
        neurochemical responses in 163-164
        self-regulation failure and 162, 164-165, 164*f*
    in Individual Zones of Optimal Functioning 201
    interdisciplinary approach to ix
    interventions for
        debriefing as 181-196
        emotional dimensions of 143-157, 162
        empirically derived model of 161-162, 164*f*
        ethical 162
        individually optimized 199-214
        interdisciplinary approach to 143-144, 154-157
        mood and self-regulation changes focus of 161-
                176, 164*f*
        Recovery-Cue as 219-225, 227-229
        training periodization and sequencing as 121-139,
                130*f*
    minimizing strategies for. *See* recovery

About the Editor

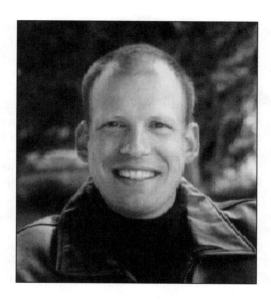

Michael Kellmann, PhD, recently accepted a position as an assistant professor in the faculty of sport science at the University of Bochum in Germany. He completed his habilitation at the University of Potsdam in Germany in January 2002. He is a member of the Association for the Advancement of Applied Sport Psychology and Psychology in High Performance Sports. He serves on the executive board of the German Association of Sport Psychology and the editorial board for *The Sport Psychologist*.

Michael's works have appeared in more than 50 publications, and he is coauthor of *Recovery-Stress Questionnaire for Athletes: User Manual*. He has consulted with and conducted research for the National Sport Centre Calgary in Canada, the Canadian national speed skating team, and the German junior national rowing team. Michael lives in Potsdam, Germany, and enjoys running and playing soccer.

Michael Kellmann, PhD
University of Bochum
Faculty of Sport Science
Unit of Sport Psychology
Stiepeler Straße 129
44780 Bochum
Germany
Tel: 001-234-32-22448
Fax: 001-234-32-14245
E-mail: Michael.Kellmann@ruhr-uni-bochum.de
http://sposerver.sportdekanat.ruhr-uni-bochum.de/sportpsych

About the Contributors

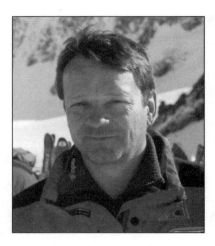

Jürgen Beckmann, PhD, is a professor of sport psychology at the University of Potsdam, Germany. He received his PhD in psychology from the University of Mannheim. Jürgen has been chief editor of the journal of the German Association of Sport Psychology, *Psychologie und Sport,* a member of the coaching team for the German Alpine Ski Team (responsible for mental training), an instructor for German ski instructors, and a psychological consultant to many German athletes. He is a member of the State Council for Education in Sport of the state of Brandenburg, the German Association of Sport Psychology, and the German Psychological Association. Jürgen has edited four books and is the author of more than 70 psychological publications.

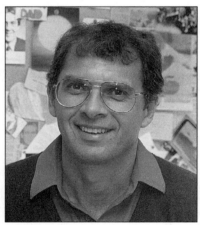

Cal Botterill, PhD, is a professor at The University of Winnipeg, Canada. He received his PhD from the University of Alberta. His research interests include peak performance, perspective, emotions, team building, and youth sport. Cal has worked with numerous professional and Olympic teams and consulted with several major companies. He has shown leadership in telecourse and on-line education and in mentoring young professionals. Cal has given more than 200 international, national, and regional keynote addresses and presentations in sport, psychology, medicine, education, and business. He has published more than 150 articles, chapters, videotapes, audiotapes, and books. Cal's wife, Doreen, and daughter, Jennifer, are two-time Olympians and his son, Jason, is a three-time world champion.

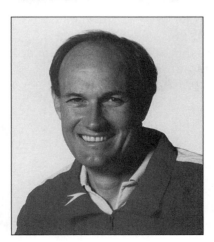

Henry (Hap) Davis IV, PhD, is a sport psychologist (AAASP Certified Consultant) and a clinical psychologist. He devotes about one-third of his time to working with athletes from his private office in Calgary, the city where he has lived and practiced since 1973. In sport, he has worked mainly with professional teams in ice hockey and with amateur athletes in many sports, including swimming, synchronized swimming, gymnastics, and equestrian sports. His publications on athlete selection, arousal, emotion, and various clinical areas reflect broad sport and clinical interests. At present he is a sport psychology consultant with the National Sport Centre Calgary, he works with a high performance swim club, and he is the National Team sport psychologist. In his free time Hap enjoys his family, his friends, and the Canadian Rockies.

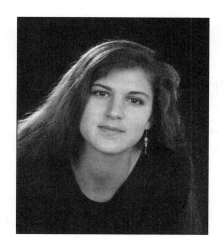

Kristen Dieffenbach, MS, is a fourth year PhD candidate in exercise and sport science and sport psychology at the University of North Carolina Greensboro. She received her MS in physical education with an emphasis in sport psychology from the University of Idaho and her BA in biology from Boston University. Her areas of concentration include performance enhancement, talent development and overtraining, staleness, burnout, and recovery. She has had applied publications in *VeloNews* and *DirtRag*. Kristin is a certified United States Track and Field coach with a level II specialization in endurance training and distance coaching and a certified expert level USA cycling coach. Currently, she coaches cycling, running, and endurance sports for individuals interested in competition and personal achievement. Kristen has competed and won awards in cross country, track and field, and cycling. Currently, she competes both on road and mountain bike, with an emphasis on endurance and ultraendurance endeavors. She is also fostering a newly discovered interest in adventure racing.

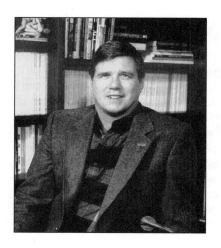

Daniel Gould, PhD, is the Bank of America Excellence Professor in the Department of Sport and Exercise Science at the University of North Carolina Greensboro (UNCG). Dan teaches graduate and undergraduate courses in sport and exercise psychology and is heavily involved in the graduate program. Actively involved in research, Dan has studied the stress-athletic performance relationship, sources of athletic stress, athlete motivation, youth sports issues, and sport psychological skills training use and effectiveness. He has consulted extensively with numerous athletes of all age and skill levels and been involved in a wide range of sports, including golf. Dan has served as a performance enhancement consultant with the U.S. Ski Team and numerous Olympic athletes. Currently, he consults with the pit crew of one of NASCAR's leading race teams. In 1994 he received UNCG's prestigious all-university Alumni Excellence in Teaching Award. In 2001 he also received the American Psychological Association Division 47 Professional Education and Training Award.

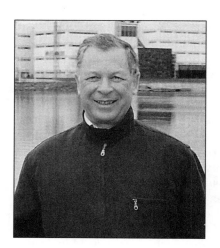

Yuri L. Hanin, PhD, DSc, is senior researcher and professor at the KIHU Research Institute for Olympic Sports, Jyväskylä, Finland. He holds PhD and DSc degrees in social psychology from St. Petersburg (Leningrad) University, Russia. His teaching, research, and consulting in sports and exercise focus on stress, anxiety, emotions and performance states; communication, leadership and optimal performance; and change, change management, and optimal performance. He is the author of four books as well as numerous book chapters and journal articles related to optimizing sports performance. His Individual Zones of Optimal Functioning model has stimulated a renewed and worldwide interest in the role of emotions in athletic performance. He is a member of the editorial board for the *International Journal of Sport Psychology, The Sport Psychologist (USA), Psychology of Sport & Exercise (UK), Revista de Psicologia del Deporte (Spain),* and *Coaching and Sport Science (Italy).* Yuri is currently serving as a FEPSAC newsletter editor and the International Association of Applied Psychology newsletter editor (Division 12–sport psychology).

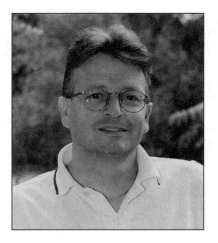

Peter Hassmén, PhD, is a professor of sport psychology at Stockholm University and Stockholm University College of Physical Education and Sports. He also received his PhD in psychology from Stockholm University. Peter has more than 20 years of experience as a researcher and has worked with elite athletes in applied settings for the same duration. He is a member of the scientific subcommittees of the Swedish Olympic Committee and the Swedish Golf Association. Peter competes in orienteering and cross-country skiing and is an active long-distance runner.

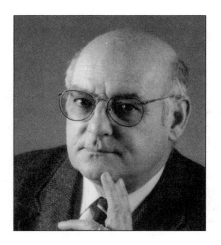

John M. Hogg, PhD, has worked as a teacher, coach, and applied sport psychologist. For over 30 years he was a successful swim coach at the club, university, and international levels and has guided many athletes to world-class competition. He pursued his interests in the field of applied sport psychology earning a master's degree (1978) and a doctoral degree (1982). John has made presentations in many countries at major conferences and congresses in both sport psychology and competitive swimming. He has published five books, contributed to book chapters, written numerous research and popular articles, and served as mentor to many young aspiring coaches in a variety of sports. In 1998 John was nominated for the Sport Medicine Council of Canada's first research award. John is currently a professor at the University of Alberta, Edmonton. He teaches applied sport psychology and performance enhancement at the graduate and undergraduate levels.

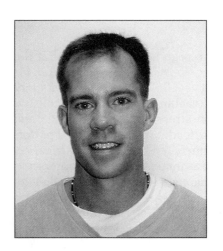

Matthew S. Johnson, PhD, is an assistant professor of sport psychology at Texas Christian University, where he teaches exercise and sport psychology and the psychology of youth sport and conducts research focusing on the quality of life for athletes using various qualitative and existential-phenomenological methodologies. Matthew is also a sport psychology consultant working with youth, collegiate, and professional athletes to enhance their athletic performance and develop their mental, physical, and spiritual balance in sport and life. Matthew is a former University of Notre Dame football quarterback. He received his MA in sport psychology from the University of North Carolina–Chapel Hill and his PhD in Sport Psychology from the University of Tennessee–Knoxville. Matthew is a member of the Association for the Advancement of Applied Sport Psychology. He has presented research on quality of life for athletes at professional conferences and is coauthor of "Personal and Participatory Socializers of the Perceived Legitimacy of Aggressive Behavior in Sport," which appeared in *Aggressive Behavior*. The article focuses on the moral perceptions of youth athletes in their sport development.

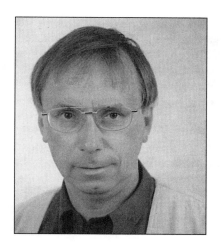

K. Wolfgang Kallus, PhD, is a full professor of work, organizational, and environmental psychology at the University of Graz in Austria, and is a member of the directorate of the Institute for Evaluation Research in Germany. Wolfgang is on the editorial board of *Neuropsychobiology,* and he is coauthor of *Recovery-Stress Questionnaire for Athletes: User Manual.* He is a member of the International Biometric Society and the Collegium Neuropsychopharmacology. His work focuses on stress, coping, and regeneration in applications as diverse as sport, work, surgery, and aviation.

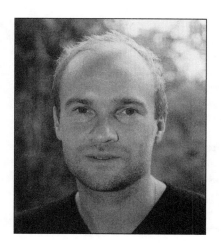

Göran Kenttä, PhD, presently works part time as a researcher in the Department of Psychology at Stockholm University and part time as a kayaking coach for the Swedish Olympic Team. His research has mainly focused on overtraining, burnout, and recovery in elite athletes and he has been invited to many sports federations to present on that subject. Göran has more than 15 years of experience as a national- and club-level coach. He received his PhD in psychology from Stockholm University. Göran won a silver medal in the Kayaking National Championships.

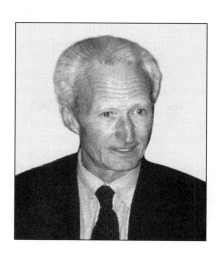

Manfred Lehmann, MD, was a professor of medicine and sports medicine at the University of Ulm and Director of the Department of Sports and Rehabilitation Medicine of the University Hospital Medical Center Ulm until his death in August 2001. His scientific work was published in more than 500 original and review papers. Manfred was an invited speaker all over the world at scientific meetings and congresses.

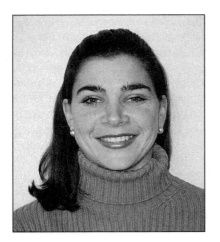

Karen MacNeill, MA, is a sport psychology consultant at the National Sport Centre Calgary and works with the National All-Around Speed Skating Team and the National Track Cycling Program. She also works at Calgary's Olympic oval and develops speed skaters, hockey players, and cyclers. She received her MA in sport psychology from the University of Ottawa and will complete her MSc in Counseling Psychology in May 2002. As a member of the Canadian National Women's Field Hockey Team for the past eight years, Karen has competed in events such as the Pan-American Games (1995/1999), the Commonwealth Games (1998), and the World Cup and Olympic Qualifiers. She is a member of National Sport Centre Calgary.

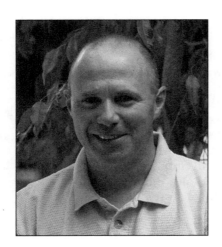

Stephen R. Norris, PhD, is a member of the multidisciplinary sport science group headed by Dr. David Smith at the University of Calgary/National Sport Centre Calgary. Originally from England, Stephen moved to Canada to pursue graduate studies. He acts as a consultant to several national sports teams, teaches and supervises graduate students specializing in applied physiology and sport science, and is involved in coach education. Stephen's research areas embrace the "umbrella" of "sustainable performance," particularly issues to do with hypoxia/hyperoxia, cardiovascular/cardiopulmonary responses to "stress," and assessing recovery and regeneration states. His focus of attention ultimately centers on the implementation of sport science into practical settings, particularly aspects to do with the planning, periodization, sequencing and monitoring of training. Stephen is primarily involved with hockey, all disciplines of skiing, luge, snowboarding, sailing, and swimming. Stephen is an avid boardsailor, snowboarder and mountain biker, and attempts to participate in squash, tennis, and golf.

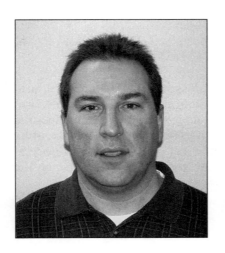

David M. Paskevich, PhD, is an assistant professor of sport and exercise psychology at the University of Calgary, Canada. His research focuses on the psychological effects of exercise and behavioral change strategies for promoting exercise adoption and adherence in chronic disease populations, specifically examining the roles played by self-efficacy, social support, and group cohesion. Currently he is researching which psychological variables may predict adherence to a lifestyle modification program for obese men as well as examining the impact of personal and social environmental factors on short- and long-term physically active behaviors in a cardiac rehabilitation program. David is also a sport psychology consultant with the National Sport Centre Calgary, and works with many local, provincial, national, international, and professional athletes. His research and applied work in sport focuses on (a) the use of mental skills and emotional management behaviors in high performance athletes and (b) the psychological effects of physical activity and behavioral change strategies to promote adoption and adherence to various training regimens. David is a member of the Canadian Society for Psychomotor Learning and Sport Psychology and the North American Society for Psychology of Sport and Physical Activity. He received his PhD in kinesiology from the University of Waterloo. David is a past recipient of the Queen's University School of Physical and Health Education Excellence in Academic Teaching Award.

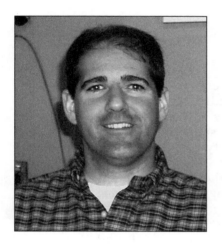

Tom Patrick, MS, is an instructor at The University of Winnipeg, Canada, where he lectures on sport and exercise psychology, the organization and administration of sport and recreation, and current issues in the areas of physical activity and sport. He is a coauthor of the book *Human Potential: Perspective, Passion and Preparation* and has published a number of articles on issues related to sport psychology and psychological skills training. Tom is a certified consultant with the Canadian Mental Training Registry and has worked with numerous top international athletes and teams in both the United States and Canada. Tom received his MS in Physical Education–Sport and Exercise Psychology from the University of Manitoba, Canada. He is completing his doctoral studies at the University of Southern Queensland in Australia.

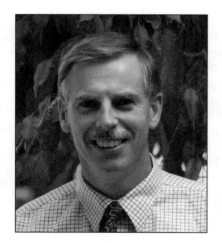

David J. Smith, PhD, is a professor of exercise physiology at the University of Calgary and sport science coordinator for the National Sport Centre Calgary. He trained as a physical education teacher in his native England then completed his PhD at the University of Alberta. Over the last 20 years, David has worked with many of Canada's top coaches in the sports of swimming, speed skating, volleyball, cross-country skiing, track and field, and synchronized swimming. His expertise lies in testing and interpretation of physiological and biochemical data combined with the design of training programs for high-performance athletes, areas in which he has widely published and presented. He has been a support staff member at five Winter and Summer Olympic Games, and athletes with whom he has directly worked have won 16 Olympic medals and achieved 35 world records. David has won numerous awards for teaching and contributions to sport science.

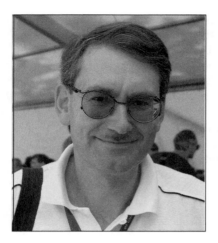

Jürgen M. Steinacker, MD, is an associate professor and vice head of the Department of Sports Medicine, University of Ulm. He is a member of the German Society of Sports Medicine, the American College of Sports Medicine (ACSM), the German Society of Cardiology, and the German Society of Internal Medicine. Jürgen has served as team physician for the German National Junior Rowing Team, as a member of the Scientific Committee of the German Society of Sports Medicine, as a Fellow of ACSM, as chief editor of *Deutsche Zeitschrift für Sportmedizin* (German Journal of Sports Medicine), and as a member of the International Rowing Federation (FISA) Medical Commission. He has published over 50 papers in reviewed journals and over 50 papers in edited books. He has served as editor of six books or special editions

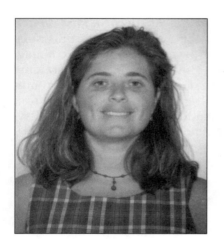

Clare Wilson, MA, is a sport psychology consultant working at the National Sport Centre Calgary and teaching sport psychology at the National Sport School in Calgary. Before moving to Calgary, Clare received her master's degree in sport psychology consulting and intervention from the University of Ottawa. Clare is presently working with a number of teams at the Olympic Oval and National Sport Centre Calgary, including the Canadian national sprint speed skating, short track speed skating, swimming, diving, and biathlon teams. In her spare time, Clare enjoys spending time in the mountains, traveling, playing ultimate, spending time with friends and family, and volunteering for the Make-A-Wish Foundation.

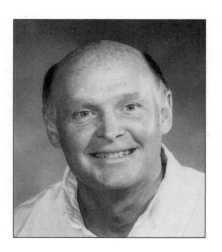

Craig A. Wrisberg, PhD, is a professor of motor behavior and sport psychology at the University of Tennessee, Knoxville. He has published numerous research articles on the topics of anticipation and timing in performance, knowledge of results and motor learning, and cognitive strategies in sport performance. He is a recipient of the Chancellor's Award for Research and Creative Achievement and the Brady Award for Excellence in Teaching. A past president of the North American Society for the Psychology of Sport and Physical Activity, Craig is a fellow of both the American Academy of Kinesiology and Physical Education and the Association for the Advancement of Applied Sport Psychology. His favorite leisure-time activities are hiking in the Great Smoky Mountains, canoeing, and playing tennis.

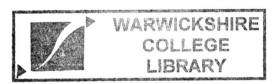